T0199927

Intervening Early in
PSYCHOSIS

A TEAM APPROACH

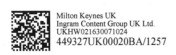

Milton Keynes UK
Ingram Content Group UK Ltd.
UKHW021630071024
449327UK00020BA/1257

Intervening Early in
PSYCHOSIS

A TEAM APPROACH

Edited by

Kate V. Hardy, Clin.Psych.D.
Jacob S. Ballon, M.D., M.P.H.
Douglas L. Noordsy, M.D.
Steven Adelsheim, M.D.

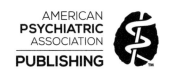

AMERICAN
PSYCHIATRIC
ASSOCIATION
PUBLISHING

Note: The authors have worked to ensure that all information in this book is accurate at the time of publication and consistent with general psychiatric and medical standards, and that information concerning drug dosages, schedules, and routes of administration is accurate at the time of publication and consistent with standards set by the U.S. Food and Drug Administration and the general medical community. As medical research and practice continue to advance, however, therapeutic standards may change. Moreover, specific situations may require a specific therapeutic response not included in this book. For these reasons and because human and mechanical errors sometimes occur, we recommend that readers follow the advice of physicians directly involved in their care or the care of a member of their family.

Books published by American Psychiatric Association Publishing represent the findings, conclusions, and views of the individual authors and do not necessarily represent the policies and opinions of American Psychiatric Association Publishing or the American Psychiatric Association.

If you wish to buy 50 or more copies of the same title, please go to www.appi.org/specialdiscounts for more information.

Copyright © 2019 American Psychiatric Association Publishing

ALL RIGHTS RESERVED

First Edition

Manufactured in the United States of America on acid-free paper
23 22 21 20 19   5 4 3 2 1

American Psychiatric Association Publishing
800 Maine Avenue SW
Suite 900
Washington, DC 20024-2812
www.appi.org

Library of Congress Cataloging-in-Publication Data
Names: Hardy, Kate V., editor. | Ballon, Jacob S., editor. | Noordsy, Douglas L., 1959– editor. | Adelsheim, Steven, editor. | American Psychiatric Association, issuing body.

Title: Intervening early in psychosis : a team approach / edited by Kate V. Hardy, Jacob S. Ballon, Douglas L. Noordsy, and Steven Adelsheim.

Description: First edition. | Washington, D.C. : American Psychiatric Association Publishing, [2019] | Includes bibliographical references and index.

Identifiers: LCCN 2019006911 (print) | LCCN 2019007351 (ebook) | ISBN 9781615372584 (ebook) | ISBN 9781615371754 (pbk. : alk. paper)

Subjects: | MESH: Psychotic Disorders—prevention & control | Early Medical Intervention | Patient Care Team

Classification: LCC RC512 (ebook) | LCC RC512 (print) | NLM WM 200 | DDC 616.89—dc23

LC record available at https://lccn.loc.gov/2019006911

British Library Cataloguing in Publication Data
A CIP record is available from the British Library.

Contents

1 Introduction: Early Intervention in Psychosis—
Beachhead for Transformational Reform in
Mental Health Care 1

*Patrick D. McGorry, A.O., M.D., Ph.D., FRCP, FRANZCP,
FAA, FAHMS, FASSA*

2 Growth of Early Intervention in Psychosis in the
United States 11

*Kate V. Hardy, Clin.Psych.D., Jacob S. Ballon, M.D., M.P.H.,
Douglas L. Noordsy, M.D., and Steven Adelsheim, M.D.*

3 Early Detection of Schizophrenia: A Population
Health Approach 23

*Maria Ferrara, M.D., Walter Mathis, M.D.,
John D. Cahill, M.D., Ph.D., Jessica Pollard, Ph.D., and
Vinod H. Srihari, M.D.*

4 Early Intervention and Policy 45

*Abram Rosenblatt, Ph.D., and
Howard H. Goldman, M.D., Ph.D.*

5 First-Person Accounts of Psychosis and
Advocacy Work 59

*Carlos Larrauri, M.S.N., APRN, PMHNP-BC, FNP-BC, and
Chantel Garrett, B.S.*

Contributors

Steven Adelsheim, M.D.
Clinical Professor, Department of Psychiatry and Behavioral Sciences, Stanford University School of Medicine, Stanford, California

Jacob S. Ballon, M.D., M.P.H.
Clinical Associate Professor, Department of Psychiatry and Behavioral Sciences, Stanford University, Stanford, California

Deborah R. Becker, M.Ed., CRC
Senior Research Associate, Westat, Lebanon, New Hampshire

Iruma Bello, Ph.D.
Assistant Professor of Psychology, Department of Psychiatry, New York State Psychiatric Institute and Columbia University Medical Center, New York, New York

Dror Ben-Zeev, Ph.D.
Professor, Department of Psychiatry and Behavioral Sciences, University of Washington, Seattle, Washington

Mary F. Brunette, M.D.
Associate Professor of Psychiatry, Geisel School of Medicine, Dartmouth College, Hanover, New Hampshire; Medical Director, Bureau of Behavioral Health, New Hampshire Department of Health and Human Services, Concord, New Hampshire

Benjamin Buck, Ph.D.
Advanced Fellow, Health Services Research and Development, VA Puget Sound: Seattle; Senior Fellow, Department of Health Services, School of Public Health, University of Washington, Seattle, Washington

Kristin Cadenhead, M.D.
Professor of Psychiatry, Department of Psychiatry, University of California–San Diego, La Jolla, California

John D. Cahill, M.D., Ph.D.
Assistant Professor, Department of Psychiatry, Yale University; Medical Director, Program for Specialized Treatment Early in Psychosis (STEP), New Haven, Connecticut

Nybelle Caruso, B.S., PSS
Co-chair, EASA Young Adult Leadership Council, Portland, Oregon

Mehak Chopra, D.O.
Student Health and Counseling Services, University of California, San Francisco, San Francisco, California

Lisa Dixon, M.D., M.P.H.
Edna L. Edison Professor of Psychiatry, New York State Psychiatric Institute, Columbia University Vagelos College of Physicians and Surgeons and New York Presbyterian, New York, New York

Robert E. Drake, M.D., Ph.D.
Vice President, Westat, Lebanon, New Hampshire

Maria Ferrara, M.D.
Postdoctoral Associate, Department of Psychiatry, Yale University; Research coordinator, Program for Specialized Treatment Early in Psychosis (STEP), New Haven, Connecticut

Chantel Garrett, B.S.
Founding Director, Strong 365, Rutherford, California

Tresha A. Gibbs, M.D.
Department of Psychiatry, Columbia University College of Physicians and Surgeons, New York, New York

Shirley M. Glynn, Ph.D.
Research Psychologist, Semel Institute of Neuroscience and Human Behavior, UCLA; Clinical Research Psychologist, VA Greater Los Angeles Healthcare System at West Los Angeles, Los Angeles, California

Howard H. Goldman, M.D., Ph.D.
Professor of Psychiatry, University of Maryland School of Medicine, Baltimore, Maryland

Michael Haines, QMHA, PSS
Lead Peer Support Specialist, PeaceHealth, Eugene, Oregon

Kate V. Hardy, Clin.Psych.D.
Clinical Associate Professor, Department of Psychiatry and Behavioral Sciences, Stanford University, Stanford, California

Jill Harkavy-Friedman, Ph.D.
Vice President of Research, American Foundation for Suicide Prevention, New York, New York

Debra R. Hrouda, Ph.D.
Director of Practice Implementation and Evaluation, Northeast Ohio Medical University, Rootstown, Ohio

Rebecca Jaynes, LCPC
Clinical Counselor, PIER Program, Maine Medical Center, Portland, Maine

Agnieszka Kalinowski, M.D., Ph.D.
Clinical Instructor, Department of Psychiatry and Behavioral Sciences, Stanford University, Stanford, California

Skylar Kelsven, M.S.
Doctoral student, San Diego State University/University of California–San Diego Joint Doctoral Program in Clinical Psychology, San Diego, California

Hyun Jung Kim, M.D.
Psychiatrist in Charge, Psychotic Disorders Division, McLean Hospital, Belmont, Massachusetts; Instructor in Psychiatry, Harvard Medical School, Cambridge, Massachusetts

David Kimhy, Ph.D.
Associate Professor and Program Leader in New Interventions in Schizophrenia; Director, Experimental Psychopathology Lab; Department of Psychiatry, Icahn School of Medicine at Mount Sinai, New York, New York; Mental Illness Research, Education and Clinical Center (MIRECC), James J. Peters VA Medical Center, Bronx, New York

Yulia Landa, Psy.D., M.S.
Assistant Professor and Director, CBT for Psychosis Research and Clinical Program, Department of Psychiatry, Icahn School of Medicine at Mount Sinai, New York, New York; Director, Advanced Psychology Fellowship Program, Mental Illness Research, Education and Clinical Center, VISN 2 South, James J. Peters VA Medical Center, Bronx, New York

Carlos Larrauri, M.S.N., APRN, PMHNP-BC, FNP-BC
Lecturer, School of Nursing and Health Studies, University of Miami, Miami, Florida

Rhoshel K. Lenroot, M.D.
Department of Psychiatry and Behavioral Sciences, University of New Mexico, Albuquerque, New Mexico

Ally Linfoot, PSS
Peer Services Coordinator, Clackamas Behavioral Health Services, Oregon City, Oregon

Rachel L. Loewy, Ph.D.
Associate Professor of Psychiatry, University of California, San Francisco, San Francisco, California

Sarah Lynch, LCSW
Director, PIER Program, Maine Medical Center, Portland, Maine

Nyamuon Nguany Machar
Peer Support Regional Coordinator, Youth Move Maine, Portland, Maine

Walter Mathis, M.D.
Assistant Professor, Yale School of Medicine, New Haven, Connecticut

Patrick D. McGorry, A.O., M.D., Ph.D., FRCP, FRANZCP, FAA, FAHMS, FASSA
Executive Director, Orygen, National Centre of Excellence in Youth Mental Health; Professor of Youth Mental Health, Centre for Youth Mental Health, University of Melbourne, Parkville, Victoria, Australia

Ryan Melton, Ph.D.
Clinical Training Director, OHSU-PSU School of Public Health, Portland Oregon

Piper Meyer-Kalos, Ph.D.
Executive Director, Minnesota Center for Chemical and Mental Health, University of Minnesota School of Social Work, St. Paul, Minnesota

Kim T. Mueser, Ph.D.
Professor, Departments of Occupational Therapy, Psychological and Brain Sciences, and Psychiatry, Boston University, Boston, Massachusetts

Tara Niendam, Ph.D.
Associate Professor of Psychiatry, University of California, Davis, Davis, California; Executive Director, UC Davis Early Psychosis Programs (EDAPT and SacEDAPT Clinics), Sacramento, California

Douglas L. Noordsy, M.D.
Clinical Professor of Psychiatry and Behavioral Sciences, Stanford University School of Medicine, Stanford, California; Professor of Psychiatry, Geisel School of Medicine at Dartmouth, Hanover, New Hampshire; Chief of Mental Health and Behavioral Science Services, Veterans Administration Medical Center, White River Junction, Vermont

Luz H. Ospina, Ph.D.
Project Director, Experimental Psychopathology Laboratory, Icahn School of Medicine at Mount Sinai, New York, New York

Jessica Pollard, Ph.D.
Assistant Professor, Department of Psychiatry, Yale University; Clinical Director, Program for Specialized Treatment Early in Psychosis (STEP), New Haven, Connecticut

Zheala Qayyum, M.D.
Assistant Clinical Professor, Department of Psychiatry, Yale University, New Haven, Connecticut

Jeffrey D. Reed, D.O.
Instructor in Psychiatry, Geisel School of Medicine, Dartmouth College, Hanover, New Hampshire; Staff Psychiatrist, West Central Behavioral Health, Affiliate of Geisel School of Medicine, Lebanon, New Hampshire

Abram Rosenblatt, Ph.D.
Associate Director, Westat, Rockville, Maryland

Megan Sage, M.S.W., LCSW
Senior Research Associate, OHSU-PSU School of Public Health, Portland, Oregon

Tamara Sale, M.A.
Director, EASA Center for Excellence, OHSU-PSU School of Public Health, Portland, Oregon

xiv Intervening Early in Psychosis

Kristen Sayles, M.S., R.N.
Nurse Manager, Adolescent Unit, Butler Hospital, Providence, Rhode Island

Vinod H. Srihari, M.D.
Associate Professor, Department of Psychiatry, Yale University; Director, Program for Specialized Treatment Early in Psychosis (STEP), New Haven, Connecticut

Gerrit Van Schalkwyk, M.B., Ch.B.
Assistant Professor (Clinician Educator) of Psychiatry and Human Behavior, Warren Alpert School of Medicine, Brown University; Unit Chief, Adolescent Unit, Butler Hospital, Providence, Rhode Island

Paula Wadell, M.D.
Associate Professor of Psychiatry, University of California, Davis, Davis, California; Medical Director, UC Davis Early Psychosis Programs (EDAPT and SacEDAPT Clinics), Sacramento, California

Barbara C. Walsh, Ph.D.
Clinical Coordinator, PRIME Clinic, Yale University School of Medicine, New Haven, Connecticut

Jian-Ping Zhang, M.D., Ph.D.
Assistant Professor, Early Treatment Program, Department of Psychiatry, Zucker Hillside Hospital, Northwell Health; [Please provide title], Department of Psychiatry, Donald and Barbara Zucker School of Medicine at Hofstra/Northwell, Glen Oaks, New York

Disclosure of Interests

The following contributors to this book have indicated a financial interest in or other affiliation with a commercial supporter, a manufacturer of a commercial product, a provider of a commercial service, a nongovernmental organization, and/or a government agency, as listed below:

Dror Ben-Zeev, Ph.D. *Intervention content licensing agreement:* Pear Therapeutics.

Carlos Larrauri, M.S.N., APRN, PMHNP-BC, FNP-BC *Consultant:* Alkermes. *Proposal review committee:* Alkermes Inspiration Grants.

Rachel L. Loewy, Ph.D. *Faculty:* Lundbeck International Neuroscience Foundation.

The following contributors have indicated that they have no financial interests or other affiliations that represent or could appear to represent a competing interest with the contributions to this book:

Deborah R. Becker, M.Ed., CRC; Iruma Bello, Ph.D.; Benjamin Buck, Ph.D.; John D. Cahill, M.D., Ph.D.; Lisa Dixon, M.D., M.P.H.; Robert E. Drake, M.D, Ph.D.; Maria Ferrara, M.D.; Chantel Garrett, B.S.; Tresha A. Gibbs, M.D.; Howard H. Goldman, M.D., Ph.D.; Jill Harkavy-Friedman, Ph.D.; Debra R. Hrouda, Ph.D.; Rebecca Jaynes, LCPC; Agnieszka Kalinowski, M.D., Ph.D.; Skylar Kelsven, M.S.; Hyun Jung Kim, M.D.; David Kimhy, Ph.D.; Rhoshel K. Lenroot, M.D.; Ally Linfoot, PSS; Sarah Lynch, LCSW; Nyamuon Nguany Machar; Walther Mathis, M.D.; Ryan Melton, Ph.D.; Tara Niendam, Ph.D.; Luz H. Ospina, Ph.D.; Jessica Pollard, Ph.D.; Zheala Qayyum, M.D.; Jeffrey D. Reed, D.O.; Abram Rosenblatt, Ph.D.; Megan Sage, M.S.W., LCSW; Kristen Sayles, M.S., R.N.; Vinod H. Srihari, M.D.; Gerrit Van Schalkwyk, M.B., Ch.B.; Paula Wadell, M.D.; Jian-Ping Zhang, M.D., Ph.D.

Foreword

THE past three decades have witnessed an exponential growth of early intervention services for people with psychosis around the globe. Early intervention has moved from research-driven clinical studies to having a significant impact on mental health service reform, with large-scale clinical implementation in many countries. This growth has not been without its challenges. The concept of early intervention to improve long-term outcomes in physical health has been common practice in medicine for many years, but early intervention in mental health has faced fierce resistance. This resistance strengthened the resolve of many early intervention clinicians and researchers to join forces across disciplines and to reach out to young people with psychosis and their families and caregivers to build a strong evidence base for early intervention. This approach has been very fruitful and has been the platform for policy changes and service reform. The debate has shifted away from disputing the concept of early intervention in psychosis, and pessimism regarding long-term outcome of young people who experience psychosis has been replaced by guarded optimism.

As early intervention is becoming more established, we still face a number of important challenges. In the United States, recent funding has been dedicated to the expansion of early psychosis care across the country, but in many other countries, service provision and implementation is still patchy and poorly funded. More research is needed to better understand the mechanisms that trigger the onset of psychosis as well as the contextual and individual factors that help build resilience and enhance recovery. It is time to further increase the participatory nature of our work and implement peer support in services. There is a need for personalized treatments that consider the personal history, strengths, and weaknesses of young people with psychosis and their families and that enable these youth to benefit from evidence-based treatments. In order to increase access to services, we need to investigate the effectiveness of new technologies in delivering interventions. These topics, and the early intervention ethos of interdisciplinary collaboration, are reflected in the content of this volume. This book will prove useful to anyone who is a policy maker, who is active clinically in early intervention, who studies or researches psychosis, who teaches about mental health, or who has experienced psychosis or cares for someone who has experienced psychosis.

Lucia Valmaggia, Ph.D., M.Sc., B.Sc.
President, IEPA–Early Intervention in Mental Health and Reader in Clinical Psychology and Digital Mental Health, Institute of Psychiatry, Psychology and Neuroscience, King's College London, London, UK

Acknowledgments

THIS book is dedicated to the many clients and families who have taught us about the transformative power of living well with, and recovery from, psychosis. We are also indebted to the many chapter authors for their gracious contributions. This book could not have happened without the intellectual stimulation within our clinic group and the support of many fine colleagues, including Nichole Olson, Agnes Kalinowski, Katie Eisen, and Justin Cheng of the INSPIRE clinic team. We owe the greatest debt of gratitude to Laura Roberts, both for her vision and leadership in forming the INSPIRE clinic and for her encouragement to create this much-needed book. Laura has long insisted that academic departments have a responsibility to be fully engaged with, and to demonstrate leadership in, addressing the pressing problems of our time, including developing and demonstrating optimal care models for people most in need, such as those at risk for and facing early psychosis.

We each have specific people in our lives to thank for their professional and personal support in guiding us toward the creation of this book:

I have been very fortunate to have benefited greatly from expert guidance, mentoring, and collaboration with numerous exceptional individuals in the field and extend my heartfelt thanks to Moggie McGowan, Anthony Morrison, Paul French, Ali Brabban, David Kingdon, Douglas Turkington, Rory Byrne, Richard Bentall, Rachel Loewy, Tamara Sale, Robert Heinssen, Kim Mueser, and David Shern. It has been a privilege to work with my coeditors, both on this book and in our clinic. Each of them brings a deep commitment and passion for working with individuals experiencing psychosis. I am humbled to learn from the many providers with whom I have had the privilege to work in community settings, who inspired the focus of this book, and who embody the ethos of a team approach in early psychosis intervention. In addition, I want to thank Bethan Reading, who taught me early on the importance of resilience, unwavering compassion, and always emphasizing the potential for recovery. On a personal note, I want to thank my parents, Rita and David Hardy, for their unerring support across two continents, my husband, Jon, for his endless patience and encouragement, and my son, Theo, for all the joy he brings.

K.V.H.

I wish to thank my first mentors in psychiatry, Steve Marder and Donna Ames, who provided me, as an undergraduate student in their research clinic, inspiration in thinking that care for people meant more than fixing symptoms. Their work in understanding the importance of treating the whole person pushed important ground for the field and laid a key foundation for the direction of my career. I am grateful for the mentoring and for the encouragement to take risks in my career that I had during my training at Stanford from Alan Schatzberg and Jennifer Hoblyn. I am also grateful for the mentorship of Jeffrey Lieberman, Scott Stroup, and Fred Jarskog, who further helped me define my voice within the academic community. I am very lucky to have the support and encouragement of my wife, Alana, in pursuing my goals and pushing me to see the world from multiple perspectives. Last, I dedicate my work in this area to my mom, Debbie, a dedicated psychiatric nurse, for providing my earliest inspiration and showing me through her passion the joy it is to work with people who have experienced psychosis.

J.S.B.

I am grateful to Bob Drake, Fred Osher, Kim Mueser, Tom Fox, Lindy Fox Smith, Chris O'Keefe ,and many others for showing me the value of multi-disciplinary, team-based, recovery-oriented care at a formative stage in my career. Their approach to engagement, mutual respect, and shared decision making have guided care for people with psychosis throughout my career. I am also grateful to Alan Green for entrusting me with a study of medication treatment for people in early psychosis and to Laura Roberts for creating the opportunity for me to join the INSPIRE clinic team. Finally, and most importantly, I am grateful to my dear wife, Mary, my beautiful children, Charlotte and Jack, and my loving family for inspiring me to strive for excellence and patiently tolerating the many hours dedicated to this volume.

D.L.N.

My professional thanks go to wonderful colleagues who provide critical education, guidance, patience, and support in educating me about the world of clinical high risk and early psychosis, allowing me to become involved in this critical effort. Thank you to Jane Lowe, Bill McFarlane, Donna Downing, Sarah Lynch, Gary Blau, Bob Heinssen, Susan Azrin, David Shern, John Kane, Delbert Robinson, Margaret Migliorati, Melina Salvador, David Graeber, Lisa Dixon, Tamara Sale, Ryan Melton, Cameron Carter, Rachel Loewy, Tara Niendam, Kate Hardy, Pat McGorry, and Laura Roberts. On a personal note, I want to thank my parents,

Marcia and Richard Adelsheim, for their lifelong support and my wife, Tara Ford, who is my daily role model and guide as I strive to hold compassion in all of my interactions. Thank you all!

S.A.

Resources:
https://med.stanford.edu/psychiatry/patient_care/inspire.html
https://med.stanford.edu/peppnet.html

CHAPTER 1

Introduction

EARLY INTERVENTION IN PSYCHOSIS— BEACHHEAD FOR TRANSFORMATIONAL REFORM IN MENTAL HEALTH CARE

Patrick D. McGorry, A.O., M.D., Ph.D., FRCP, FRANZCP, FAA, FAHMS, FASSA

The Challenge

Even in high-income countries, only a small minority of people with mental illness obtain access to evidence-based care in a timely way and in cultures of care that are welcoming and effective. The human and economic consequences of this global neglect are enormous (Bloom et al., 2011), especially because mental disorders begin largely in young people on the threshold of productive life, and the damage extends across decades of adult life (Insel and Fenton 2005). Therefore, the opportunity to save lives, restore and safeguard futures, and strengthen the global economy is correspondingly huge (The Economist 2014). The evidence-based reform of early intervention in psychosis, pioneered around the world for the last two to three decades, represents a blueprint and launch pad for dissolving the barriers that have constrained effective mental health care for so long, paves the way for early intervention across the full spectrum of disorders affecting young people, and fundamentally strengthens societies across the globe.

Optimism in mental health care has always been in short supply. Mental disorders have been hidden from public gaze, permeated by fear, discrimination, and maltreatment. Even today most people fail to realize how common and treatable these illnesses actually are. This is due to a toxic mix of flawed concepts, prejudice, learned helplessness within professional groups, and funding neglect. Nowhere is this better illustrated than in the phenomenon of dementia praecox, later schizophrenia, which was deliberately associated conceptually by Emil Kraepelin and his contemporaries with an essentially hopeless future. This was a serious conceptual and strategic mistake, one that has still to be corrected, and the corrosive pessimism it reinforced was to sabotage the care of people with psychosis for over a century. There have been challenges to this orthodoxy, but it is particularly tenacious, sustained as it has been by deep and pervasive neglect of those with mental illness, which in turn has reinforced the "clinician's illusion" that the prognosis is much worse than it truly is (Cohen and Cohen 1984).

The facts soon began to get in the way of the Kraepelinian paradigm, with recovery proving more possible than had been allowed (Bleuler et al. 1976). However, even the advent of effective antipsychotic drugs, developed in the 1950s, and the rise of community psychiatry failed to dispel this pessimism. It was not until the 1980s that focus turned to the early stages of psychotic illness and the notion of early diagnosis would become a realistic proposition. Initially, this was driven by a research agenda, which correctly proposed that studying individuals with first-episode psychosis free of the many confounding variables that were present in chronic and multi-episode samples would shed more light on etiological questions. At the outset it was unforeseen that this research agenda, which led to the establishment of streamed, or discrete, early psychosis programs in the 1980s and 1990s, would also reveal the clinical imperatives of both viewing psychosis from a harm reduction perspective and providing an opportunity for reductions in premature death and disability and more complete functional recovery.

This was certainly our own experience in Melbourne, Australia, where in 1984 we established a 10-bed clinical research unit for patients with first-episode psychosis (Copolov et al. 1989; McGorry 1985). Their clinical needs were starkly different from those of older multi-episode patients. These young individuals were typically propelled into the hospital after a prolonged period of untreated psychosis as a result of a suicidal or behavioral crisis, usually with police involvement. They were terrified by their Dickensian surroundings and the confrontation in the admission ward with an acutely disturbed cohort of much older chronically mentally ill individuals. Deep pessimism regarding their future was communicated to them on every level, directly by psychiatrists and nursing staff true to the Kraepelinian traditions of the time and subtly reinforced by the compelling, yet illusory, evidence of the chronicity of the illness that surrounded them in the form of their older co-patients (Cohen and Cohen 1984). These acute units were dangerous and frightening places (sadly, even in the general hospital settings of today, they all too often still are). Not only were their fellow patients disorganized, frightened, and often aggressive; this was the era of rapid neuroleptization, and young, drug-naïve people with first-episode psychosis were at risk of receiving vastly more medication than they needed to achieve remission. Their families were equally shattered by these experiences.

The task was simple. First, we had to reduce or prevent the harm that patients were exposed to by separating them from the longer-term patients and the toxic messages and treatments that were draining hope and optimism for the future and then find the minimally effective dose of antipsychotics that would result in remission with no, or minimal, side effects. Second, we had to develop and evaluate psychosocial interventions for both these young people and their families that were truly relevant for their stage of illness and psychosocial development and that would promote recovery (McGorry 1992). Third, we had to build cultures of care that were capable of guaranteeing safe, humane, and effective care and scale them up to replace the existing system.

An Idea Whose Time Has Come

Growing research interest in first-episode psychosis that had begun at Northwick Park in London (Crow et al. 1986) and Hillside Hospital in New York (Kane et al. 1982; Lieberman et al. 1992) and the seminal paper by Richard Wyatt assembling the evidence demonstrating the destructive impact of treatment delay (Wyatt 1991) created the context for the exponential growth not only in early psychosis research but in new treatments and models of care that were to follow. With the benefit of hindsight, it is often said of an idea that has spread that "its time had come." However, many such ideas fail to flourish and spread. Powerful ideas must also be actively spread or translated into reality, a process that requires many additional ingredients other than mere vision, creativity, or even research evidence. Key among these is the demonstration that the idea can work in a real-world setting and that it can subsequently be scaled up in many other locations. Thanks to a phalanx of inspirational leaders and early adopters around the world, this adaptation and scaling-up process gained momentum during the late 1990s and early 2000s. This reform was powered by a new global community, the International Early Psychosis Association (IEPA), which has held 11 conferences from 1996 to 2018 to drive research, clinical care, and service reform. Another catalyst has been the journal *Early Intervention in Psychiatry*, founded in 2007 as the official journal of the IEPA, which has successfully helped to grow capacity and evidence transdiagnostically in the early intervention field.

The scientific literature in early psychosis has expanded exponentially over the past 20 years, and many textbooks have appeared as well. The neurobiology of onset became much better understood, and the evidence base for optimal treatment and culture of care is much stronger. More than 60 nations are represented at IEPA conferences, and hundreds of early psychosis services, first-episode centers, and clinical high-risk centers have been developed in many countries. These have typically been local initiatives, and they vary in terms of fidelity to a core or optimal model (Table 1–1). However, some nations have scaled up services more systematically, some even with widespread or full national coverage. The latter include England, Canada, Denmark, Hong Kong, Singapore, and Australia.

Although U.S. researchers have played a leading role in first-episode research (Kirch et al. 1992; Lieberman et al. 1992), especially neurobiological research, because of the limitations of the U.S. health care system, service reform has been piecemeal until recently. Oregon has been the pioneer in service reform, with a statewide commitment to early psychosis care for several years based on the Early Assessment and Support Alliance model (Tamara Sale and colleagues, www.easacommunity.org). The Recovery After an Initial Schizophrenia Episode (RAISE) Project (Kane et al. 2016) has been a game changer that is catalyzing a nationwide wave of service reform. The National Institute of Mental Health under the directorship of Dr. Tom Insel and the inspired and strategic yet unassuming leadership of Dr. Robert Heinssen in assembling and nurturing national early psychosis research collaborations and using the data to leverage new federal funding have been absolutely crucial in ensuring that early intervention has now been placed at the apex of U.S. mental health reform.

Resistance to Reform: Genuine Skeptics or Merchants of Doubt?

Despite this wave of evidence-based reform, progress has been slower than ideal. When one surveys the landscape of premature death, preventable suffering, and multiple risks and the blighted lives and the recoveries against the odds despite the often harmful, poor quality, and at best patchy care on offer in most traditional settings for psychotic illness and contrasts this with the effectiveness and cost-effectiveness of expert care for early psychosis when it is provided and sustained, one might wonder why early care has not been scaled up even more rapidly and why a small cadre of critics, especially in the United Kingdom and

---

TABLE 1–1.   Core components of a specialized early psychosis service

---

Core components can be loosely grouped according to their function within the service, with certain components operating across the whole model and others more closely aligned to one of the three key functions of early detection, acute care, and recovery. This allows for a flexible yet comprehensive service that is able to respond quickly and appropriately to the individual needs of the young person and his or her family.

Early detection

1. **Community education** to improve awareness of young people's mental health issues among the general public and those who work closely with young people

2. **Easy access to the service** through one clear entry point with a "no wrong door" policy and guaranteed referral for those who do not meet entry criteria

3. **Home-based assessment and care** available via a mobile multidisciplinary team able to provide triage, assessment, crisis intervention, and home-based acute treatment 24 hours a day, 7 days a week

Acute care

4. **Acute phase care** delivered in the community by the mobile team or, when necessary, in a dedicated youth-friendly inpatient unit

5. **Access to subacute care** for additional support after an acute episode

Continuing care

6. **Case management** with an individual case manager who provides an individually tailored treatment approach as well as support with practical issues

7. **Medical interventions**, primarily low-dose pharmacotherapy

8. **Psychological interventions**, including psychoeducation, individual psychotherapy, and cognitive-behavioral therapy

9. **A functional recovery program** with an emphasis on returning to full social, educational, and vocational functioning

10. **Group programs** to enhance psychosocial and functional recovery; focus should be on topics of interest to young people, ranging from health-related issues such as stress management, coping with anxiety, and reducing drug use to study, school, and work issues, as well as social and leisure activities such as music, art, and outdoor adventure

11. **Family programs and family peer support** for the families and friends of young people with early psychosis

12. **Youth participation and peer support** for maintaining youth friendliness and accountability to young people in these services

---

TABLE 1–1.   Core components of a specialized early psychosis
                   service *(continued)*

---

13. **Mobile outreach** for those young people with complex issues who have
    difficulty engaging with services

14. **Partnerships** with other organizations that can enhance the support for
    young people with mental health issues

15. **Workforce development** to create highly skilled and clinically expert
    mental health professionals specializing in youth mental health

16. **Ultra-high-risk young people** should be treated within a specialized
    service, with the aim of minimizing symptoms and distress and
    maintaining a normal functional trajectory to prevent further deterioration
    in functioning and thus to prevent a first episode of psychosis

---

Source.   Adapted from Hughes et al. 2014.

Australia, has fiercely resisted its advance. Although the safety of
screening and proactive early treatment in cancer and elsewhere has
been debated in a logical fashion, the debates concerning early intervention in psychosis have taken on a more strident and, at times, emotional, even personal, tone (e.g., Frances 2011).

Skepticism and debate are, of course, crucial scientific processes to
guide and safeguard effective reform. However, extreme or excessive
skepticism, especially in relation to a reform with strong face validity
and strong, if incomplete, evidence, should prompt an analysis of mo-
tives because vested interests and ideological groups have been known
to misuse science to undermine valid change and reform (Oreskes and
Conway 2010). The timing of this skepticism appears to coincide with a
shift of momentum from pure research studies to substantial new in-
vestment in early psychosis services. To an extent, this resistance is understandable in the context of the neglect of the mental health care of
even people with severe and persistent illnesses. Clinicians working in
these underfunded and low-morale cultures of care, barely beyond the
shadows of the asylum, genuinely feel that more must be done to relieve the suffering of their patients and their families, especially when
this neglect is leading to homelessness and the widespread incarcera-
tion of the mentally ill in prisons. These clinicians fear that early intervention will divert scarce, finite, and precious resources from these
neglected patients to notionally less deserving patients, often citing the
experience of the 1960s, when this did, in fact, occur in the United
States.

However, the fundamental fallacy that these well-intentioned, yet
essentially simplistic, emotion-based critiques promote is that this is a
zero-sum game, that substantial growth in funding for mental health

care is not an achievable goal and that only one focus should be pursued—a classic false dichotomy. Yet, compellingly, the evidence that early intervention actually saves money in all kinds of ways means that it is almost certainly part of the solution in relation to better funding for longer-term care (McCrone et al. 2010; Mihalopoulos et al. 2009). The notion that individuals with prolonged and severe mental illness should receive sole priority until their care is truly optimal is part of the mantra of many critics, yet it is not a principle that has been accepted in cancer and cardiovascular medicine. In these illnesses, we do not see the trivialization of the needs of patients in earlier stages or with less severe or persistent forms of illness as the "worried well" or the fanning of fears of labeling and overtreatment. In cancer, we do not see palliative care being pitted against early diagnosis. It is important that these conversations, debates, dilemmas, and choices are faced honestly and openly in the light of the facts and the evidence and that they are not buried, distorted, or hijacked by ideologues, vested interests, irresponsible journalists, or even misguided humanitarians. Complex scientific and sociological forces must be understood within the cycle of innovation and reform.

Next Wave of Reform: Beyond Psychosis

The clinical epidemiology of the onset of mental disorders is more or less the mirror image of that seen in physical illness, with 75% of mental and substance use disorders emerging for the first time by age 25. Some of these disorders, notably neurodevelopmental disorders and some behavioral and anxiety disorders, commence in childhood before age 12; however, the dominant and potentially persistent and disabling mental and substance use disorders of adult life are a phenomenon of adolescence and emerging adulthood. Until recently, there has been no sense of urgency to intervene to alter their course and outcome. This obviously has to change.

A conceptual underpinning of this change is the wider application of early intervention beyond psychosis to all emerging disorders, particularly, but not only, in young people. This conceptual framework will be difficult to progress given the silos present in psychiatric research and the organization of specialist clinical care. However, buttressed by more flexible research and diagnostic approaches such as the Research Domain Criteria (Insel et al. 2010) and clinical staging (McGorry 2007a), a transdiagnostic focus for early intervention (McGorry and Nelson 2016) sits alongside a new wave of service reforms in youth mental health in an increasing number of countries (McGorry et al. 2013, 2014). These reforms aim to create a comprehensive, fully integrated youth mental health service stream for young people that offers seamless mental health care from puberty to mature adulthood up to around age 25 years, with soft transitions at either boundary with child and older adult mental health care. Such a vertically integrated system embraces the reality of dynamic biopsychosocial development and recognizes the complexity of the challenges faced by young people as they become independent adults, as well the burden of disease imposed on this age group by mental ill health. It responds by blurring the distinctions and borders between the tiers of primary and specialist care in recognition of the complexity of the presentation of much of the mental ill health apparent in young people, allowing a flexible and appropriate response for each individual (McGorry et al. 2013, 2014). A corresponding increase in flexibility and sophistication is required on the diagnostic side of the endeavor (McGorry and Nelson 2016; Nelson et al. 2017).

The foundations for reform in mental health must be built on the principles of demonstrable need, capacity to benefit, and evidence-informed care, including indicative evidence of value for better health outcomes and value for money, which, given the timing of morbidity, is likely to trump almost any other domain of health and social care (McGorry 2007b; McGorry et al. 2011). Youth mental health is emerging as a new professional field, and more evidence will be created as the field evolves. However, we can be optimistic here, not least because of the success of the early psychosis paradigm, which not only has provided proof of concept for early intervention but has largely driven the current transformation of psychiatry toward a more preventive and personalized focus, analogous to the approach now widespread in physical medicine. Early intervention, the essential element of preemptive psychiatry, is now being explored across the full diagnostic spectrum, and this exciting new field promises human, economic, and public health benefits on a much larger scale than could have been envisioned even a decade ago.

References

Bleuler M, Huber G, Gross G, Schüttler R: Long-term course of schizophrenic psychoses: joint results of two studies [in German]. Nervenarzt 47(8):477–481, 1976 822365

Bloom DE, Cafiero ET, Jane-Llopis E, et al: The Global Economic Burden of Non-Communicable Disease. Geneva, Switzerland, World Economic Forum, 2011

Cohen P, Cohen J: The clinician's illusion. Arch Gen Psychiatry 41(12):1178–1182, 1984 6334503

Copolov DL, McGorry PD, Keks N, et al: Origins and establishment of the schizophrenia research programme at Royal Park Psychiatric Hospital. Aust N Z J Psychiatry 23(4):443–451, 1989 2610645

Crow TJ, MacMillan JF, Johnson AL, Johnstone EC: A randomised controlled trial of prophylactic neuroleptic treatment. Br J Psychiatry 148:120–127, 1986 2870753

The Economist: Mental Health and Integration. London, The Economist, 2014

Frances A: Australia's reckless experiment in early intervention. Psychology Today, May 21, 2011. Available at: www.psychologytoday.com/au/blog/dsm5-in-distress/201105/australias-reckless-experiment-in-early-intervention. Accessed February 18, 2 019.

Hughes F, Stavely H, Simpson R, et al: At the heart of an early psychosis centre: the core components of the 2014 Early Psychosis Prevention and Intervention Centre model for Australian communities. Australas Psychiatry 22(3):228–234, 2014 24789848

Insel T, Cuthbert B, Garvey M, et al: Research domain criteria (RDoC): toward a new classification framework for research on mental disorders. Am J Psychiatry 167(7):748–751, 2010 20595427

Insel TR, Fenton WS: Psychiatric epidemiology: it's not just about counting anymore. Arch Gen Psychiatry 62(6):590–592, 2005 15939836

Kane JM, Rifkin A, Quitkin F, et al: Fluphenazine vs placebo in patients with remitted, acute first-episode schizophrenia. Arch Gen Psychiatry 39(1):70–73, 1982 6275811

Kane JM, Robinson DG, Schooler NR, et al: Comprehensive versus usual community care for first-episode psychosis: 2-year outcomes from the NIMH RAISE Early Treatment Program. Am J Psychiatry 173(4):362–372, 2016 26481174

Kirch DG, Lieberman JA, Matthews SM (eds): First-episode psychosis (special issue). Schizophr Bull 18(2):159–336,1992

Lieberman JA, Alvir JM, Woerner M, et al: Prospective study of psychobiology in first-episode schizophrenia at Hillside Hospital. Schizophr Bull 18(3):351–371, 1992 1411327

McCrone P, Craig TK, Power P, Garety PA: Cost-effectiveness of an early intervention service for people with psychosis. Br J Psychiatry 196(5):377–382, 2010 20435964

McGorry PD: The Aubrey Lewis Unit: The origins, development and first year of operation of the clinical research unit and Royal Park Psychiatric Hospital. Dissertation for membership of the Royal Australian and New Zealand College of Psychiatrists. Melbourne, Victoria, Australia, Royal Australian and New Zealand College of Psychiatrists, 1985

McGorry PD: The concept of recovery and secondary prevention in psychotic disorders. Aust N Z J Psychiatry 26(1):3–17, 1992 1580883

McGorry PD: Issues for DSM-V: clinical staging: a heuristic pathway to valid nosology and safer, more effective treatment in psychiatry. Am J Psychiatry 164(6):859–860, 2007a 17541042

McGorry PD: The specialist youth mental health model: strengthening the weakest link in the public mental health system. Med J Aust 187(7)(suppl):S53–S56, 2007b 17908028

McGorry P, Nelson B: Why we need a transdiagnostic staging approach to emerging psychopathology, early diagnosis, and treatment. JAMA Psychiatry 73(3):191–192, 2016 26765254

McGorry P, Bates T, Birchwood M: Designing youth mental health services for the 21st century: examples from Australia, Ireland and the UK. Br J Psychiatry Suppl 54:s30–s35, 2013 23288499

McGorry PD, Purcell R, Goldstone S, Amminger GP: Age of onset and timing of treatment for mental and substance use disorders: implications for preventive intervention strategies and models of care. Curr Opin Psychiatry 24(4):301–306, 2011 21532481

McGorry PD, Goldstone SD, Parker AG, et al: Cultures for mental health care of young people: an Australian blueprint for reform. Lancet Psychiatry 1(7):559–568, 2014 26361315

Mihalopoulos C, Harris M, Henry L, et al: Is early intervention in psychosis cost-effective over the long term? Schizophr Bull 35(5):909–918, 2009 19509308

Nelson B, McGorry PD, Wichers M, et al: Moving from static to dynamic models of the onset of mental disorder: a review. JAMA Psychiatry 74(5):528–534, 2017 28355471

Oreskes N, Conway E: Merchants of Doubt. London, Bloomsbury, 2010

Wyatt RJ: Neuroleptics and the natural course of schizophrenia. Schizophr Bull 17(2):325–351, 1991 1679255

CHAPTER
2

Growth of Early Intervention in Psychosis in the United States

Kate V. Hardy, Clin.Psych.D.
Jacob S. Ballon, M.D., M.P.H.
Douglas L. Noordsy, M.D.
Steven Adelsheim, M.D.

A Brief History of Early Intervention in Psychosis

Throughout medicine, it is generally considered the best practice to initiate treatment as early in the course of an illness as possible. The Framingham risk criteria help predict the likelihood of heart disease, and numerous screening tools, such as colonoscopy or mammography, try to identify the earliest signs of otherwise occult cancers. In psychiatry, however, early identification often proves difficult because there are no definitive tests to identify the precise onset, or definitive at-risk state, to guide decisions about when to initiate treatment. Concerns over potentially stigmatizing diagnoses further necessitate diagnostic precision at the onset of symptoms.

Psychiatric diagnosis has certainly evolved over the decades. The publication of the first *Diagnostic and Statistical Manual of Mental Disorders* (DSM) in 1952 (American Psychiatric Association 1952) came before the commercial release of chlorpromazine, the first antipsychotic medication, and it was written with a psychoanalytic mindset reflective of the time in which it was developed. The third edition of DSM first brought the concept of diagnostic criteria to the mainstream in 1980 (American Psychiatric Association 1980). It was with DSM-III that a person could be diagnosed as having schizophrenia if he or she experienced a subset of the listed symptoms, including hallucinations, delusions, and decrease in functioning. The shift to a diagnostic framework based on observable symptoms marked a change in how and when treatment was expected to initiate. In concert with the cultural changes, the onset of the medication era also changed the available modes of treatment from primarily psychoanalytic to include psychopharmacology and other biologically based treatments and heralded the medical model that became the dominant paradigm for that era.

Notably, it was in the DSM-III that the concept of a *prodrome* to schizophrenia was put forth as a formal component of diagnosis. However, this was not the first time that the concept of a prodrome, or high-risk state, was first posited. Early work, including that by Chapman (1966), showed a premorbid increase in symptom severity without treatment. Notably, it was in this time that it was initially reported that a longer duration of untreated psychosis (DUP) related to a worsened prognosis overall.

This recognition about DUP, along with revisions to the diagnostic classifications of schizophrenia overall, led to a need to better characterize the nature of the earliest stages of psychotic illness. Additionally, a greater emphasis on prevention led to a greater recognition of the putatively prodromal, or clinical high-risk state, and the value of defining interventions for this population of people with early symptoms of schizophrenia. McGorry et al. (2006) developed a clinical staging model, described in the section "Staging Model," that serves as an effective framework for marking the stages of development in psychotic illness. Delineating this model effectively set the stage for a line of research focused on the earlier phases of illness.

Transitioning From Chronic Care to Early Intervention

Research on the pathophysiology, diagnosis, and treatment of psychosis has predominantly focused on advanced phases of disease. Prominent psychiatrists who defined schizophrenia spectrum disorders, such as Emil Kraepelin, Eugen Bleuler, and Kurt Schneider, identified manifestations of florid psychosis, including first-rank psychotic symptoms, catatonia, and cognitive decline. Treatment during the compassionate care era of the nineteenth and twentieth centuries centered on long-term hospital-based care communities for people with psychoses. With the advent of medications and changes in attitudes toward civil rights, there was a shift toward deinstitutionalization beginning in the 1960s. Over the past 50 years, the effects of moving people out of long-term hospitals have changed the focus of care for people with severe mental illness to community-based treatment programs.

Although this change in focus has not come without challenges, people with psychosis primarily live immersed in their communities, and therefore the goal of care had to shift to one that supports individuals with advanced disease to adapt to life outside a hospital. Unfortunately, the effects of long-term institutionalization had contributed to beliefs about schizophrenia as an inevitably disabling disease. Pervasive among providers were attitudes about the chronicity of schizophrenia and a belief in the need for paternalistic protection and involuntary treatment. Psychosocial rehabilitation interventions were developed to counter the effects of institutionalization and negative symptoms on social functioning but were typically viewed as only partially ameliorative. The pioneering work of Harding et al. (1987) identified that many people with schizophrenia go on to achieve remission of psychosis. This work set the stage for changes in the perceived potential prognosis for people with psychotic disorders by identifying variability of outcomes and the bias inherent in selective attention to people seen in institutional treatment settings. This experience is similar to the recognition that if a clinician saw only patients with stage 4 skin cancer, by analogy, that clinician's perception of the prognosis of skin cancer on all people's lives would be distorted.

Another line of work began to identify the impact of DUP at the outset of psychosis on long-term outcomes. Documentation of higher rates of response to antipsychotic medication treatment and remission among people in their first episode of psychosis compared with those with multiple episodes also heightened interest in focusing on early stages of illness (Robinson et al. 1999). These observations led to the development of specialized clinical programs focused on intervening early in psychosis in both Australia and across Europe. These programs provided both invaluable clinical experience and an essential evidence base from which further developments in the field have grown (Amminger et al. 2011, Melle et al. 2008). Collectively, this work generated recognition that early psychosis was an evolving process and that there might be an opportunity to intervene early in the progression of symptoms and delay or even potentially prevent the movement toward more serious psychiatric illness. The early intervention movement had arrived.

Principles of Intervening Early in Psychosis

The introduction of early intervention in psychosis represented a paradigm shift in the field of mental health care. In particular, this shift encouraged providers, researchers, consumers, families, and society at large to reconsider how emerging serious mental health problems are assessed, treated, and conceptualized and shifted the focus from understanding psychosis as a chronic and debilitating illness to embracing the potential for early intervention and recovery. As such, a number of key principles unite the early intervention in psychosis movement internationally. These principles provide a foundation on which, arguably, all early psychosis services are developed and offer guidance regarding multiple aspects of service provision, including workforce development and training, the breadth of interventions offered, and overall ethos of the service.

In 2005 the World Health Organization issued the seminal consensus statement on early intervention (Bertolote and McGorry 2005). Within this consensus document, five key principles were highlighted, and the core values and vision for early intervention were described. The five key principles are 1) raising community awareness, 2) improving access and engagement, 3) promoting recovery, 4) encouraging family engagement and support, and 5) providing workforce training. The principles are outlined below in the following subsections and are elaborated on in later chapters of this book.

Raising Community Awareness

A key tenet of early intervention is community education to support the early identification of individuals who may be experiencing early signs of psychosis. There are multiple community education initiatives that draw on innovative means of reaching the target audience (e.g., via social media, advertisements in movie theaters, information outreach talks to key stakeholders) and provide information on early psychosis at an appropriate level. Taking the approach of going into the community and educating stakeholders (e.g., young people, educators, family members, primary care doctors) contrasts with the traditional approach of many mental health centers that rely on established referral pathways for consumers to access treatment. However, this traditional approach has been associated with delays in accessing care, resulting in an extended DUP, shown to result in poorer long-term outcomes (Kane et al. 2016). Another important element of raising community awareness is the opportunity to provide up-to-date, accurate information about psychosis symptoms, address misconceptions about mental health, and address head-on the stigma that is often associated with acknowledging mental illness in our homes and families.

Improving Access and Engagement

The very essence of early intervention is ensuring that individuals access treatments shown to be effective for early psychosis in a timely manner. As such, ensuring that services are accessible, responsive, and prioritize engaging the young person is essential to this approach. In the United States the median of duration of untreated psychosis is 74 weeks (Addington et al. 2015). This time frame far exceeds the internationally recommended standard of 12 weeks. Although the reasons for an extended duration of psychosis are multifaceted, this principle of easy and early access encourages early psychosis teams to respond rapidly to referrals (including developing models for triaging referrals and supporting waitlist management) and ensuring that services are offered in youth-friendly settings to aid overall engagement.

Promoting Recovery

The third principle emphasizes that the focus should be on recovery, healing, functioning, and shared decision making rather than disability and illness management. This core principle permeates all aspects of an early psychosis service, including medication management, individual and family psychosocial interventions, peer support, and support for education and employment. It is essential that all members of the early intervention team have a full understanding of this principle and that they adhere to this recovery frame in their interactions with the client, the family, and other stakeholders. Recovery is a concept typically defined by the client on the basis of the goals and values that they identify and helps to drive treatment in order to support the individual in reaching those goals.

Encouraging Family Engagement and Support

Given the age at onset of early psychosis, many symptomatic individuals are often still closely connected to or living with their family or other support systems. As such, family members should have access to information regarding psychosis and how best to support their loved one. The developmental needs of this young population also need to be considered in service development. In contrast to traditional adult mental health services, families are generally actively engaged in the treatment process. Early psychosis programs may need to consider how best to support family members, navigate family dynamics, and ensure that information provided on psychosis is culturally salient.

Providing Workforce Training

One element of early psychosis treatment has been a dedication to providing evidence-based treatments. This principle requires commitment to training providers in these specialized approaches and ensuring ongoing, sustainable consultation to help practitioners access cutting-edge treatments and stay abreast of the field. As such, early psychosis services should consider training at multiple levels, including preimplementation planning, training implementation, ongoing consultation, and repeating training efforts to respond to staff turnover.

Developmental Framework

The first episode of psychosis typically occurs in late adolescence or early adulthood. This time frame spans a key developmental period from 16 to 24 years, with individuals of this age range often referred to as transitional-age youth (TAY). This developmental stage can challenge mental health services that are traditionally divided into services for children (up to age 18) and adults (ages 18 and older). Because individuals with early psychosis generally span two different systems of mental health care, it is critical to consider how best to support navigation of these two often disparate systems.

The needs of the TAY population vary greatly from those of children or adults. Consideration should be given to the developmental needs of each of these populations, and services should be adapted accordingly. This reality requires workforce training in developmental approaches, recognition of the different medication and physical health needs of individuals younger than 18 years, consideration of medicolegal issues of consent and confidentiality, adaptation of evidence-based individual and family therapy approaches, and the importance of supporting continued educational attainment through specialized services designed specifically for secondary school and higher education. In addition, the environment of the clinical space needs to reflect this developmental stage, and services should be encouraged to develop youth-friendly environments. Providers must also recognize these young people as a dynamic and changing age group who are evolving in terms of their personality, sexuality and gender orientation, sense of autonomy and independence, and social supports. In particular, the role of the family may change over the course of providing care for an individual receiving services for early psychosis. Chapter 22, "Care for Adolescents on the First-Episode Psychosis Continuum," provides more information on developmental approaches for this population.

Staging Model

McGorry and colleagues developed a clinical staging model that serves as an effective framework for marking the stages of psychotic illness development (Fusar-Poli et al. 2017; McGorry et al. 2006). This model, which is based on the model of staging other developing and/or chronic illnesses such as cancer or osteoporosis, sets benchmarks for delineating the steps through which an individual might progress in moving from very early symptoms to a full psychotic disorder. The stages range from stage 0, which occurs without symptoms but with elevated risk for psychosis, to stage 1, with the first identification of concerning symptoms, through stage 2, which is the first episode of psychosis, stage 3, with relapses of the first episode, and ultimately, stage 4, which is a fully established, more chronic disorder. Not everyone progresses through each stage, but the stages are designed to help better understand the nature of the current state for the individual and to guide stage-specific treatment to help provide appropriate levels of intervention.

Clinical staging can be useful in guiding treatment selection and determining potential impacts of an intervention. Preventive, neuroprotective interventions are indicated in stages 0–1, whereas specific therapeutic interventions are indicated in stages 2–4 (Fusar-Poli et al. 2017). As in cancer, therapeutic interventions have the highest opportunity for efficacy in earlier stages of disease, and relapse raises the need for more complex care. These relationships serve to advance understanding that one of the most important ways that our field can improve the efficacy of interventions for psychosis is to apply them in an early, timely, and consistent manner, before tertiary disease develops. There may be as much potential gain from efforts to improve the timing of application of existing treatments as there is in trying to develop new, more efficacious treatments. This reality has implications for both the design and availability of clinical services and for public health efforts to ensure broad public awareness of psychosis.

Historical Context of United States Early Intervention Support and Funding

Although intervening early in the course of psychosis has been broadly adopted in Australia and several European countries over the past two decades, the United States was a relative latecomer to the systematic implementation of early psychosis service models. Challenges related to funding services, access through insurance, and a lack of a coordinated infrastructure to support widespread implementation all acted as initial barriers to the growth of this approach in the United States and hampered policy development that would have otherwise supported implementation.

Initial early psychosis programs in the United States were developed at either a community level (e.g., Early Assessment and Support Alliance [EASA], Portland Identification and Early Referral [PIER]), through community-academic partnerships (e.g., Prevention and Recovery in Early Psychosis [PREP; Hardy et al. 2011]), or in an academic setting (e.g., Specialized Treatment Early in Psychosis [STEP; Srihari et al. 2014]) and drew on early psychosis models prevalent in Australia and the United Kingdom. These models often integrated evidence-based practices for psychosis with local adaptations reflecting cultural and geographical needs. In addition to this grassroots development, the National Institute of Mental Health (NIMH) sponsored both the North American Prodromal Longitudinal Study (NAPLS) and Recovery After an Initial Schizophrenia Episode (RAISE) studies. NAPLS is now in its third iteration, focusing on people with elevated risk for psychosis. Critical results include refinement of the components of the at-risk state, leading to the recent development of a risk calculator for determining the risk of conversion to psychosis from the clinical high-risk state (Carrión et al. 2016).

In addition, the RAISE studies are the largest clinical trials to focus on people in their first episode of psychosis (Dixon et al. 2015; Kane et al. 2016). Research into the optimal treatment for the first episode of schizophrenia in general has been difficult to undertake in large numbers for many reasons. Despite difficulty in initiating treatment for many people, once an individual is identified as having an early psychotic illness, treatment is often initiated before potential enrollment in pretreatment research can be arranged. Further, the effects of medication in the first episode are rapid, and the timing of initial treatments, or delay of recognition for initiating treatment, can have a profound impact on the later course of illness. Furthermore, recruitment and retention of research subjects in this stage of illness are challenging, and alignment between clinicians and clients and families on the need for treatment is often difficult to achieve.

One important outcome of RAISE was the development and validation of the coordinated specialty care (CSC) model for comprehensive treatment of people experiencing an initial episode of psychosis and the importance of interdisciplinary teams to partner with both clients and family members on service implementation. This CSC approach was implemented within community mental health centers across the United States to allow for evaluation of this approach in a real-world setting and trained staff in these centers to deliver the interventions.

In addition, the Robert Wood Johnson Foundation funded the Early Detection, Intervention, and Prevention of Psychosis Program (EDIPPP) clinical high-risk study at six U.S. sites (McFarlane et al. 2015). Whereas the RAISE studies focused on early interventions for persons with psychotic illness, others, such as NALPS and EDIPPP, focused on broad outreach and case finding to bring those at clinical high risk for psychosis in for early intervention, with the hope of delaying or possibly preventing the movement to a first psychotic episode.

The success of RAISE and other early psychosis services in the United States contributed to the federal decision to allocate an additional 5% to each state's Mental Health Services Block Grant for early psychosis recognition and treatment, which was doubled to 10% in 2016. These funds are dedicated to the development and provision of programs for young people experiencing early psychosis. This expansion has resulted in the exponential growth of early psychosis programs across the United States, with approximately 200 programs across 40 states in EASA at this time (EASA Center for Excellence 2016). In 2018 the Substance Abuse and Mental Health Services Administration released the first funding for programs supporting persons at clinical high risk for psychosis, thereby expanding the potential continuum of federal funding support for early psychosis programs nationally.

Coordinated Specialty Care in the United States

The NIMH sponsored the RAISE studies to establish that effective early intervention services for psychosis could be broadly implemented in the United States (Dixon et al. 2015, 2018; Kane et al. 2016). The CSC model was developed on the basis of evidence-based care strategies previously implemented with people with chronic psychosis, as well as successful global early intervention models. CSC was designed to provide comprehensive treatment for people experiencing an initial episode of psychosis, including case management, psychotherapy, pharmacotherapy, family intervention, and supported education and employment. Care is delivered by interdisciplinary teams that provide services to both clients and their family members. Although most early intervention studies are not designed to test the individual components of CSC or similar models, multidisciplinary, team-based care has been shown to be effective in reducing symptom severity and improving functional outcomes for people in first-episode psychosis. Multimodal care models are used in effective early intervention programs across the globe and are now considered the standard of care.

Throughout the chapters of this book, you will find details on specific interventions and modalities of care. It is important to be mindful that these interventions are intended for use within a team-based care program and may not be as effective in isolation. Intervening early in psychosis works best in a team approach with coordination between multiple disciplines and stakeholders and strong partnerships with clients and their support network. We encourage you to consider how you can incorporate an early and comprehensive range of interventions, delivered in a multidisciplinary setting, in partnership with individuals with early psychosis and their families.

KEY CONCEPTS

- Traditionally, mental health services took a watch-and-wait approach to psychosis, with a focus on managing chronic psychotic symptoms.

- International efforts to intervene early in the course of psychosis have provided guiding principles for the development of early intervention services in the United States.

- In the United States, these international guiding principles were integrated into models of early psychosis care called coordinated specialty care (CSC).

- There has been a growth in the availability of CSC services across the United States over the past decade.

- A developmentally based approach to working with individuals with early psychosis and their family is critical for treatment success.

Discussion Questions

1. Where is your closest CSC service?

2. How is an individual experiencing a first episode of psychosis, and his or her family, currently provided with evidence-based interventions for early psychosis in your area?

3. What resources are locally available to support the growth of CSC in your area?

Suggested Readings

Articles and Reports

Dixon LB, Goldman HH, Srihari VH, et al: Transforming the treatment of schizophrenia in the United States: the RAISE initiative. Annu Rev Clin Psychol 14(1):237–258, 2018

Heinssen RK, Goldstein AB, Azrin ST: Evidence-Based Treatments for First Episode Psychosis: Components of Coordinated Specialty Care. Bethesda, MD, National Institute of Mental Health, April 14, 2014. Available at: www.nimh.nih.gov/health/topics/schizophrenia/raise/nimh-white-paper-csc-for-fep_147096.pdf. Accessed September 27, 2018.

Sale T, Fetzer P, Humensky J, et al: The Integration of Early Psychosis Services in a System of Care Framework: Opportunities, Issues, and Recommendations. Stanford, CA, Stanford Medicine, April 2018. Available at: http://med.stanford.edu/content/dam/sm/peppnet/documents/Integration-of-Early-Psychosis-Services-in-SoC-Framework-Final.pdf. Accessed January 18, 2019.

Website

Prodrome and Early Psychosis Program Network (PEPPNET): https://med.stanford.edu/peppnet.html

References

Addington J, Heinssen RK, Robinson DG, et al: Duration of untreated psychosis in community treatment settings in the United States. Psychiatr Serv 66(7):753–756, 2015 25588418

American Psychiatric Association: Diagnostic and Statistical Manual: Mental Disorders. Washington, DC, American Psychiatric Association, 1952

American Psychiatric Association: Diagnostic and Statistical Manual of Mental Disorders, 3rd Edition. Washington, DC, American Psychiatric Association, 1980

Amminger GP, Henry LP, Harrigan SM, et al: Outcome in early-onset schizophrenia revisited: findings from the Early Psychosis Prevention and Intervention Centre long-term follow-up study. Schizophr Res 131(1–3):112–119, 2011 21741219

Bertolote J, McGorry P: Early intervention and recovery for young people with early psychosis: consensus statement. Br J Psychiatry Suppl 48:s116–s119, 2005 16055800

Carrión RE, Cornblatt BA, Burton CZ, et al: Personalized prediction of psychosis: external validation of the NAPLS-2 psychosis risk calculator with the EDIPPP project. Am J Psychiatry 173(10):989–996, 2016 27363511

Chapman J: The early symptoms of schizophrenia. Br J Psychiatry 112(484):225–251, 1966 4957283

Dixon LB, Goldman HH, Bennett ME, et al: Implementing coordinated specialty care for early psychosis: the RAISE connection program. Psychiatr Serv 66(7):691–698, 2015 25772764

Dixon LB, Goldman HH, Srihari VH, et al: Transforming the treatment of schizophrenia in the United States: the RAISE initiative. Annu Rev Clin Psychol 14(1):237–258, 2018 29328779

EASA Center for Excellence: Program Directory of Early Psychosis Intervention Programs. Salem, OR, Early Assessment and Support Alliance, 2016. Available at: https://med.stanford.edu/content/dam/sm/peppnet/documents/easa-program-directory-2017.pdf. Accessed September 27, 2018.

Fusar-Poli P, McGorry PD, Kane JM: Improving outcomes of first-episode psychosis: an overview. World Psychiatry 16(3):251–265, 2017 28941089

Harding CM, Brooks GW, Ashikaga T, et al: The Vermont longitudinal study of persons with severe mental illness, II: Long-term outcome of subjects who retrospectively met DSM-III criteria for schizophrenia. Am J Psychiatry 144(6):727–735, 1987 3591992

Hardy KV, Moore M, Rose D, et al: Filling the implementation gap: a community-academic partnership approach to early intervention in psychosis. Early Interv Psychiatry 5(4):366–374, 2011 22032550

Kane JM, Robinson DG, Schooler NR, et al: Comprehensive versus usual community care for first-episode psychosis: 2-year outcomes from the NIMH RAISE early treatment program. Am J Psychiatry 173(4):362–372, 2016 26481174

McFarlane WR, Levin B, Travis L, et al: Clinical and functional outcomes after 2 years in the early detection and intervention for the prevention of psychosis multisite effectiveness trial. Schizophr Bull 41(1):30–43, 2015 25065017

McGorry PD, Hickie IB, Yung AR, et al: Clinical staging of psychiatric disorders: a heuristic framework for choosing earlier, safer and more effective interventions. Aust N Z J Psychiatry 40(8):616–622, 2006 16866756

Melle I, Larsen TK, Haahr U, et al: Prevention of negative symptom psychopathologies in first-episode schizophrenia: two-year effects of reducing the duration of untreated psychosis. Arch Gen Psychiatry 65(6):634–640, 2008 18519821

Robinson DG, Woerner MG, Alvir JM, et al: Predictors of treatment response from a first episode of schizophrenia or schizoaffective disorder. Am J Psychiatry 156(4):544–549, 1999 10200732

Srihari VH, Tek C, Pollard J, et al: Reducing the duration of untreated psychosis and its impact in the U.S.: the STEP-ED study. BMC Psychiatry 14(1):335, 2014 25471062

CHAPTER 3

Early Detection of Schizophrenia

A POPULATION HEALTH APPROACH

Maria Ferrara, M.D.
Walter Mathis, M.D.
John D. Cahill, M.D., Ph.D.
Jessica Pollard, Ph.D.
Vinod H. Srihari, M.D.

Case Example

Langston is a 21-year-old African American male who has lived with his mother since being asked to take a leave of absence from a 4-year college. While a freshman 3 years ago, he was taken to the college counseling center by his roommate because he was displaying disorganized thinking and experiencing auditory hallucinations. After assessment by a primary care physician and psychiatrist, Langston was diagnosed with a primary psychotic disorder. His mother recalls that, aside from mild "clumsiness" as a child, he had met usual developmental milestones on time. She remembered noticing, a year or so prior to the psychotic episode, that Langston appeared less interested in socializing with friends and that he would sometimes become preoccupied with the notion that his peers at school were talking about him. She is worried about whether her son will be able to return to college as he wishes. She blames herself for not acting sooner on his behalf to get help and has a lot of questions about Langston's current medications and how to manage his frequent requests to stop treatment.

The schizophrenia spectrum disorders (henceforth *schizophrenia*) are a family of illnesses with diverse etiologies that can exert their impact over an extended period of neurodevelopment (from pregnancy through early adulthood) and cause varied clinical presentations and courses. Despite this heterogeneity, much is known about the course and treatment of schizophrenia. Over the past 20 years, the early intervention services (EIS) paradigm has brought two conceptually overlapping approaches to improve the lives of those afflicted and their family members: early detection seeks to reduce delays to care, and first-episode services (FES), the provision of packages of empirically based interventions by specialty teams, has emerged as a best practice. FES can improve a variety of outcomes in the first few years after psychosis onset. Called coordinated specialty care (CSC) in the United States, these teams are equipped to provide a range of relevant services to clients like Langston (e.g., medication treatment, psychotherapy, vocational assistance) and his mother and other caregivers (e.g., education, support) (Srihari et al. 2012). The delivery of CSC care is detailed in the rest of this book; in this chapter we focus on early detection and specifically on how FES services can conceptualize and implement approaches to shortening delays to care.

The onset of frank psychotic symptoms, usually in late adolescence or early adulthood, can be a distressing and confusing experience. The proactive involvement of humane and competent health care professionals can significantly reduce unnecessary suffering for affected clients and families. This is reason enough to advocate changing the status quo of unacceptably long delays to best practice FES. There is also strong evidence linking prolonged delays in providing care, with poorer long-term outcomes. This association has been consistent across many health care systems and many methods of measuring the time between onset of full-blown psychosis and initiation of appropriate treatment, operationalized as the duration of untreated psychosis (DUP; (Perkins et al. 2005). Furthermore, tests of early detection strategies to reduce DUP have demonstrated reductions in suicidality and symptom severity at presentation to care and improvements in outcomes that are measurable up to 10 years later (Hegelstad et al. 2012). Shorter DUP is associated with reduced social isolation, unemployment, and homelessness. Hastening access to care may also reduce the community burden of suicides and homicides among early psychosis populations (Srihari et al. 2014).

Efforts toward reducing DUP should be contextualized in the rich and longstanding literature pointing to the severe human costs of delayed and inadequate care. Prospective studies of schizophrenia spectrum disorders suggest that most of the clinical and psychosocial deterioration occurs within the first 2–5 years after psychosis onset (Birchwood et al. 1998). This is also a high-risk period for suicide, highest in the first year after first hospitalization for psychotic disorder. In the first 12 months after a psychosis diagnosis, mortality rates were 24 times higher than those of an age-matched cohort in the U.S. general population (Simon et al. 2018b).

This early, turbulent period is usually followed not by progressive decline but rather a plateau in symptoms and impairment, even under usual systems of care. Reassuringly, 75% or more of individuals in treatment for first-episode psychosis (FEP) experience symptomatic remission within the first year (Lieberman et al. 1993; Tohen et al. 2000), but this is often followed by treatment discontinuation and relapse, and less than one-third achieve minimal age appropriate employment or educational functioning in the first few years after frank psychosis has emerged (Menezes et al. 2006). EIS holds the promise of significantly improving on these outcomes of usual care.

Duration of Untreated Psychosis or Duration of Untreated Illness?

Case Example *(continued)*

When asked about when he first noticed a change, Langston was able to recall a period 2 years before his first hospitalization when he felt more sensitive to sounds. Occasionally, other people's voices sounded louder than usual, and, at other times, he heard his name being called but turned around and realized it might have been his imagination. These experiences were infrequent and resolved after a few months, but after this he started hearing whispers. He began to feel "on edge," especially around other people. His mother recalled that during this period he appeared more distracted and was less interested in spending time with his friends after class. Langston also reported that his teachers used "more and more words" he could not follow, and his grades began to drop.

Psychotic symptoms that are severe enough to warrant clinical care are usually preceded by months to even years of prodromal abnormalities in thought (e.g., mild or attenuated positive symptoms), feeling, or behavior (e.g., social withdrawal). There are also measurable declines in cognitive performance and social and school functioning. However, these changes are often apparent only in retrospect as precursors to schizophrenia. The first episode of frank psychosis remains the most reliable way of identifying the presence of a disorder that will likely require chronic treatment. The first episode of psychosis is thus best understood not as the true beginning but rather as the *end of the beginning* of a complex biopsychosocial process wherein vulnerabilities (e.g., genetic, in utero exposures) interact with a wide range of environmental factors to drive progression toward diagnosable illness. Reliable identification of individuals during the pre-FEP phase is an area of active research, and promising possibilities have been tested to prevent or delay progression to full blown psychosis (Millan et al. 2016). Nevertheless, the state of the art for early detection, at the time of this writing, remains focused on targeting FEP (to reduce DUP).

The actions of individuals in a wide variety of roles both within and outside health care agencies (e.g., police, educators, youth and family organizations, clergy) can make a substantial impact on DUP. First-episode services or CSC services need to engage with these stakeholders to implement early detection. In the next section, we provide a conceptual model for such efforts.

Population Health for Early Intervention

Case Example *(continued)*

Langston is of African American descent and the youngest of three siblings raised by their mother, a high school principal. His father had been incarcerated for a drug-related offense and lost contact with the family during Langston's childhood. His older brother, also a schoolteacher, lives nearby with his wife and 3-year-old daughter and helps pay for Langston's living expenses. Langston's sister, the middle sibling, is a physician and has been a strong source of support and a role model for Langston, who attended the same college that she did.

Population health is the goal of "achieving measurable improvements in the health of a defined population" (Kindig et al. 2008, pp. 2081–2083). This perspective turns a critical eye to the definition and measurement of health outcomes (dependent variables) as well as the determinants of health, construed broadly (independent variables). Importantly, there is an embedded concern with social justice; assessing differences in outcomes within the target population—health disparities—is integral to population health. This model can be visualized in a table with mortality and morbidity paired with disparities measured across race and ethnicity, socioeconomic status, geographic location, and sex (Kindig et al. 2008). In our adaptation of Kindig et al.'s (2008) conceptualization, Figure 3–1 lists examples of determinants for early psychosis to illustrate factors that EIS should consider. In addition, quality of life in Kindig's original formulation is enlarged to include a variety of measures of morbidity that are relevant to schizophrenia.

The weighting or relative importance given to various *population health outcomes* should be determined by the *social valuation* of local stakeholders. This means that the list of outcomes chosen for the mor-

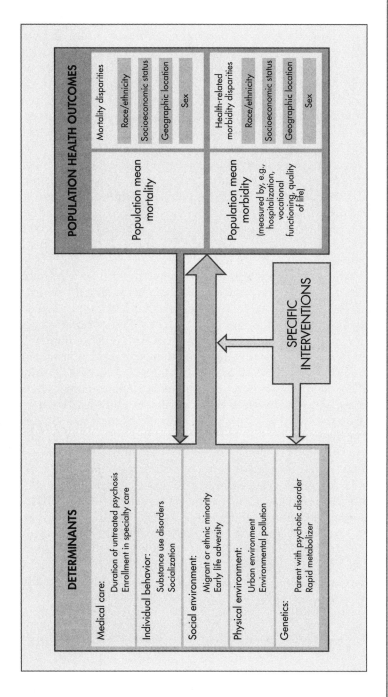

FIGURE 3–1. Population health and early intervention services for schizophrenia.

Source. Adapted from Kindig et al. 2008.

bidity cell can vary across regions. In contrast, the weighting of the relative impact of the *determinants* should be derived empirically (i.e., not by social valuation). The Evans-Stoddart model (Evans et al. 1994) proposes five broad categories of determinants: medical care, individual behavior, social environment, physical environment, and genetics. Factors within these categories can interact with each other in complex ways, limiting inferences about the independent impact of individual determinants. Additionally, these determinants can have differential impacts on different subgroups, contributing to health disparities. For example, minority racial status and residence in a high-crime neighborhood can lead to aversive pathways to care (e.g., via the criminal justice system) that, if not assertively addressed, can contribute to poor engagement with FES and poorer outcomes. As these interactions are better understood, they can be leveraged as targets for specific interventions.

Interventions to improve outcomes can be aimed at moderating the effects of determinants on outcomes (e.g., care models that intentionally intersect with criminal justice agencies [Wasser et al. 2017]), or modifying the determinants directly (e.g., reducing delays to care). Such approaches may require collaboration with diverse community stakeholders because many determinants are not within the direct control of clinics and will need to address a wide mix of population needs that may also have distinct regional profiles. The population health model thus provides a bridge between the poles of the traditional public health focus on more distal determinants of health in mostly non-ill populations (e.g., fortification of salt with iodine, promotion of seat belt use) and the clinical focus on more proximal factors in samples already enrolled in care. For FES staff, the population health framework provides a way to "step out" of the clinic and engage local stakeholders in impacting determinants that operate earlier in the pathway to care, as well as to influence responsiveness to treatment. Geopolitical areas rather than simple geographic zones have been recommended in using the population health framework because funding decisions and regulations are inherently political in nature (Dawn and Teutsch 2012).

How can this framework be made operational by clinics that are seeking to reduce delays to care in their localities? In the next section, we offer a vocabulary for population health–informed early detection and examples and lessons from the application of this approach by an EIS in southern Connecticut, the program for Specialized Treatment Early in Psychosis (STEP).

Pathways, Networks, and Systems: A Vocabulary for Population Health–Based Early Detection

Case Example *(continued)*

When Langston's mother first heard about his difficulties in college, she was mostly concerned that his academic performance not suffer and worried aloud to him that his reduced enthusiasm and social withdrawal in the last year of high school might have persisted into college. She saw this largely as a problem he could address with more effort. She encouraged Langston to seek out more tutoring. When he raised concerns—which he was unable to clearly articulate—about his safety on campus, she suggested that these worries were likely unfounded and advised him to speak to his resident advisor. Instead, Langston repeatedly called the campus police, who were unable to find any evidence to substantiate his concerns and grew increasingly wary of his phone calls.

Over the course of the semester, Langston began going to classes in an increasingly disheveled state, wearing sunglasses even while indoors, and was seen talking to himself in the dormitory corridors. When his sister talked to him on the phone, she grew concerned about his mental state and requested that his roommate accompany him to the college counseling center. This was Langston's first experience of mental health care and resulted in the recommendation that he withdraw from college to attend to his health. Although there was an appointment scheduled in 1 month's time with the primary care physician, Langston's mother was able to arrange for him to be evaluated earlier by a psychiatrist, who diagnosed him with a schizophrenia spectrum disorder and prescribed antipsychotic medication.

After Langston returned home, he asked to stop seeing the psychiatrist. He noted feeling safe at home and said that the medication made him feel "emotionally flat." He did not think his psychiatrist understood his concerns; "he just wants me to take the medications." Eventually, Langston prevailed in his wishes to stop seeing the psychiatrist and to discontinue antipsychotic medication. After he discontinued treatment, he appeared indifferent about most of his prior interests, including playing the guitar (a long-standing passion), and seemed content to stay in his room. His brother sometimes found him staring at the wall and grew frustrated after trying repeatedly to get him to spend more time with his family or go out with friends from high school.

Six months later, when Langston again started paying less attention to his personal hygiene, as he had before his first psychotic episode, his mother grew more concerned. Langston became increasingly irritable and voiced suspicions that the neighbors were watching him and sending him messages through their shared wall. One evening, his mother had to call the police after he pushed her to the floor. The police officer found Langston to be markedly disheveled, loudly alleging that "[the neighbors are] messing with my business" and that his mother "does not believe me." The officer had to threaten him with arrest to have him agree to an evaluation at the local emergency department.

Langston arrived at the hospital upset and refusing to cooperate with the psychiatric evaluation. He was placed in soft leather restraints and given involuntary intramuscular tranquilizing medications after he threw his food tray at a staff member and attempted to run out of the emergency room. After a brief hospitalization of 6 days, during which he agreed to take antipsychotic medications and follow up with after-care, Langston was discharged with a referral to a local clinic. However, he did not arrive for this visit, explaining to his mother that he now felt better and saw no need for care.

One week later, Langston was sent back to the emergency department from a local community college where, per the police report, he was found "wandering on campus" in a severely disorganized state. After two more involuntary hospitalizations, he was referred to a local FES, the STEP clinic. This was 18 months after the onset of the psychotic symptoms that had led to his leaving college.

Langston's journey (a composite of many individual narratives) is marked by inordinate delay, lost opportunities for referral and engagement with FES, and aversive interactions with criminal justice and involuntary medical care. However, this journey to FES can also be viewed as involving many community members with important roles in this young person's life who can be empowered to assist his passage to optimal care and eventual return to a full role in these communities. In the next subsection, we seek to provide a set of useful concepts and approaches toward this goal.

Pathways and Networks: Essential Concepts for Early Detection

A diverse group of actors are often involved in a young person's journey, or *pathway*, to FES. Psychotic illnesses can cause behavioral disruptions in many settings, but perhaps unlike other public medical events (e.g., cardiac arrest, seizures), these behaviors can be met with combinations of fear of violence, aversion, or shaming responses from uneducated observers. This means that a network of care needs to extend beyond traditional clinical settings to include all who might be expected to facilitate pathways to and through FES.

Langston's pathway to care can be divided into two periods that constitute the DUP: the *demand* side (illness identification and attempts to access health care) and *supply* side (diagnosis of psychosis, initiation of treatment, and referral to FES) (Srihari et al. 2014). The demand side of DUP includes all the actors, events, and opportunities that emerge in the window of time that begins with the onset of frank psychosis and ends with contact with a health care provider or facility with the ability to initiate treatment and referral to best practice care. The supply side begins with such contact and ends with entry into best practice care or FES. Delays in both the demand and supply sides are implicated in prolonged DUP.

A heuristic model of Langston's pathways to FES, as used by the STEP program, is provided in Figure 3–2. The dashed line depicts the demand side of delay, which in this client's case intersected with at least five distinct groups (family, friends, college staff, police, and mental health services) before engagement with STEP. In Langston's case, there was a delay between the onset of symptoms and signs and the recognition of a need for professional care (at college counseling). Rather than entry into FES, this resulted in visits to an available psychiatrist covered by Langston's mother's health insurance plan. Although this ended the demand side of the journey, it certainly did not mark the end of DUP. Rather, this was the beginning of the supply side of delay. The needs of individuals with FEP and their families for education and iterative, extended attempts at engagement into care proved beyond the capacity of the private psychiatrist. However, when the psychiatrist was unable to provide needed care, effective referral to local FES was not made. After disengagement with this provider, Langston unfortunately reentered the medical system in a manner that required the intervention of the police. This aversive, involuntary process likely led to an understandable reluctance on Langston's part to engage with psychiatric services after discharge from the hospital. Thus, even when best practice care is locally available, supply-side delays can be considerable and can be mediated by a dynamic mix of factors, including a lack awareness of the client of the need for care, the potentially alienating experience of involuntary care, and the various ways in which providers may be unaware of, or unable to make, appropriate referrals to FES.

How can this inform an early detection strategy? An FES that takes a population health approach to early detection will need to decide on a target region and then consider how to intervene on these variables to shorten DUP. One way to begin is to consider who the relevant actors may be in the local network. Figure 3–3 depicts eight stakeholder groups identified in the planning phases of STEP's early detection strategy, which is focused on a geopolitical catchment of 10 towns, with approximately 400,000 residents. The list was prepared by consulting the literature as well as clinicians and administrators with tenure in the region of interest. These categories can help organize a strategy and can be expanded or narrowed as data are gathered on actual local pathways. These data can be gathered passively from electronic health records of integrated health care networks and/or claims databases (Simon et al. 2018a) or, ideally, national registries (Srihari 2018) that can inform the FES on the distribution of contacts that clients with FEP have

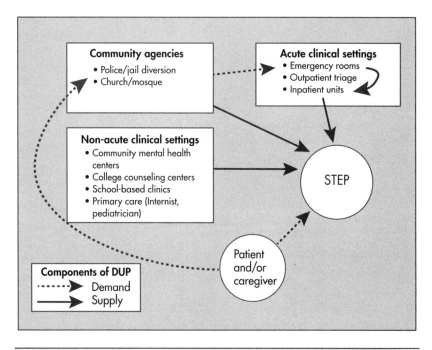

FIGURE 3–2. Heuristic model for DUP in STEP's catchment.

Abbreviations.   DUP=duration of untreated psychosis; STEP= Specialized Treatment Early in Psychosis.

Source.   Adapted from Srihari et al. 2014.

made, within and outside the health care sector. Additionally, the FES can use structured questionnaires to query entrants about all their prior help-seeking attempts, which allows the FES to gather information about contacts outside formal systems of care. However, these data will suffer from a sampling bias by being able to include only clients who have been able to enroll at the service. Such questionnaires (Judge et al. 2005) can nevertheless provide the FES with useful information about local referral partners and targets for professional outreach.

Information gathered about local pathways will raise the need for a response. For example, long delays on the demand side may suggest that individuals with FEP and their families are waiting too long to seek care. This may reflect a low degree of awareness in the community of the common signs and symptoms of psychosis. Information campaigns, such as those tested by the Norwegian Early Treatment and Intervention in Psychosis (TIPS) investigators using print, broadcast, and online media, were partly directed at this possibility (Johannessen et al. 2001). Such delays, however, could also be due to the relative inaccessibility or unattractiveness of available care. A few of the interventions that can

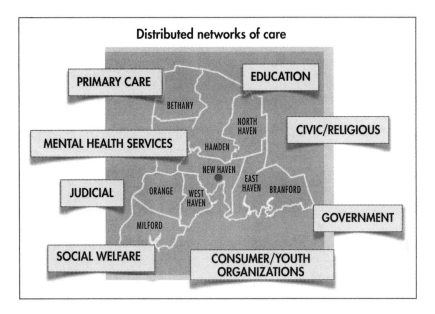

FIGURE 3–3. Understanding local networks to transform pathways to early intervention services.

have an impact include quick, flexible responses to requests for help; the ability to conduct assessments in familiar (e.g., homes, college campuses) or acute care (e.g., emergency departments, inpatient units) settings; and the lowering of structural barriers to care access (e.g., insurance coverage, age restrictions, transportation costs).

To shorten the supply side of DUP, interfacing with members of the local referral network (i.e., individuals and agencies that are or can be influential on local pathways to care for FEP) emerges as a key task. Conducting educational workshops with provision of continuing education credits that are ideally followed up by recurring visits to places of work can be used as a platform to build relationships wherein the FEP is more likely to be detected early in the pathway (e.g., by the college counseling staff who are worried but yet uncertain about a psychosis diagnosis). There is also a need for quick and welcoming responses to calls for consultation from these colleagues. Many of these calls may not concern eligible clients, but responding to them promptly will establish networks that enable rapid identification of other individuals experiencing FEP. Local groups that have not generated referrals (e.g., primary care clinics) may require proactive outreach efforts from the FES.

Finally, delays on the supply side can happen at the "front door" of the FES. The time between receipt of an appropriate referral and entry into FES care can be prolonged by a collusion of many factors, including the common ambivalence of the client to entering treatment, the work-flow of busy clinicians who may struggle to prioritize new assessments over established clients, and myriad other factors that are often idiosyn-cratic to each case. The use of a dedicated *early detection team* tasked with the mission of reducing DUP can help assure good customer service to all calls for assistance and arrange rapid assessments for eligibility. In order to facilitate rapid enrollment into care, program leadership is vital to en-sure careful handoff to the clinicians on the FES team. Regular audits of times between referral and enrollment, within a performance improve-ment ethos and under oversight by program leadership, can help the team discover sources of delay that might require more systematic atten-tion, while also ensuring organizational learning about how to respond in a more personalized manner to modifiable and client-specific sources of delay. It is vital to avoid the enactment of implicit waitlists for FES.

The list of tasks needed to enable early detection can be culled from approaches used by systematic efforts to reduce DUP but can also be developed over time by an FES that is gathering knowledge of local pathways. Early detection can be a resource-intensive project, and there is a related paradox that will confront an FES that seeks to shorten DUP: although most clinicians can easily recall cases where any of a variety of efforts demonstrably reduced delays and improved the experience of entry for particular clients, it can be difficult to demonstrate this at a population level. Reviews of prior research point to the challenges of ef-fecting measurable reductions in regional DUP (Oliver et al. 2018), with a plethora of factors likely implicated in these delays. The fact that all of these factors cannot be feasibly addressed by an FES or even multiple agencies within the health care sector is a sobering reality.

Some features of U.S. health care, including fragmented payment and delivery and the lack of established gatekeepers to specialty care, make early detection more challenging. The multifactorial and dynamic nature of these interactive factors necessitates the use of many strategies at once. Furthermore, the distribution of factors across geopolitical regions will vary, along with their relative responsiveness to intervention: what works in one region may not work in another. Campaigns that have succeeded in-cluded multiyear strategies targeting multiple sources of delay in demand and supply. The seminal Norwegian TIPS study used an intensive media campaign along with early detection teams that could rapidly assess refer-rals in the community. STEP's ongoing early detection effort (the MindMap campaign; Srihari et al. 2014) has acted on this insight to implement a *so-cioecological* approach that targets a very wide range of putative levers for DUP reduction that are generalizable as categories across diverse U.S. health care ecologies but engages actors who are specifically salient within the targeted geopolitical region.

Given these challenges, FES providers may reasonably worry about the diversion of limited resources from the treatment of already admitted patients toward early detection efforts. However, the reduction of DUP can reduce unnecessary suffering in a community, may reduce suicide and violence during a critical period of elevated risk, and has been shown to have durable effects on long-term outcomes (Hegelstad et al. 2012). Allocating resources between these two components (early detection and FES) of EIS presents a difficult trade-off. One way to navigate this tension is to conceptualize the role of the clinical service as an *integrator of a local network of actors* wherein the work of improving population outcomes becomes a shared task. This is taken up in the next section.

Building Systems for Early Intervention Services

We prefer to use *system* to refer to a set of activities with a common set of objectives to contrast with the common usage of the term to connote the fixed features of some aggregation of health care agencies or actors. Our putative population health systems include the dynamic caregiving activities of a wide and variable group of actors (in Langston's case, his peers in college, campus security, his family, and college instructors) who may or may not be coordinating efforts or even be aware of themselves as assisting help seeking, are mostly outside the formal health care sector, and may have limited prior experience with accessing FES. Along with health care agencies, such de facto regional *networks* determine the quality and speed of clients' *pathways* to and through the health care system and the resources available for recovery (Figure 3–4). The hosting and self-aware integration of such a regional network should become a priority for FES staff who wish to provide a regional system of EIS.

When services are organized into a functioning system of care (Srihari et al. 2016), the following occurs:

1. There is a common overall *aim*.
2. Objectives are drawn from a list of outcomes that, per the population health framework, have been prioritized on the basis of the social valuation of local stakeholders.
3. These objectives are tied to "achievable" *standards* of what is feasible locally and continually aspire to what has been accomplished in best practice international EIS. The *objectives* are explicit and linked to outcome *measures* that are client centered but also include measures of relevance to other agents who are important for optimal pathways to care and can be leveraged to become active stakeholders in this system.

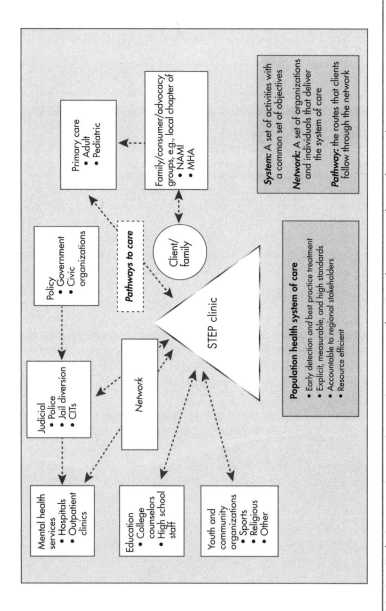

FIGURE 3–4. Early intervention services as integrators of regional systems of care for psychosis.

Abbreviations. CITs=crisis intervention teams; MHA=Mental Health America; NAMI=National Alliance on Mental Illness.

One working example of such a system specification from the STEP program is depicted in Table 3–1.

The generation of a list of objectives (which is dynamic) involves iterative and systematic querying of local stakeholders, conversion of their values to rigorous and feasible measurement protocols, and establishing a culture of practice within the clinical service that respects such measurement and welcomes changes in care processes to respond to gaps between achievable and aspirational standards. The description of how to do this is beyond the scope of this chapter, but we seek here to highlight the need for local ownership of the system and the role of the clinic in hosting the generation of a system specification that can hold the EIS accountable to local stakeholders but also engage them in collaborative efforts to improve outcomes of shared interest.

Regular auditing (e.g., in an annual report or actively maintained dashboard) of progress toward espoused standards can drive refinements of care within an iterative process. This requires flexibility, creativity, responsiveness, and collaboration from all stakeholders—there are no recipes or key ingredients that will deliver improvement across all valued outcomes. In this way, the mission of early detection is embedded as one objective within the overall goal of improving outcomes for early psychosis populations, and each objective can be prioritized on the basis of measured performance of a particular EIS. Baseline assessments of pathways to care for FES enrollees might suggest opportunities for improvement with traditional plan-do-study-act cycles. For example, to address poor rates of follow-up from inpatient referrals, providers of the STEP program have used brief visits to meet patients on referring inpatient units to effectively decrease no-shows for first appointments.

The development and use of reliable measurement procedures for these or other outcomes is an important consideration but beyond the scope of this chapter. Some combination of passive harvesting from electronic health records (when possible), with dedicated and trained staff to administer a limited number of measures (e.g., the Positive and Negative Syndrome Scale [PANSS]), would meet the needs of most EIS that wish to demonstrate impact to their stakeholders. As we have argued elsewhere (Pollard et al. 2016; Srihari et al. 2016), keeping this end in mind should be part of the implementation of new services rather than an afterthought. Although there are no consensually accepted measures for DUP, early detection efforts can begin by choosing one of several available conceptualizations (Polari et al. 2011) and investing resources over time to improve reliability.

TABLE 3–1. System specification for STEP's population health–based early intervention services in southern Connecticut

Objective[a]	Measure	Standard
Access		
Rapidity	DUP 1 <3 months[b]	Achievable (30%); aspirational (75%)
	DUP 2 <12 months[c]	Achievable (50%); aspirational (75%)
Equity	Proportion of females	Achievable (20%); aspirational (30%)
	Ratio of ethnic groups	Aspirational: matches census percentages
	Ratio of towns of residence	Aspirational: matches percentage of towns
	Proportion ages <18	Achievable (5%); aspirational (10%)
Coverage	Number annually offered STEP care/expected annual incidence in the zone	Achievable (15%); aspirational (80%)
Pathways to care	Proportion of individuals admitted to STEP after psychiatric hospitalization	Achievable (<60%); aspirational (<30%)
Engagement		
Overall engagement	In contact with FES at 12 months postadmission	Achievable (70%); aspirational (90%)
Exposure to family education and support	Family participation in at least one qualifying event in first month	Achievable (75%); aspirational (90%)
Exposure to specialized, empirically based psychotherapy	Engagement in qualifying event in first month	Achievable (75%); aspirational (90%)
Outcomes		
Hospitalization	Psychiatric admission in months 1–6 and 7–12	Achievable (<25%); aspirational (<10%)
Suicide prevention	Patients making attempt in first year of admission	Achievable (<10%); aspirational (<1%)

TABLE 3–1.   System specification for STEP's population health–based early intervention services in southern Connecticut *(continued)*

Objective[a]	Measure	Standard
Outcomes *(continued)*		
Remission	PANSS positive subscore <3 at 6 months	Achievable (70%); aspirational (85%)
	PANSS positive subscore <3 at 1 year	Achievable (80%); aspirational (90%)
Recovery	GF: Role scale level 8 or better	Achievable (70%); aspirational (85%)
	GF: Social scale level 8 or better	Achievable (70%); aspirational (85%)
Vocational engagement	Not in labor market (NEET full or part time; not a full-time caregiver)	Achievable (<10%); aspirational (<5%)
Cardiovascular risk		
Smoking	New smokers at 6 months	Achievable (<20%); aspirational (<10%)
	Smoking rate at 6 months	Achievable (<60%); aspirational (<30%)
Overweight or obese	BMI <25 at 12 months	Achievable (30%); aspirational (75%)
	Normal BMIs retained at 12 months	Achievable (60%); aspirational (75%)
Disposition	Successfully transitioned to mainstream health care services at or before 2 years	Achievable (70%); aspirational (80%)

[a]The overall aim of population health system for early intervention is to "transform outcomes of all individuals within the first 3 years of psychosis onset within a catchment zone of 10 surrounding towns" (extracted from the program for Specialized Treatment Early in Psychosis [STEP] in New Haven, Connecticut).
[b]DUP 1: time between psychosis onset and first antipsychotic medication trial.
[c]DUP 2: time between psychosis onset and enrollment in STEP.
Abbreviations.   BMI=body mass index (calculated as weight in kilograms divided by height in meters squared); DUP=duration of untreated psychosis; FES=first-episode services; NEET=not in education, employment, or training; GF=Global Functioning: Role and Social Scale; PANSS=Positive and Negative Syndrome Scale; STEP=Specialized Treatment Early in Psychosis.
Source.   Adapted from Srihari et al. 2016.

Early Detection and the Future
of Early Intervention Services

Case Example *(continued)*

Soon after entering the STEP clinic, Langston expressed a strong wish to
return to college and added that he experienced his visits to the clinic
and his interaction with psychiatric care in general as an interruption in
his education and planned trajectory to train to become a nurse.
Langston's clinician connected him to the vocational counselor on the
CSC team, who first helped him navigate his way out of liability for
most of his tuition for his last semester. She also helped him prepare an
application to a local community college.

Two months after enrollment, Langston accepted a low dose of an
antipsychotic medication and reported that it helped him sleep and was
not causing him to feel emotionally dulled. He continued to voice concerns about his neighbors but learned to not bring up his concerns directly with them but rather to discuss them with his clinician.

Six months after entering the STEP clinic, Langston was able to return
part time to a local community college with a plan to eventually transfer to
a nearby state university, where he planned to work toward a bachelor's
degree in nursing. He has allowed regular contact with his family, especially his sister, and his mother and brother have visited individually with
clinic staff and attended workshops with other family members.

The first few years after the onset of frank psychosis can be turbulent ones for those affected and for their caregivers, along with the
many other community members who are also typically involved. In
usual care systems, this period is marked by elevated risks for suicide,
aggression, and cycles of treatment discontinuation and symptomatic
relapse that can exact a disproportionate toll on long-term functioning
by derailing educational and vocational trajectories at a developmentally vulnerable period of young adulthood. Conversely, the provision
of EIS can address many modifiable prognostic factors at once and can
achieve gratifying results for all stakeholders. This is an optimistic time
for early psychosis care in the United States: leadership from the National Institute of Mental Health and the Substance Abuse and Mental
Health Services Administration has catalyzed the establishment of multiple new CSC services across the country (Dixon et al. 2018). These
could serve as a platform for adding early detection to further maximize population health impact.

As knowledge of the pre-psychotic phases of schizophrenia evolves,
the population health systems we advocate for in this chapter could
also serve to implement earlier intervention to potentially delay or even
prevent FEP. In the interim, these EIS can participate in necessary re-

search to better delineate the trajectory of prodromal states and to test preventive approaches.

KEY CONCEPTS

- The period between psychosis onset and entry into care is associated with significant suffering, disability, risk for violence, suicide, and the emergence of comorbidities (e.g., substance abuse).

- Evidence from worldwide early detection studies to shorten the duration of untreated psychosis (DUP) and efforts by first-episode services (FES) or, in the United States, coordinated specialty care (CSC) suggest that many of these sources of suffering, disability, and premature mortality are modifiable, and the early period after emergence of psychosis is a particularly important window of opportunity.

- Early detection efforts focused on shortening DUP offer a way to further improve on outcomes of established FES or CSC teams.

- Population health approaches to early detection can help transform community-based FES or CSC into comprehensive EIS programs.

- FES or CSC teams can have a powerful influence on local systems of care while attempting to reduce DUP and improve pathways to care.

Discussion Questions

1. Which geopolitical region do you wish to target for early detection efforts?

2. Who are the key stakeholders in this region, and what are their expectations of your EIS? How can you make common cause with them on your goals?

3. Which population outcome benchmarks are you hoping to meet with your EIS? How will you include your local network as full stakeholders in these outcomes?

4. What barriers to early detection do you expect within your FES or health care agency?

5. How do you envision integrating emerging knowledge about detection of prodromal states into your service?

Suggested Readings

Birchwood M, Todd P, Jackson C: Early intervention in psychosis: the critical period hypothesis. Br J Psychiatry Suppl 172(33):53–59, 1998. An excellent summary of observational data supporting the critical period hypothesis that continues to provide a useful organizing principle for early intervention services.

Kane JM, Robinson DG, Schooler NR, et al: Comprehensive versus usual community care for first-episode psychosis: 2-year outcomes from the NIMH RAISE early treatment program. Am J Psychiatry 173(4):362–372, 2016. Multisite cluster randomized trial of a first-episode service that established the feasible application of this model of care across multiple nonacademic clinical settings in the United States.

Srihari VH, Cahill JD: Early intervention for schizophrenia: building systems of care for knowledge translation, in Youth Mental Health: Vulnerability and Opportunities for Prevention and Early Intervention. Strüngmann Forum Rep Vol 28. Edited by Uhlhaas PJ, Wood SW. Cambridge, MA, MIT Press, 2019. An elaboration of the population health–based model for national implementation that invokes the concept of learning health care systems.

Srihari VH, Shah J, Keshavan MS: Is early intervention for psychosis feasible and effective? Psychiatr Clin North Am 35(3):613–631, 2012. Picking up from Birchwood's summary of observational data, this paper reviews subsequent experimental data from randomized trials of first-episode services from around the world prior to the U.S. STEP and RAISE trials.

Srihari VH, Tek C, Pollard J, et al: Reducing the duration of untreated psychosis and its impact in the U.S.: the STEP-ED study. BMC Psychiatry 14(1):335, 2014. Details of the rationale and design of the first U.S. attempt to adapt and replicate the TIPS study.

Srihari VH, Tek C, Kucukgoncu S, et al: First-episode services for psychotic disorders in the U.S. public sector: a pragmatic randomized controlled trial. Psychiatr Serv 66(7):705–712, 2015. First randomized controlled study of a first-episode service in the United States, which showed effectiveness of specialty team–based care within a public-academic collaboration.

Srihari VH, Jani A, Gray M: Early intervention for psychotic disorders: building population health systems. JAMA Psychiatry 73(2):101–102, 2016.The STEP program's vision for population-based early intervention services.

References

Birchwood M, Todd P, Jackson C: Early intervention in psychosis: the critical period hypothesis. Br J Psychiatry Suppl 172(33):53–59, 1998 9764127

Dawn MJ, Teutsch S: An Environmental Scan of Integrated Approaches for Defining and Measuring Total Population Health by the Clinical Care System, the Government Public Health System, and Stakeholder Organizations. Washington, DC, National Quality Forum, June 2012. Available at: www.qualityforum.org/Publications/2012/06/An_Environmental_Scan_of_Integrated_Approaches_for_Defining_and_Measuring_Total_Population_Health.aspx. Retrieved September 27, 2018.

Dixon LB, Goldman HH, Srihari VH, et al: Transforming the treatment of schizophrenia in the United States: the RAISE Initiative. Annu Rev Clin Psychol 14:237–258, 2018 29328779

Evans RG, Barer ML, Marmor TR: Why Are Some People Healthy and Others Not? The Determinants of Health of Populations. New York, Aldine de Gruyter, 1994

Hegelstad WT, Larsen TK, Auestad B, et al: Long-term follow-up of the TIPS early detection in psychosis study: effects on 10-year outcome. Am J Psychiatry 169(4):374–380, 2012 22407080

Johannessen JO, McGlashan TH, Larsen TK, et al: Early detection strategies for untreated first-episode psychosis. Schizophr Res 51(1):39–46, 2001 11479064

Judge AM, Perkins DO, Nieri J, et al: Pathways to care in first episode psychosis: a pilot study on help-seeking precipitants and barriers to care. J Ment Health 14(5):465–469, 2005

Kindig DA, Asada Y, Booske B: A population health framework for setting national and state health goals. JAMA 299(17):2081–2083, 2008 18460667

Lieberman J, Jody D, Geisler S, et al: Time course and biologic correlates of treatment response in first-episode schizophrenia. Arch Gen Psychiatry 50(5):369–376, 1993 8098203

Menezes NM, Arenovich T, Zipursky RB: A systematic review of longitudinal outcome studies of first-episode psychosis. Psychol Med 36(10):1349–1362, 2006 16756689

Millan MJ, Andrieux A, Bartzokis G, et al: Altering the course of schizophrenia: progress and perspectives. Nat Rev Drug Discov 15(7):485–515, 2016 26939910

Oliver D, Davies C, Crossland G, et al: Can we reduce the duration of untreated psychosis? A systematic review and meta-analysis of controlled interventional studies. Schizophr Bull January 24, 2018 [Epub ahead of print] 29373755

Perkins DO, Gu H, Boteva K, Lieberman JA: Relationship between duration of untreated psychosis and outcome in first-episode schizophrenia: a critical review and meta-analysis. Am J Psychiatry 162(10):1785–1804, 2005 16199825

Polari A, Lavoie S, Sarrasin P, et al: Duration of untreated psychosis: a proposition regarding treatment definition. Early Interv Psychiatry 5(4):301–308, 2011 22032548

Pollard MJ, Cahill DJ, Srihari HV: Building early intervention services for psychotic disorders: a primer for early adopters in the U.S. Curr Psychiatry Rev 12(4):350–356, 2016

Simon GE, Stewart C, Hunkeler EM, et al: Care pathways before first diagnosis of a psychotic disorder in adolescents and young adults. Am J Psychiatry 175(5):434–442, 2018a 29361848

Simon GE, Stewart C, Yarborough BJ, et al: Mortality rates after the first diagnosis of psychotic disorder in adolescents and young adults. JAMA Psychiatry 75(3):254–260, 2018b 29387876

Srihari VH: Working toward changing the duration of untreated psychosis (DUP). Schizophr Res 193:39–40, 2018 28779850

Srihari VH, Shah J, Keshavan MS: Is early intervention for psychosis feasible and effective? Psychiatr Clin North Am 35(3):613–631, 2012 22929869

Srihari VH, Tek C, Pollard J, et al: Reducing the duration of untreated psychosis and its impact in the U.S.: the STEP-ED study. BMC Psychiatry 14:335, 2014 25471062

Srihari VH, Jani A, Gray M: Early intervention for psychotic disorders: building population health systems. JAMA Psychiatry 73(2):101–102, 2016 26747524

Tohen M, Strakowski SM, Zarate C Jr, et al: The McLean-Harvard first-episode project: 6-month symptomatic and functional outcome in affective and nonaffective psychosis. Biol Psychiatry 48(6):467–476, 2000 11018220

Wasser T, Pollard J, Fisk D, et al: First-episode psychosis and the criminal justice system: using a sequential intercept framework to highlight risks and opportunities. Psychiatr Serv 68(10):994–996, 2017 28859587

CHAPTER 4

Early Intervention and Policy

Abram Rosenblatt, Ph.D.
Howard H. Goldman, M.D., Ph.D.

SIGNIFICANT advances in the early treatment of psychosis occur in the nexus of numerous challenges for contemporary mental health policy formulation in the United States. Adolescents and young adults typically develop psychosis in the transitional age range of 15–25 years, when services must bridge child- and adult-focused delivery systems. Effective constellations of services for early psychosis require a broad range of therapeutic treatments, psychosocial interventions, and educational or vocational services. By definition, early treatment often requires providing preventive-based services before young people fully meet specific diagnostic and disability criteria. Evidence-based service delivery models for early psychosis are most effectively applied to those persons for whom the interventions were originally developed. To maximize their effectiveness, these services require fidelity and quality monitoring as well as sufficient training and ongoing supports. All the policy-relevant aspects of financing and delivering services for the early treatment of psychosis transpire against the backdrop of a continually shifting health policy landscape, especially with the Affordable Care Act (ACA) facing ongoing legislative and administrative modifications.

In this chapter, we focus on policy considerations pertinent to the early treatment of psychosis within the broader context of contemporary challenges for health and mental health policy. Financing effective early treatment services remains at the core of policy formulation, with the overall goal of providing affordable and accessible health insurance coverage (Goldman 2017). Although financing is a necessary condition for humane policy formation, it is far from sufficient in assuring access to services (Saloner et al. 2017) or in enhancing the effectiveness and efficiency of service delivery (Dixon et al. 2018). Additional challenges for policy development include fragmentation in categorically based service delivery systems, translating and implementing evidence-based services in community settings, monitoring fidelity and quality, establishing a sufficient workforce, and addressing discriminatory attitudes and practices.

Financing Early Psychosis Treatment

Coordinated Specialty Care

In the United States, individuals with schizophrenia have high rates of morbidity and mortality. People with psychotic disorders, including schizophrenia, die an average of 11 years earlier than the general population, and up to 10% die by suicide (Druss et al. 2011). Individuals have a three times higher rate of mortality in the 3 years following an initial diagnosis of psychosis when compared with a general outpatient population (Simon et al. 2018). By any measure, schizophrenia constitutes a serious public health problem. The emergent understanding of schizophrenia as a modifiable illness, with the initial onset of symptoms representing an optimal time for intervention, underlies current early intervention treatment approaches that carry the promise of clinical and functional recovery for persons with schizophrenia (Dixon et al. 2015). Current evidence establishes that early intervention in psychosis, specifically coordinated specialty care (CSC), can improve symptoms and functioning when compared with usual care (Dixon et al. 2018).

CSC is a team-based intervention developed for persons with first-episode psychosis that fosters recovery and strives to prevent disability, focusing particularly on the first episode of psychosis. It combines various well-established evidence-based treatments, including assertive case management, individual or group psychotherapy, supported employment and education services, family education and support, and, as necessary, low doses of antipsychotic medications. These services are also closely coordinated with primary health care (Azrin et al. 2015). In addition to its multidisciplinary team-based approach, CSC relies on a suite of recovery-oriented person-centered treatment approaches combined in a shared decision-making framework. This approach is designed to engage young people in treatment and keep them participating while respecting their preferences and treatment goals. When appropriate, CSC engages the individual's close friends, family members, or peer supports as active participants (Dixon et al. 2018).

A series of studies (e.g., Dixon et al. 2018) demonstrates the feasibility, acceptability, and effectiveness of CSC in U.S. community mental health settings. Yet the adoption of the model is far from universal, largely because of a lack of adequate financing (Lieberman et al. 2013). Financing first-episode psychosis (FEP) services is complex and difficult, requiring funding an array of services that are not typically covered by public or private health insurance (Shern et al. 2017). Medicaid can fund psychotherapy, case management, family support and education, medication, and, in some states, supported employment and education or peer support. However, Medicaid does not cover community outreach and the full cost of supported employment and education services, among other program costs. Commercial health insurance programs are more restrictive, allowing for billing of psychotherapy, case management, and medication while leaving other services unreimbursed. Consequently, states rely on additional local funding sources for CSC program implementation, including highly variable state general funds. Some states, such as Oregon and New York, are using Section 1115 waiver demonstrations to address early psychosis. These demonstrations originate from Section 1115 of the Social Security Act, which allows the U.S. Department of Health and Human Services to approve experimental, pilot, or demonstration projects that further the objectives of Medicaid and the Children's Health Insurance Program (CHIP). Waiver demonstrations allow for the flexibility to design and improve programs; demonstrate and evaluate policy approaches; and use innovative service delivery systems to improve care, increase efficiency, and reduce costs.

Adding to the complexity is the age at onset for psychosis, which often falls during late adolescence or early adulthood. Funding for services to children and adolescents who are 21 years of age and younger includes options that have no comparable adult funding mechanisms. Medicaid-eligible children with a mental health diagnosis that meets medical necessity criteria are federally entitled to receive mental health services through the Early and Periodic Screening, Diagnostic, and Treatment (EPSDT) program. This program includes young people in the dependency and juvenile justice systems. EPSDT is relatively comprehensive, funding a wide variety of services, including some of those that are necessary for CSC.

Although usually underfunded and difficult to access, special education enabled through the Individuals with Disabilities Education Act (IDEA) also provides a federal entitlement to mental health services to assist children in achieving educational benefits. IDEA eligibility ends at age 21. In addition, civil rights law (Section 504) prohibits discrimination on the basis of disabling conditions such as psychosis by schools benefiting from federal financial assistance. Unfortunately, the criteria for identification, eligibility, appropriate education, and due process procedures vary between IDEA and Section 504, complicating transitions in educational services. Similarly, as youth younger than age 21 who are in the early stages of psychosis transition to the adult mental health system, they may lose coverage for a range of services consistent with CSC. Additionally, when youth become adults, those youth who are not Medicaid eligible must typically meet a means test and stringent mental illness criteria to access public services.

The ACA improved funding opportunities for CSC services through both expanded private insurance and increased Medicaid coverage. Prior to the passage of the ACA, youth were removed from parental health insurance unless they were full-time students, lost insurance if they left the workplace, and were potentially excluded from insurance because their mental illness was considered a preexisting condition (Goldman et al. 2013). Under the ACA, many individuals younger than age 26 remain on parental insurance even if they are not full-time students. The removal of preexisting condition limitations allows individuals to purchase insurance on the health exchanges even though their FEP would previously have been considered a preexisting condition. More individuals now qualify for Medicaid in Medicaid expansion states, even if they are not yet disabled and receiving Supplemental Security Income. Preventive services and essential health benefits are expanded. A state can also modify its Medicaid plan to include CSC under the 1915i provisions of the ACA (Goldman et al. 2013). Yet with all of these positive changes, states still need to supplement CSC services and provide resources for staff training as well as outreach and engagement (Goldman and Karakus 2014).

Also potentially relevant to funding CSC services, the ACA included provisions for the establishment of health homes. Health homes are intended to improve the treatment of chronic conditions, including for individuals with schizophrenia and other mental health disorders, by providing flexibility in both the array and intensity of services provided. States have considerable flexibility, but the provisions for these health homes do not allow for funding the provision of direct, individual treatment services. Potential supports such as information technology, training, and oversight can be funded. States are currently experimenting with implementing CSC services within health homes (Shern et al. 2017).

The Substance Abuse and Mental Health Services Administration (SAMHSA) provides essential support for FEP services, including the implementation of CSC. Community Mental Health Block Grants allow states to implement models across a continuum, including those that are required for CSC. SAMHSA's Mental Health Services Block Grants (MHBGs) are noncompetitive and provide funding for community-based mental health services for adults with serious mental illness or children with serious emotional disturbance. A 5% allocation set aside for CSC programs began in 2015 and was doubled to 10% in 2016, providing $50 million that states can use to develop CSC programs. Currently, 36 states are implementing one or more CSC programs. The 21st Century Cures Act reinforces the allocation, requiring states to use at least 10% of their block grant funds on CSC for individuals with early psychosis. SAMHSA, in collaboration with the National Institute of Mental Health (NIMH) and Office of the Assistant Secretary for Planning and Evaluation, contracted with a research corporation (Westat) to lead an evaluation of this Mental Health Block Grant 10% SetAside. This national evaluation will provide information on the implementation and outcomes of FEP sites funded through the MHBG (Rosenblatt 2018).

In 2017, SAMHSA also awarded funding to eight states to participate in a 2-year demonstration project to expand access to behavioral health services in community-based settings (Shern et al. 2017). Participating states receiving the funding will develop certified community behavioral health clinics (CCBHCs), which will receive enhanced Medicaid reimbursement rates to better align with the costs of providing community-based care. The services provided through the CCBHCs are suitable for providing CSC and include crisis services; screening, assessment, and diagnosis (including risk assessment); client-centered treatment and planning; outpatient behavioral health services; outpatient primary care screening and monitoring; targeted case management; psychiatric rehabilitation services; peer support and family support services; and intensive community care for veterans and members of the armed forces. CCBHCs prioritize 24-hour crisis services, evidence-based practices, care coordination, and the integration of physical and behavioral health care.

In 2018, SAMHSA broadened funding opportunities to include awards for services delivered to youth who are at clinical high risk for psychosis (the Community Programs for Outreach and Intervention With Youth and Young Adults at Clinical High Risk for Psychosis Grant Program, CFDA 93.243). The purpose of this program is to identify youth and young adults up to age 25 who are at clinical high risk for psychosis and provide evidence-based interventions to prevent the onset of psychosis or lessen the severity of psychotic disorder. NIMH is expected to announce funding availability for researchers studying and evaluating the effectiveness of these programs and interventions, and SAMHSA is encouraging partnerships between funded sites and researchers to conduct such studies.

Financing Patchwork

As is evident from the discussion to this point, there is little that is comprehensive or coordinated about the financing of early intervention services for psychosis, including CSC. The capacity to use Medicaid

effectively depends in part on states, which have latitude in implementing the program, including whether to participate in the expansion per-
mitted by the ACA. Adolescents and young adults often find their
coverage under Medicaid shifting dramatically simply by virtue of ag-
ing out of the EPSDT program. Private health insurance does not cover
the full range of services required to implement CSC. SAMHSA funding,
including the MHBG and, to a lesser degree, CCBHCs, serves to drive reform and leverage Medicaid and private insurance while providing
funds for development and implementation. Nonetheless, SAMHSA
funds are appropriation based and are insufficient to fully fund CSC services nationally. For the foreseeable future, funding CSC programs will
require using a patchwork of state and federal funds to fill in the funding
gaps in Medicaid and private health insurance.

Access and Quality of Care

Providing access to services, which is inextricably linked to funding,
comes with a unique set of policy-related concerns. Goldman (2017)
strikes a cautionary note regarding the limitations of improved insurance coverage. For example, using data from the National Survey on
Drug Use and Health (NSDUH), Saloner et al. (2017) found that health
insurance coverage increased subsequent to the implementation of the
ACA, yet utilization of services for treating substance use disorder did
not improve, and there was limited, if any, increase in other behavioral
health services use. This finding is consistent with prior studies of improvements in health insurance coverage such as parity, in which utilization of behavioral health services does not increase with improved
coverage. This dilemma is not due to lack of need; the NSDUH study
and others demonstrate that need continues to exceed use. As Goldman
(2017) and Dixon (2017) explain, providing coverage for services does
not fully address the problem of access to services. Stigma; lack of
trained providers and appropriate referral mechanisms; and fragmentation between schools, social service organizations, law enforcement
and justice systems, and child and adult services systems all conspire to
establish barriers to timely care, even when coverage is available.

Providing sufficient quality of care literally begins with timely referral and access to services. The Recovery After an Initial Schizophrenia
Episode Early Treatment Program (RAISE-ETP) study (Kane et al. 2015)
demonstrated that individuals with a shorter duration of untreated
psychosis (less than 74 weeks) had better outcomes than those with a
longer duration of untreated psychosis. Clinical quality reporting programs are required though the CHIP Re-authorization Act of 2009
(CHIPRA), the Health Information Technology for Economic and Clinical Health Act of 2009 (HITECH), and the ACA. The Centers for Medi-

care and Medicaid Services adopted a core set of children's and adult health care quality measures for Medicaid and CHIP participants, including measures focused on behavioral health. This brief set of measures includes follow-up after hospitalization for mental illness for both children and adults. Other measures relate to suicide risk; attention-deficit/hyperactivity disorder; depression medication; and cessation and treatment for tobacco, alcohol, and other drugs. In addition, pursuant to the ACA, SAMHSA developed the National Behavioral Health Quality Framework and the National Quality Forum. SAMHSA grantees report a range of child and adult behavioral health–related outcomes through the national outcomes measures resulting from the Government Performance and Results Modernization Act. Finally, many states use a range of performance monitoring and quality measures, with limited consistency between states and sometimes even within states.

These performance measures are not specific to CSC and the early treatment of psychosis, although they do result in indicators that could conceivably be compared across different types of mental health programs. Fidelity to CSC as a model is a different matter, falling somewhere between more global quality indicators of behavioral health care and specific fidelity measures used in effectiveness studies. The First-Episode Psychosis Services Fidelity Scale (FEPS-FS) (Addington et al. 2016), for example, is brief and feasible and has demonstrable reliability and validity. This scale is designed to be used to assess adherence to evidence-based practices for FEP services across a range of service delivery settings. Taking a somewhat different approach to pragmatically assessing fidelity, Essock et al. (2015) used measures commonly available in existing data sets linked to billing practices, combined with interviews with clients, to assess fidelity of key components. This approach illustrates that fidelity to CSC models can be assessed using existing data sets and minimally intrusive performance monitoring methods. Methods and measures exist to maintain fidelity to CSC in public and private service delivery agencies. Federal, state, and local policy can all encourage or even mandate their use.

Training, Workforce, and Service Delivery Systems

Numerous broader challenges related to training, the workforce, and the existing structure of service delivery systems can, in part, be addressed through ongoing and future policy making at federal, state, and local levels. With regard to child and adolescent behavioral health services, over the past three decades, federal and state policy has focused extensively on improving the organization, coordination, and delivery of children's mental health services. The systems of care approach that emerged from these efforts involves collaboration across agencies with youth and families to provide an array of effective, community-based, culturally and linguistically appropriate services and supports for children, youth, and young adults with or at risk for behavioral health challenges and their families (Stroul and Blau 2008). Behavioral health services to adults with severe mental illness also historically address the problem of systems integration and coordination, including, but not limited to, more recent work on integrating behavioral health and primary care.

The considerable progress made toward understanding methods for better coordinating and integrating care for adults with severe mental illness and children and youth with severe emotional disturbance is relevant to the effective and efficient delivery of early intervention services for psychosis, including CSC. Of special note, however, is the problem of the transition between the child and adult service systems. Children and adolescents may experience severe emotional disturbances that seriously hinder functional capacities across age ranges. Adolescents and young adults experiencing FEP, however, are typically in the 15- to 25-year age range considered transitional age. This stage of life encompasses life changes that are especially difficult for those youth living with a serious mental health condition, resulting in struggles to complete high school, enroll in and complete college, and establish adult work lives. Transitional-age youth with serious mental health conditions also receive services in multiple public child and adult systems, including mental health, justice systems, foster care, and vocational rehabilitation. Each of these service systems is organized by inconsistent age groups. Child welfare services may be provided up to age 18 or 21, whereas adult mental health services usually begin at age 18 and special education services may continue up to age 21 (Davis et al. 2018). Varying eligibility criteria, funding streams, accountability structures, staff training, and service cultures add to system fragmentation.

This gap between the adult- and child-focused service systems has numerous implications for early psychosis treatment and CSC. The most obvious is the problem discussed earlier in the section "Financing Early Psychosis Treatment" of the lack of continuity between financing systems that create confusion and gaps in coverage and service delivery during a crucial developmental stage, particularly for persons experiencing FEP. Little is actually understood about programs that collaborate across this age divide, especially with regard to transitional-age youth with severe mental health conditions (Davis et al. 2018). As Dixon (2017) noted, however, there are other less direct but equally important concerns. Clinicians, for example, are typically trained to work with children and adolescents or to work with adults. Treatments for children and adolescents are often different from those for adults, and especially at the younger age ranges are typically not focused specifically on severe mental illness. Family members are commonly integral parts of service delivery for children and adolescents and may be less directly involved in adult services. Legal responsibility changes dramatically when a young person becomes an adult, and service organizations are usually specialized to work within individual age groups. Consequently, working with transitional-age youth requires unique skill sets that are generally not taught in the professional training of social workers, psychologists, psychiatrists, and other providers.

Also important, particularly with regard to legislative and other policy-related activities, are the gaps between the advocacy communities for children and adolescents and those for adults. Historically adult-focused organizations such as the National Alliance for the Mentally Ill are different from child-focused organizations such as the Federation of Families for Children's Mental Health and Youth MOVE National. In part, this is because the advocacy needs for children and adolescents with severe emotional disturbance vary from those of adults with severe mental illness. Lived experience can have diverse meanings, and many youth receiving services within the public child and adolescent behavioral health service system who are experiencing potentially serious and significantly disabling emotional disturbances do not develop or have a history of specific severe mental illnesses such as schizophrenia and bipolar disorder. Transitional-age youth and their families, particularly those experiencing FEP, may navigate varying advocacy and self-help organizations and structures. Such divides and potential confusion can dilute the strength of advocacy efforts and hamper activating the policy voice of young people experiencing early psychosis.

Implementation of Coordinated Special Care: California

Federal legislation and national initiatives provide an essential backdrop and an array of financial and policy guidance that significantly influence the provision of services to individuals experiencing FEP. Services are, nonetheless, provided primarily at the local level, and states retain considerable flexibility in the implementation of service delivery and the application of federal guidelines and funding requirements. State and local policies provide essential contours and detail regarding the overall landscape for CSC programs. The variability across all U.S. states and territories precludes an adequate summary in this chapter. Nonetheless, California, as the nation's most populous and diverse state, provides an illustrative example of the complexities inherent at the state level along with an example of how state initiatives can profoundly influence service delivery to individuals experiencing FEP.

Behavioral health services in California are administered largely through the 58 individual county health and behavioral health systems. Although there are some exceptions, eligibility for services is tied to counties, and service recipients can lose or gain eligibility for specific services by moving—in some cases just a few miles or less—across county lines. Because of California's sheer size (39.5 million residents in 2017), federal initiatives such as Mental Health Block Grant 10% Set-Aside funding often result in relatively small allocations at the county level, requiring counties to significantly supplement MHBG funds to establish local FEP programs. The challenges to funding CSC programs outlined throughout this chapter apply to California counties in varying ways, depending on county composition and size.

In 2004, advocates and legislators in California, recognizing the limitations of existing funding streams for individuals with serious mental illness, including those experiencing FEP, succeeded in using the initiative process in the state to pass Proposition 63, the Mental Health Services Act (MHSA), which placed a 1% state tax on incomes over 1 million dollars to transform and expand the reach of the state's mental health services. The MHSA mandates that counties spend between 75% and 80% of the funds allocated for community services and supports for people in immediate mental health crisis and between 15% and 20% on prevention and early intervention. Counties can also allocate up to 10% of the funding for innovative practices. In 2017, Assembly Bill 1315 established an advisory committee to the Proposition 63 Mental Health Services Oversight and Accountability Commission, which was designed to encourage the expansion of detection and intervention services for early psychosis and mood disorder.

The MHSA, although variable in implementation and overall success, nonetheless resulted in a plethora of experimentation and innovation at the county level in the provision of mental health services. This included the establishment and ongoing funding of FEP programs, mostly using the prevention and early intervention or innovative practice components of the MHSA. Some MHSA-funded programs emerged as state and national models (e.g., the Sacramento Early Diagnosis and Preventative Treatment [Sac-EDAPT] clinic). Many of these programs combined available patchwork funding, including Medicaid, EPSDT, and MHBG resources, with substantially more flexible and generous MHSA resources to establish and sustain their CSC programs.

The flexibility in county implementation of the MHSA promoted variability and innovation. However, limited guidance on how MHSA dollars are allocated and used also allowed for variation from established fidelity, training, and quality improvement practices. Consequently, behavioral health services, including CSC and other FEP programs, may not be consistently implemented or available across counties. Other aspects of CSC implementation beyond funding, such as training, availability of providers, stigma, and broader systemic issues in the adult- and child-focused behavioral health systems, can remain barriers in implementing effective CSC programs even with the availability of relatively flexible MHSA funds. A central lesson from the implementation of MHSA in California to date mirrors those discussed earlier: adequate and flexible funding, although essential and potentially promoting innovation, is nonetheless not sufficient for assuring efficient, equitable, and effective service delivery, including CSC, for individuals with FEP.

KEY CONCEPTS

Evidence strongly suggests that providing effective early psychosis services, including coordinated specialty care (CSC), constitutes an important component to addressing the significant public health problem posed by schizophrenia. There are numerous key policy concerns that emerge in considering how to promote the wide-scale implementation of these services, including the following:

- Financing CSC programs is currently complex and difficult. Public financing, mostly provided through Medicaid, does not cover all the necessary components of CSC. Private insurance covers even fewer components. Consequently, states currently rely on a combination of state general funds and federal grants and waivers to cover CSC services. States vary with regard to both how widely Medicaid is implemented under the ACA and how extensively they use local funds or apply for waivers and grants. Legislative changes or administrative modifications to the ACA could serve to roll back gains made by the legislation, including expanded Medicaid services; extended commercial insurance options for youth younger than age 26 who are covered by parental plans; and the protection afforded individuals with preexisting conditions, including schizophrenia.

- The transition of adolescents with psychosis from child-serving behavioral health and related systems to adult service systems creates particular policy challenges for this population. Funding options exist for children and adolescents that do not have comparable adult mechanisms. The gap between adult- and child-serving systems also creates problems for continuity of care, for consistency in the skills of providers and organizations, and for advocacy on behalf of youth and young adults with psychosis.

- Access to services and quality of care both have unique policy concerns that extend beyond financing. Increased coverage does not directly translate to increased access. Stigma, inadequate referral mechanisms, workforce issues, and service system fragmentation all may create barriers to accessing services. Services also may be provided without sufficient fidelity and to populations beyond those experiencing first or early episodes of psychosis for which they were not originally intended, reducing their potential effectiveness.

- Creating and maintaining a well-trained workforce who can address the special needs of transitional-age youth experiencing psychosis requires bridging adult and child modalities; drawing from different therapeutic and training traditions; and modifying curricula, practicum, and continuing education requirements. Creating teams dedicated to treating early psychosis may prove difficult in areas with small populations and/or low population density and in more remote locations.

- Mobilizing for policy change is essential and remains potentially difficult for adolescents and young adults experiencing psychosis. Child- and adult-focused advocacy organizations vary in perspective and approach. The involvement of young adults, adolescents, and families can be hampered by stigma and competing interests for scarce resources. Provider groups similarly vary, potentially creating additional confusion among policy makers and administrators.

Discussion Questions

1. How can policy for early treatment of psychosis create more seamless funding options across the child- and adult-focused services systems while addressing the existing gaps in funding for CSC services so that the existing patchwork financing quilt is more coherent?

2. What policies best address the need to improve access, fidelity, and quality of care and at what level should they be implemented? For example, are federal or state guidelines more likely to impact local service delivery?

3. What can professional organizations, institutions of higher education, and accrediting bodies do to improve the workforce of providers skilled in the treatment of early psychosis?

4. How can advocates across the child- and adult-serving systems unite to bring a coherent youth and family voice to the policy debate?

5. What is the optimal role of temporary, allocated, or leveraged funding such as waivers and block grants in creating sustainable and effective service delivery systems for young people experiencing a first or early episode of psychosis?

Suggested Readings

Addington DE, Norman R, Bond GR, et al: Development and testing of the first-episode Psychosis Services Fidelity Scale. Psychiatr Serv 67(9):1023–1025, 2016

Dixon LB, Goldman H, Srihari VH, et al: Transforming the treatment of schizophrenia in the United States: the RAISE initiative. Annu Rev Clin Psychol 14:237–258, 2018

Essock SM, Nossel IR, McNamara K, et al: Practical monitoring of treatment fidelity: examples from a team-based intervention for people with early psychosis. Psychiatr Serv 66(7):674–676, 2015

Goldman HH, Karakus M, Frey W, et al: Economic grand rounds: financing first-episode psychosis services in the United States. Psychiatr Serv 64(6):506–508, 2013

Shern D, Neylon K, Kazandjian MA, et al: Use of Medicaid to Finance Coordinated Specialty Care Services for First Episode Psychosis. Alexandria, VA, National Association of State Mental Health Program Directors, 2017. Available at: www.nasmhpd.org/sites/default/files/Medicaid_brief_1.pdf. Accessed September 27, 2018.

References

Addington DE, Norman R, Bond GR, et al: Development and testing of the first-episode Psychosis Services Fidelity Scale. Psychiatr Serv 67(9):1023–1025, 2016 27032665

Azrin ST, Goldstein AB, Heinssen RK: Early intervention for psychosis: the Recovery After an Initial Schizophrenia Episode project. Psychiatr Ann 45(11):548–553, 2015

Davis M, Koroloff N, Sabella K, et al: Crossing the age divide: cross-age collaboration between programs serving transition-age youth. J Behav Health Serv Res 45(3):356–369, 2018 29417359

Dixon L: What it will take to make coordinated specialty care available to anyone experiencing early schizophrenia: getting over the hump. JAMA Psychiatry 74(1):7–8, 2017 27851843

Dixon LB, Goldman HH, Bennett ME, et al: Implementing coordinated specialty care for early psychosis: the RAISE connection program. Psychiatr Serv 66(7):691–698, 2015 25772764

Dixon LB, Goldman H, Srihari VH, et al: Transforming the treatment of schizophrenia in the United States: the RAISE initiative. Annu Rev Clin Psychol 14:237–258, 2018 29328779

Druss BG, Zhao L, Von Esenwein S, et al: Understanding excess mortality in persons with mental illness: 17-year follow up of a nationally representative US survey. Med Care 49(6):599–604, 2011 21577183

Essock SM, Nossel IR, McNamara K, et al: Practical monitoring of treatment fidelity: examples from a team-based intervention for people with early psychosis. Psychiatr Serv 66(7):674–676, 2015 25555176

Goldman HH: Maintaining ACA's gains in insurance coverage and improving access to behavioral health care. Psychiatr Serv 68(6):529, 2017 28566039

Goldman HH, Karakus MC: Do not turn out the lights on the public mental health system when the ACA is fully implemented. J Behav Health Serv Res 41(4):429–433, 2014 24807644

Goldman HH, Karakus M, Frey W, et al: Economic grand rounds: financing first-episode psychosis services in the United States. Psychiatr Serv 64(6):506–508, 2013 23728599

Kane JM, Schooler NR, Marcy P, et al: The RAISE early treatment program for first-episode psychosis: background, rationale, and study design. J Clin Psychiatry 76(3):240–246, 2015 25830446

Lieberman JA, Dixon LB, Goldman HH: Early detection and intervention in schizophrenia: a new therapeutic model. JAMA 310(7):689–690, 2013 23989167

Rosenblatt A: Preliminary findings of the MHBG 10% Set Aside National Evaluation: overview. Presented at the 24th NIMH Mental Health Services Research Conference, North Bethesda, MD, August 2018

Saloner B, Bandara S, Bachhuber M, et al: Insurance coverage and treatment use under the Affordable Care Act among adults with mental and substance use disorders. Psychiatr Serv 68(6):542–548, 2017 28093059

Shern D, Neylon K, Kazandjian MA, et al: Use of Medicaid to finance coordinated specialty care services for first episode psychosis. Alexandria, VA, National Association of State Mental Health Program Directors, 2017. Available at: www.nasmhpd.org/sites/default/files/Medicaid_brief_1.pdf. Accessed September 27, 2018.

Simon GE, Stewart C, Yarborough BJ, et al: Mortality rates after the first diagnosis of psychotic disorder in adolescents and young adults. JAMA Psychiatry 75(3):254–260, 2018 29387876

Stroul BA, Blau GM (eds): The System of Care Handbook: Transforming Mental Health Services for Children, Youth, and Families. Baltimore, MD, Paul H Brookes, 2008

CHAPTER 5

First-Person Accounts of Psychosis and Advocacy Work

Carlos Larrauri, M.S.N., APRN, PMHNP-BC, FNP-BC
Chantel Garrett, B.S.

AN often overlooked aspect of the recovery process is the shift in both an individual's perspective about his or her own identity and that of family and close friends. Changing the way we perceive experiences of psychosis and learning that we are not alone in them is nearly as critical as clinical intervention because it is often stigma—both self-imposed stigma and societal misconceptions—that serves as the first barriers to early intervention. Stigma promotes isolation, lack of information, and shame. The ignorance and apathy that stigma breeds also constrain funding for much-needed innovation in preventing and treating psychosis. In our own personal journeys, we have found that the impact of stigma is perhaps the biggest barrier to full functional recovery.

One of the most powerful tools we possess for chipping away at the harmful effects of stigma is the sharing of personal narratives that support new, empowering notions about what it looks like to experience mental illness (Rüsch et al. 2005). Connection—whether virtual or personal—with those who have fought for recovery has inspired each of us along our own recovery paths. This chapter is meant to illuminate many of the challenges that we faced and insights gained along this path to help bring a more nuanced understanding of the power that peers, strong support networks, and community support wield in the recovery process.

The Role of Community and Family Support in My Recovery

Carlos Larrauri

My Family and Childhood Years

I am the first-born son of Cuban immigrants and a child of the American Dream. My mother's family came to the United States having crossed the Rio Grande River when she was 6 years old. She crossed the river in a rubber raft at the mercy of the people her family were paying to smuggle them in. My father's family immigrated from Cuba to Venezuela. He studied medicine in Spain and returned to Venezuela to practice; however, facing economic and political uncertainty, he decided to come to the United States. He started his career over in his late thirties as a landscaper and used car salesman. My parents and their families faced tremendous challenges as immigrants, but they nevertheless achieved the coveted American Dream that we often spoke of in aspiring and revered tones.

My mother worked 35 years as a graphic journalist for the *Miami Herald*. My father continued to simultaneously work and study, becoming first a registered nurse and then a physician assistant. My parents inculcated the expectation among my two brothers and myself that anything was achievable and that much of the rest of the world did not have the privilege of such economic or political security. Hundreds of thousands of people leave their homes and family, risk their lives and health, all for the opportunities we were born into. My parents worked hard and made necessary sacrifices so that we could be raised within the security and comfort of a middle-class life.

As a child I was happy and sociable. I enjoyed school work, and my mother nicknamed me the mini-mayor for my outgoing personality. My parents enrolled me in Little League Baseball and paid for piano and guitar lessons, but I was mostly interested in playing Super Mario and Donkey Kong. We spent summers at the beach watching Shark Week and playing dominoes. I remember my grandmother in the kitchen frying *croquetas* and my grandfather drinking whiskey and smoking his pipe. We spent winter vacations on road trips to the Great Smoky Mountains, the closest place from Miami where we could see snow, and there were several family vacations to European castles and monuments.

By all measures I had an extremely privileged childhood. The only darker memories of my childhood were the occasional instances of corporal punishment for a poor grade or fighting among my brothers. In retrospect, it was within the context of what is normal for my parents' culture and generation, but I do recall them as frightening experiences. Otherwise, I am grateful for a fortunate and delightful childhood.

Adolescence and Prodromal Period

It was by the end of my eighth-grade summer that a shift began to occur in my behavior and mood. I was introduced to weed by my older cousin, and shortly thereafter, the focus of most of my efforts in high school was on figuring out how to get high. I would meet a fellow student on my walk to school, poke holes in a soda can and smoke weed, and then we would start our day at school. On some days I would take our half-hour lunch break to smoke cigarettes or a joint on my walk home after school.

Toward the later years of high school, I experimented with harder drugs. I would take ecstasy and dance all night at rave parties or trip on mushrooms and LSD with friends at musical festivals or house parties. There were a handful of times I tried cocaine and prescription medications such as Xanax and Valium. I identified with party subcultures such as the rave and electronic music scene or hippie and psychedelic music, but it was always weed that was the most frequent and consistent drug I used to cope or connect with people. There were long periods of time when I was smoking weed every day or several times a day and getting high with friends or alone.

Nevertheless, I was a good student throughout high school. I was in mostly AP and Honors courses, and I graduated summa cum laude, partially attending a dual enrollment program, where I earned college credits at the local community college. The best opportunity I had available after finishing high school was to attend an Early Admission Placement program at the Ohio State University College of Medicine. At 18 years old, I was offered a seat in medical school, and as long as I could maintain a reasonable 3.2 GPA, I could avoid taking the dreaded MCAT. It was a great opportunity that also included great expectations and pressures as the first-born son in an immigrant family.

Crisis During the College Years

In hindsight, I may have gone through an untreated episode of depression during my freshman year at Ohio State. In my first couple of semesters, I skipped classes, slept in for 10–12 hours, and gained 20–30 pounds, and my GPA dropped to a 1.80. I remember for the first time feeling like a minority person now that I was no longer among mostly Hispanic people like at home in Miami. Furthermore, I had not yet developed the study skills or coping skills to succeed in a more competitive environment, so I struggled without knowing whom to talk with or reach out to. I befriended a few other minority people in the program, and we quickly became stoner buddies who spent most of our time in the dorm room, sheltered away from the unforgiving Midwest winter, getting high and playing video games.

By the end of my second semester, I called my mom and told her I wanted to come back home. She remembers that when she saw me for the first time since going away for college, she was struck by how I had let my beard grow unkempt. I came back home, started working, and studied for a couple semesters at the local community college. With a renewed sense of momentum, I left home to complete a bachelor's degree, this time at New College of Florida. I was moving forward with completing my studies, but I continued to struggle academically and was placed on academic probation.

I can recall what was initially trouble with concentration and performing school work. I would sit at my computer desk to write my senior year thesis, but I would either space out or find it impossible to focus. I also had increasing difficulty sleeping and would stay up until the early hours in the morning, talking or rhyming to myself as if in a spoken word contest. I began my studies at New College of Florida as a literature major, with the reasoning that I could write well, so I should develop this skill, but by my senior year I was taking mostly religious coursework and becoming increasingly preoccupied with reading religious texts.

At the time, I felt something was off, so I went to see the school psychologist. We had several visits and talked about the pressure of writing a senior-year thesis, but we failed to intervene or identify the growing severity of the situation. I continued to develop a profound sense that I was having a religious experience. I started hearing whispers assuring me I was a prophet and an angel being initiated into a greater realm of spiritual existence. The voices grew louder and began saying, "You are so good…you are so beautiful…." What started as whispers grew into a noisy cacophony of conversations and chaos. I started to believe that the religious text I was reading was speaking directly to me and telling me that I would live to a hundred years or that I would be rewarded with great financial prosperity. There were nights when I would lie down to smoke a cigarette and watch with wonder and awe as the smoke from my cigarettes and clouds in the night sky coalesced to form crucifixes, doves, and other religious imagery. I was experiencing what felt like the heavens directly opening up, and it was driving me toward incessant tears, laughter, and joy.

Psychosis is an enigmatic experience that can be challenging to understand because it can be simultaneously profound, bizarre, and terrifying. On one occasion I stayed up all night, wrapped in a bed sheet in front of my dorm room, posing and gesturing in mannerisms like the Virgin Mary, and all the while, groundskeepers and students walked by and proceeded with their day normally. I also became sexually preoccupied and would loudly play pornographic material in the middle of the day with my doors and windows wide open. I was sure I could smell a woman's vagina everywhere I went and would crudely say, "Do you smell that? I smell pussy!" At times famous athletes or musicians such as Dwayne Wade or Pitbull would talk to me through the radio or television and say, "What's up, Tino?" or "What's happening, man?"

Most of all, there was a growing sense of fear and confusion. I remember experiencing what felt like my mind beginning to fail at processing my environment. One day, I was sitting in class when my brain could not understand the conversations of my classmates. The words coming from their mouths became garbled sounds, and their gestures grew distorted and menacing. As they talked over each other, their conversations grew louder and louder, and I became overwhelmed by what felt like a torrent of environmental stimuli. It felt as if my identity was beginning to disappear and disintegrate into this chaos. I was unable to express what was happening to me, so I left the classroom, feeling confused and disoriented, and found somewhere isolated to smoke a cigarette. On several nights, when the assault of the senses grew too intense, I would find a few hours of comfort cradled in the fetal position in a dorm room shower.

My friends and family were growing increasingly perplexed. Their observations from this time noted that I began to talk incessantly about Jesus Christ, and my gaze was fixated toward the sky like the martyr or saint figures in Counter-Reformation paintings. I would laugh nervously to myself and say, "Ah, good shit, man" in response to most social situations. My behavior grew increasingly inappropriate, and I received several conduct violations at school, including an accusation of having exposed myself to roommates in the dorms. By the end of my senior year, I was nearly isolated from my college community and in a state of florid psychotic hallucinations. I was eating meals out of the cafeteria trash cans, smoking cigarette butts off the floor, and wandering the campus at odd hours as I rambled incoherently to myself.

A close family friend I had known since high school, who was also attending New College, called my mother and said, "Something in Carlos has changed that isn't just stress or drug use. You need to speak with Carlos right away." My parents came to campus the following day and we met with my academic advisor, who said, "Carlos, you are an adult, and you have the right to privacy, and as such we don't have to discuss any of the academic or conduct violations that have occurred on campus." Seeing the desperation and frustration on my mother's face, I said, "With all due respect, Dr. Clark, I have a Cuban mother; I have never had the right to privacy." This moment was a turning point that opened the way for an honest conversation about my mental health challenges at college.

The Right Diagnosis and Right Treatment

I was asked to leave campus but was allowed to finish my senior-year thesis at home. I came back home, and my mother and I proceeded to meet with nearly a dozen mental health professionals. I received several diagnoses in the process of getting help. One psychiatrist, in his toxic machismo, simply stated I was fine and needed to *cortar caña*, or do hard labor.

During this period, my mother was in contact with a family friend, Dr. Joseph Gonzalez-Heidrich, who is an Assistant Professor of Psychiatry at Harvard Medical School. Joe asked my mom, "Is Carlos still playing music? How is his academic performance? How is his hygiene?" She said my guitar playing had turned into droning, as if I were getting stuck on a chord or note, and that my hygiene and school performance had deteriorated. I developed the habit of rolling my own cigarettes and smoking them down to my fingers, so the tips of my fingers had turned yellow and orange from nicotine. Trying to get me to sit down and finish writing my thesis was a source of conflict. Joe didn't provide a diagnosis but suggested we see providers for an appropriate diagnostic workup.

We saw a team of mental health professionals for several months, but all the while, my behavior was continuing to deteriorate. I had an incessant manic energy and would exercise for hours at a time. I was routinely jogging down the streets and singing at the top of my lungs. I would go to the park to play basketball in the middle of the night, all the while loudly cursing and laughing to myself. My mom, convinced I would be arrested, quietly followed behind me in her minivan to be sure I was really going to the park to play basketball or going for a midnight jog. During a fight with my youngest brother, I broke a glass window with my fist, and he retaliated by throwing broken glass back at me. My father, in his own state of denial, was starting to call my mom the crazy one for taking me to find treatment.

Five months into the evaluation process, my mother called the institution conducting the evaluation one early December day and said that she would hold them liable if my behavior worsened or if I hurt myself or somebody else. The next day, roughly 2 weeks shy of my 22nd birthday, we received a 12-page clinical evaluation that concluded with the diagnosis of *adult-onset schizophrenia*.

Recovery in the Community

I remember seeing my provider after reading the report of my diagnosis. The provider was an incredibly accomplished man, with both an M.D. and a Ph.D. He looked me in the eyes and with complete seriousness said, "Carlos, this isn't good shit, man. We think you have schizophrenia." I said, bewildered and still in denial, "Doctor, what does this mean? Will I be able to go to graduate school or work?" He said, "We don't know, Carlos. It's up to you to take your medication and engage in your recovery to see if your goals are possible."

I was confused and unsure of what was going to happen next, and I had my own expectations and prejudices of what it meant to be diagnosed with schizophrenia. I thought this meant I would stay at home collecting disability, smoking cigarettes, and spacing out or talking to the television. The roller-coaster ride of psychosis took me from the highs of grandeur, where I thought I was Jesus Christ, to the lows of being labeled and belonging to the most stigmatized group in society. I felt as if I had been branded with a scarlet letter that would forever haunt my life, define who I was, and further incapacitate me.

Dr. Gonzalez-Heydrich, who had suggested that we get the diagnostic workup, also suggested that we connect with our local chapter of the National Alliance on Mental Illness (NAMI). NAMI is the largest grassroots organization that advocates and supports individuals with mental illness and their families. My mother encouraged me to attend the support groups, and at a support group meeting I met Judith Robinson, a mental health advocate with 50 years of experience in Miami's mental health system. She took me under her wing and provided much-needed guidance and direction. On her recommendation, I received training to facilitate support groups and was encouraged to get involved with the Board of Directors. The NAMI community supported me as I attempted to make sense of my suffering and experience by helping others with similar experiences. I was encouraged to share my story at every opportunity and always felt safe and welcomed in doing so. The community helped to normalize the experience, and I was able to form several close friendships with peers and professional mentors who had had similar adversities. With the support of family, friends, and my NAMI community, I decided early on that I wanted to become a mental health professional to work with others going through psychosis or schizophrenia.

In the beginning phases of my recovery, my father would literally hand me the medication and take me by the hand to enroll in community college courses. This required me to get out of the house and navigate my recovery in the community. I had to learn to cope with hearing voices on the bus and in the classroom. I had to learn how to remain calm and composed, even with the occasional flare-up of psychotic symptoms. It felt like I was having to start my life over at 22 years old; I had to develop a new sense of identity, purpose, and community. Eventually, my volunteer efforts in the Miami mental health community led me to a job interview with Cindy Schwartz from the Jail Diversion Program (JDP) spearheaded by Judge Stephen Leifman. They earnestly asked me about my lived experience with schizophrenia.

Cindy said, "It's great that you went to a good school, but tell me about what you went through. What was it like going through your episode?" We talked about my experience with psychosis not in hushed or shameful tones but as if it were a valuable asset that I would bring to the table with future clients of their program. They also employed peer support specialists and were vocal proponents of the recovery model, rooted in the notion that when people get the right treatment, recovery is the natural and expected outcome with mental illnesses. Clients of JDP were being diverted from criminal justice system involvement and into community-based treatment with medication, outpatient therapy, case management, and peer support, and my job was to help to bring in the federal dollars by helping clients apply for Social Security disability insurance. It was wonderful to help people in a practical and concrete way, but I wanted to keep studying and had greater aspirations, so I enrolled in nursing school, with the goal of becoming a psychiatric mental health nurse practitioner.

I completed an accelerated registered nursing program and began working the night shift at a maximum-security forensic hospital. I routinely cared for the psychiatric and medical needs of up to 28 patients with serious mental illness and pending criminal charges. The hospital was rife with an undercurrent of violent and racial tension because many of the patients were poor and minority individuals, and the risk of assault was a daily reality. It was an eye-opening experience to witness the sad reality of the treatment of individuals with serious mental illness in a public system.

I resigned after a coworker took a controlled substance out of the medication administration system under my name and wouldn't resolve the issue with me. Furthermore, the shift work and long hours were starting to take a toll on my mental health. On several occasions, I had been asked to work double shifts of 16 hours because of short staffing and had to administer hundreds of medications and continue to respond to crisis situations between staff or patients. It was an ethically precarious situation to be part of, and I was complicit in a system that was profiting from society's sickest individuals, so I decided to leave the job and refocus on my initial goal of going to graduate school.

I was experiencing burnout while working the night shift, and my mother began recognizing another mental health decompensation. She asked that I speak with Dr. Gonzalez-Heydrich, who had previously guided us toward a correct diagnosis and NAMI. He said, "You're going to start graduate school, and it would help to hunker down, so look at your medication like this: something that is dynamic in response to your stressors and workload. You've chosen a challenging career as a fellow clinician, so why not increase the risperidone to 1 mg?" Over a period of several years, I had weaned down to 0.25 mg of risperidone to see if I could maintain my recovery on the lowest amount of medication or whether stopping medication was possible, but I could also recognize that I was beginning to struggle again. After failing the first several exams of graduate school, I increased my dosage, and sure enough, my academic performance, sleeping, and behavior began to steadily improve once more.

Advocacy and Future Aspirations

I have been able to live my life in a much more productive and fruitful way since engaging in recovery. I see the need to maintain a low-dose medication regimen, possibly for the rest of my life, and continue to check in with therapists and clinicians. Otherwise, I try to lead a generally normal and healthy life, avoiding drugs and alcohol, staying physically active, and finding meaning and sense of my experience through work and helping others. I'm currently a board-certified family nurse practitioner and practice in a child, adolescent, and adult psychiatric practice. I treat patients in both English and Spanish and work in a collaborative setting with several nurse practitioners, licensed mental health counselors, psychologists, and psychiatrists. I am pursuing a second board certification as a psychiatric mental health nurse practitioner at the University of Miami so that I may practice at the full extent of my education and training. Nevertheless, I plan to continue to practice in a collaborative and team-based approach because this leads to the best outcomes for patients.

I am currently serving on the Board of Directors for NAMI, both at the local community level with NAMI-Miami Dade County and in a 3-year term at the national level. At the local level, we are a growing nonprofit organization, offering free support groups and education courses for family members and people with mental health issues. NAMI should be considered a crucial part of care for people with psychosis because it provides family support services and a welcoming community. At the national level, I developed an agenda focused on continuing to change the conversation surrounding mental health by sharing the stories of people in recovery and with lived experience, focusing on early intervention with the adolescent and young adult population and developing an understanding of the financial and policy-related skills necessary to successfully advocate and create systems-level change.

I continue to share my story with students at local universities and colleges, police officers in training academy, and health care professionals at community events. I hope the sharing of my story in this context will help inform and shape the narrative surrounding early intervention services for psychosis in some positive and productive way. I hope to run for a second term with NAMI and build organizational partnerships with professional nursing, Latino/Hispanic, and youth organizations, as well as increase the representation and voice of diverse perspectives and lived experience with mental illness at the highest echelons of our society and government.

Embracing my identity as an individual in recovery has helped me to manage an immensely challenging illness. It took a terrifying diagnosis of schizophrenia for me to form a healthy identity and develop a strong sense of resiliency, but I am now able to find a deep gratification and purpose in helping others overcome their own struggles with mental illness. My recovery would not have been feasible without the impromptu team of people who have supported me along the way. Now more than ever, we must continue to advocate for funding and services that surround young people with support and care during the early phases of this illness. To this end, I intend to pursue further graduate education in either health policy or public health or to assist communities and organizations in developing systems for the prevention and treatment of mental illness in youth. I am filled with gratitude and forever indebted to the friends, family, and community who have supported me in this journey through recovery and well-being.

My Brother's Road to Recovery: A Sister's Perspective

Chantel Garrett

Note: This narrative was written with the consent of my brother, Nate, who wishes to be identified by his first name.

I will never forget the day that my brother was diagnosed with schizophrenia. I was 22 at the time, having just started a career in financial services in San Francisco. My brother, Nate, 16 months my junior, was in the Active Marine Corps Reserve program, living on base in San Diego. After months of concern over strange behavior that our family couldn't make sense of, I got a call from my mom at work saying my brother was in the hospital and had been diagnosed with paranoid schizophrenia.

The mouthful of those two words hung heavy in the space between us. None of us saw schizophrenia coming. I remember vague images of movie characters portraying what I thought could have been schizophrenia flashed through my mind. *What is it, anyway?* Were recreational drugs to blame? Stress? What will this mean for his health, his future? How did this happen? And will it happen to me, too?

Nearly 20 years later, even with all of the learning, advocating, and progress we've made as a family, it hasn't gotten much easier to recount this story. But the unnecessary isolation and shame bred by the experience of supporting a loved one through psychosis motivates me to share our experience. If nothing else, I want mothers, fathers, sisters, and brothers to know that if their parent, sibling, or child is suffering in a way that they could never have imagined, they are not alone. This is our family's story of navigating the bumpy, winding road of seeking recovery alongside my brother.

Growing Up

Nate and I grew up in San Diego with my mom, a single parent for most of our childhood. The fact that our parents were divorced and lived a couple of hours from one another was only made more apparent by the intact family units we observed in our friends' homes; neither of us can form a mental picture of our parents in one room together, let alone in love. In the summer and for a school year or two during our childhoods, we spent time in the country with my dad and his family, offering us a diverse set of experiences—being immersed in San Diego's beach and surf culture, gaining an appreciation for the performing arts through our mom's singing career, and time spent with our dad getting lost on horses and quad bikes on back country roads.

Nate recently told me that the first time he heard voices he was about 6 years old. He remembers he and I playing in the living room of my grandparents' home and hearing the first clear outsider's voice speak to him. It would be another 14 years until changes in his brain manifested into a full-blown psychotic break. Changes that, unbeknownst to him or any of us, had been slowly manifesting since he was a small child.

Now that I know that early psychosis is highly treatable, I can't help but wonder what would have happened had Nate shared his experiences as a child or adolescent. What would have happened if my parents had been aware of what these early experiences could foreshadow, especially given a family history of psychotic disorders?

Family History

It wasn't until my brother was diagnosed and I began to learn about schizophrenia that I began to see my maternal grandmother's behavior through a lens of mental disorder. Fragments of hushed-tone conversations that I had overheard as a child replayed in my mind: a midlife nervous breakdown...hysteria...commitment to a psychiatric hospital...electric shock therapy. A picture of my grandma's struggle as some form of a psychotic disorder began to take shape. I started to realize that her extreme obsession with microscopic bugs that tormented only her and that no one else could see was a form of a hallucination. Her intense suspicion of neighbors flashing lights in her windows and putting streaks of water on her driveway were delusions. The elaborate daily system of combating the bugs over a period of many years and my grandfather's unwavering support enabled her to cope with her symptoms. Never in our upbringing was my grandmother's mental health addressed or discussed openly. Even today, I don't think that many of our extended family members understand the depths of her quiet struggle that persisted for decades.

First Signs

As I look back at our high school years, I can see the first signs of my brother's illness. Nate was formerly the wittiest guy in the room, but his behavior became erratic in his sophomore year and he began to pull away from his friends. His grades dropped precipitously. He holed himself up in his room with his guitar, became obsessive about a girl he had a crush on, and managed to teach himself Portuguese so that he could speak with her in her native tongue. While he was at it, he became fluent in Spanish as well. Drugs were definitely part of the equation. I didn't know how much, but at the time, I assumed that drugs were the reason for Nate's shift in behavior and his disinterest in school. My reaction was similar to my mom's: *Get your act together!*

I was away at my first year of college when Nate abruptly left high school in his senior year and joined the Marines. It was extremely out of character and not something he had ever talked about previously. With the benefit of hindsight, I believe that he could have been trying to find stability as he found the rigors of high school and the college application process more difficult given the deterioration of his mental health and was navigating an increasingly stressful situation at home.

First Hospitalization

I remember visiting Nate during that first hospitalization. There was my brother, barely 20 years old. I was relieved that he was safe, that he seemed less agitated. But where was he? He sat hunched over, a pale shadow of himself, unable to speak, unable to make eye contact. His left hand trembled lifelessly along his thigh. He was worn out from the trauma of being held in the hospital against his best efforts to convince everyone to let him go, from lack of sleep, and from his brain attempting to adjust to heavy medication.

His doctors spoke of the grave outcomes we should expect with paranoid schizophrenia. His social worker swiftly filed for medical discharge from the military and set him up to receive long-term disability benefits, referring him to a local group home to live in with other veterans who were disabled by mental illnesses.

Months passed. Nate was no longer in a crisis state but did not show many signs of improvement. He slept most of his days away. The few friends he had left slowly faded away. He hated the medication, but it was the only thing offered to him. There was no ongoing form of treatment or therapy. My mom was told to call 911 if things got really bad, and Nate would be taken to the hospital by police. A few months later, that is exactly what happened.

Living With Schizophrenia: The Early Years

Over that first year, without knowing it, I began the process of grieving the person I'd grown up with. I didn't tell many people about Nate's health because most people appeared visibly uncomfortable by the conversation, tripping over comforting words as they looked as confused as I once was about schizophrenia. This only reinforced how alone I felt in our family's suffering, on top of deep sadness and feeling overwhelmed. Despite going to family education classes and group therapy, opening up to people outside of my inner circle with relative grace and confidence would take years of practice.

My brother's well-being was exhausting to think about when our family was not in immediate crisis (which was rare in the first few years), so I tried not to. I went to therapy to try to cope with what felt like a devastating loss and more stress than I could bear. In the first 10 years of his illness, Nate went through intermittent, sometimes long, periods of opting not to take medication that took the roughest edges off his symptoms but left him feeling that life was not worth living. He regularly cycled in and out of hospitals—often at the hands of police. He was held in jail cells for days at a time with no medical attention while every hospital bed was full. After being restrained in hospital beds and injected with sedatives, it's no wonder that he once leaped from a moving car in order to avoid hospitalization. He was kicked out of his church for behavior they couldn't understand. He was routinely the victim of fraud. He was stolen from and taken advantage of by landlords and roommates time and time again.

One of our earliest struggles was that Nate could not live at home because it was extremely triggering for him; those closest to him were the root of most of his delusions. Unfortunately, he didn't do well in group homes, either. Nate found himself alienated and depressed against a dreary backdrop. Most of his housemates, all of whom lived with psychosis, were substantially older than he was. When they weren't smoking, they were usually watching TV or sleeping. Nearly all had been long forgotten by family and friends. A few times each year, a housemate would quietly pass away, most often decades before the average expected lifespan for a healthy American man. Within days, a new veteran in need of supported housing would promptly take his spot. All of this understandably terrified Nate, a 21-year-old who just 1 year earlier seemed to have his whole life and full potential ahead of him. Nate decided he was not going to be labeled a castaway disabled Marine who would eventually be left to die a lonely death alongside his peers.

About 3 years into Nate's diagnosis, he went missing. When we found him, he was living in a commune-like setting in rural New Jersey, in a "natural treatment center" that held the promise to take him off his medication and replace it with healthy food. To my brother, this sounded like exactly the miracle cure he had been waiting for. They had taken thousands of dollars from him—his entire life savings—to fulfill this promise, which was quickly made impossible when, like clock-work, he slipped into severe psychosis on stopping his medication and ended up hospitalized for several months. Despite our pleas and legal threats, he was never reimbursed for his few weeks of "treatment." The paperwork he signed covered the center for all liabilities.

When my dad and I flew out to bring Nate home on hospital discharge, the three of us went for a walk before the return home. I'll never forget the conversation I had with Nate that day, seated on a bench on a glorious spring morning on the Princeton University campus. He told us that his medication made him feel like he was drowning. He said that not one doctor had yet attempted to listen to how he felt or offer any hope of a future that he could envision for himself. He plainly stated that he would rather be homeless or dead than take the medication or endure any more treatment. It was the first time I was struck by this reality—and I would be struck by it again and again over the years: as much as I wanted my brother to be safe, happy, and well, I could not force him to accept treatment.

It was then that I realized that although we could lead Nate down a path and provide possibilities, the decision to take control of his wellness had to be his. He had to see treatment as valuable—a decision that was now exceedingly challenging because his association with treatment was painful, disempowering, and even traumatic. All I could do in that moment was offer him love, compassion, deepest respect, and even awe because the seemingly endless path of suffering that he had been walking for the past several years was not something I would ever understand first hand. I would never know what it was like to hear multiple voices that try to cut me down throughout the day.

I wondered how we were going to hold on to hope that Nate would be able to surmount these obstacles. I also felt more driven than ever to find better treatment and support and show Nate that there was hope. But I also knew that if it was going to work, he would have to be the one to forge his path toward recovery.

Turning Point

After about 11 years of cycling in and out of hospitals, my brother finally surrendered. It did not mean he found a more meaningful life—it meant that he couldn't endure hospitalizations anymore, so he bitterly took his medication every day and resolved to rarely step foot out of his group home. He suffered long periods of grave depression and harbored intense anger at his situation. We especially worried about his will to keep going during this especially dark time. This went on for another six fairly miserable years, until, through mental health advocacy work focused on prevention and early intervention that I had begun, I was introduced to a U.S. Veterans Administration (VA)–based treatment program in San Diego geared specifically toward people living with psychosis.

The program, a partnership between the University of California, San Diego and the San Diego VA, has been a game changer for my brother. The program's focus is cognitive-behavioral social skills training, which is exactly what it sounds like—a mix of cognitive-behavioral therapy and social skills training. It focuses on real-world functional recovery, primarily through classes and group therapy aimed at helping participants learn how to deal with all aspects of living with schizophrenia.

For the first time since his diagnosis, my brother is now in a very supportive living situation. And for the first time in more than a decade, he now gets out into the community, is playing his guitar again and studying online, and is making friends and seeking out things he is passionate about, like music. He recently told me that he is happier than he's been in a very long time, even though he is still frustrated with his medication. This was surely a sign of breaking new ground; for as long as I could remember, he had very rarely shared a hopeful or positive thought about himself.

Reflection

I have often thought about what the past 18 years might have looked like had Nate been able to access specialty care at the outset of his symptoms. Instead, our road was longer, but the impact of family, community, and (although late stage) a specialized treatment team supported Nate into wellness. I would like to believe that part of what led Nate to finally accept the support of a treatment team was our family's continued faith in him, leading him to finally conclude what we had known all along: that despite illness, he had so much to offer the world and, likewise, that engaging in the world had a lot to offer him—and that was worth fighting for. He saw that we believed in him, the treatment program practitioners and fellow participants believed in him, and his new "house mom" and roommates believed in him. In the end, it took a village to remind him of his remarkable strength, his wit, and numerous talents. I have observed this virtuous cycle: his small daily victories are noticed by others, offering him a motivation boost to step out and try new things—to show himself that he can do even more. Ultimately, he had to decide that it was time and make the effort to walk down a new path. Finally, after 16 years of considerable struggle, he went for it.

Our family's story is one of hope, endurance, and radical acceptance. If nothing else, it reinforces that it is never too late. Recovery is not a linear path. It takes massive determination, persistence, and inner strength. It also takes at least one person to not give up on you and keep being patient and present, even when it seems impossible or hopeless.

Holding on to hope required me to proactively educate myself about schizophrenia and to learn how to establish a relationship on equitable terms with my brother. Most of all, it required finding a larger capacity in myself to love unconditionally, to see myself in his suffering and to recognize our shared infinite potential. My personal mission through the nonprofit project I founded, Strong 365, is all about empowering people with the tools to take that next step, no matter where they are in their recovery journey.

If I knew at the outset of my brother's first episode what I know now, I might have been able to at least question whether changes in my brother's behavior were related to changes in his brain, especially given a well-established history of mental illness in our family (which, as in most families, was rarely discussed). I might have understood the importance of treatment that aimed beyond simply muting my brother's delusions and hallucinations but also focused on regaining cognitive function and social skills—the things that would have allowed him to retain his identity, confidence, and independence sooner.

With the current standard of care, we underestimate the major side effects of antipsychotic drugs and undervalue some of the greatest deficits that psychosis-bearing illnesses often carry with them: difficulty relating socially and expressing emotion—core skills necessary for maintaining relationships and contributing meaningfully to a community. For my brother, becoming well enough to be discharged from an inpatient unit meant that he was interested in living and showed fewer outward symptoms of psychosis. Hospital discharge also came with heavy doses of medication that left him feeling numb or, in his words, like he was "constantly drowning" and included no follow-up care or support. It did not mean he was prepared to go to college, or apply for a job, or regain his friendships; nor did he believe that these things were possible, as we were repeatedly told by his many doctors that they were not.

Today, we can offer young people much-improved care focused on prevention and early intervention. In order to ensure that more young people can benefit from specialty psychosis care, we must spread awareness and humanize and destigmatize these experiences.

Advocacy

When I first learned about the promise of early intervention for psychosis, I felt as though I had just been let in on the greatest, most elaborate secret in health care. How was it possible that early intervention existed, while families like mine suffered on the rough road to recovery or never found it at all? The question haunted me, so much so, that I applied my experience as a corporate marketer to establishing a youth-led nonprofit project that meets young people where they are (online) to connect them earlier to mental health treatment and support.

Nearly 20 years after my brother was diagnosed, a lot has changed for the nine million Americans (Perälä et al. 2007) like my brother who are living with serious brain health challenges, but not nearly enough. It is well understood that mental illness is the chief health issue for teens and young adults: one in five young adults ages 18–25 are affected by a mental health condition (National Institute of Mental Health 2017). Psychiatric disorders are the number one disease burden for young people ages 10–24 (Benyamina et al. 2012). Untreated mental health problems put us at risk for a myriad of life-threatening health issues, including suicide, the second leading cause of death for 15- to 24-year-olds in the United States (Xu et al. 2016).

Yet only half of teens and young adults get the treatment they need and deserve (Substance Abuse and Mental Health Services Administration 2015). My family's story—and the hundreds of others I have met in doing this work who have walked similar paths—inspires me to be a small part of changing young lives through early intervention.

KEY CONCEPTS

- It is essential that narratives of individuals with lived experience of psychosis are shared with consumers, families, and health care providers. These narratives demonstrate the rich experience of recovery, represent diverse cultural and ethnic experiences, and offer hope to all stakeholders.

- There is need for a team that provides psychosocial services in addition to medical care. Although medication is often necessary, it is not sufficient. Psychosocial services such as peer support, family education, and supportive work or school environments get people back into the community and functioning.

- Advocacy is necessary to ensure reduction of harmful stigma that keeps young people and their families from seeking help and to increase funding for services and research. In addition, it provides a pathway in recovery for people to help others, create meaning from their experience, and leverage their lived experience in a career in the helping profession (e.g., peer support, counselor, clinician).

- The presentation of an acute crisis may be years after the onset of subtle behavioral changes or even longer from the onset of neurodevelopmental abnormalities. Early intervention is crucial for curbing the impact of untreated psychosis. We must create a pathway to care from a systems-level perspective so people can engage care before an acute crisis that disrupts the family and community life.

Discussion Questions

1. What has been your experience with psychosis or with psychosis of a loved one?

2. How do you draw on this experience in the work that you do?

3. How will you advocate for team-based care and/or care that incorporates psychosocial services, family, or community involvement in recovery?

4. How is your team equipped to develop and share personal narratives of recovery?

Suggested Readings

CureSZ Foundation: Schizophrenia Survivors, https://curesz.org/resources/schizophrenia-survivors

National Alliance on Mental Illness: Early Psychosis and Psychosis, https://www.nami.org/earlypsychosis

OnTrackNY: www.ontrackny.org/Videos—personal stories of recovery

The Stability Network: Our Stories: Testimony to the Power of Healing, www.thestabilitynetwork.org/ourstories

Strong 365: www.strong365.org—online resource for information on early psychosis, treatment, online peer chat and personal stories

Time to Change: www.time-to-change.org.uk/personal-stories—personal stories of recovery

References

Benyamina A, Blecha L, Reynaud M: Global burden of disease in young people aged 10–24 years. Lancet 379(9810):29, 2012 22225669

National Institute of Mental Health: Mental illness: prevalence of any mental illness. Bethesda, MD, National Institute of Mental Health, November 2017. Available at: www.nimh.nih.gov/health/statistics/mental-illness.shtml#part_155771. Accessed September 28, 2018.

Perälä J, Suvisaari J, Saarni SI, et al: Lifetime prevalence of psychotic and bipolar I disorders in a general population. Arch Gen Psychiatry 64(1):19–28, 2007 17199051

Rüsch N, Angermeyer MC, Corrigan PW: Mental illness stigma: concepts, consequences, and initiatives to reduce stigma. Eur Psychiatry 20(8):529–539, 2005 16171984

Substance Abuse and Mental Health Services Administration: Behavioral Health Barometer: United States, 2014 (HHS Publ No SMA-15-4895). Rockville, MD, Substance Abuse and Mental Health Services Administration, 2015

Xu J, Murphy SL, Kochanek KD, et al: Deaths: final data for 2013. Natl Vital Stat Rep 64(2):1–119, 2016 26905861

CHAPTER 6

Engaging Families and Individuals in Care

Sarah Lynch, LCSW
Rebecca Jaynes, LCPC
Nyamuon Nguany Machar

PSYCHOTIC disorders, including schizophrenia spectrum and mood disorders with psychosis, can cause severe functional impairment, high rates of mortality, and comorbid illnesses, reducing life expectancy (Breitborde et al. 2017). It is now clearly established that treatment as early as possible in the course of psychosis is associated with significant improvement in clinical and functional outcomes (Breitborde et al. 2017). A treatment delay of 1–3 years is common with psychosis onset, and there is an 80% dropout rate within the first year of treatment (Dixon et al. 2016). That said, treatment adherence is only the tip of the iceberg in the world of engagement, which is multifaceted and complex.

The National Alliance on Mental Illness arrived at a definition of engagement that incorporates diverse perspectives: "Engagement is the strengths-based process through which individuals with mental health conditions form a healing connection with people that support their recovery and wellness within the context of family, culture and community" (National Alliance on Mental Illness 2016, p. 6). Engagement should emphasize these contexts of family, culture, and community, and we present a three-stage model that ensures engagement at all levels. The three stages of engagement are 1) increasing early detection and intervention by engaging the community with education and outreach; 2) working with participants and families in treatment through a prolonged, individualized, and creative engagement phase; and 3) maintaining active engagement with participants and family members through all phases of recovery with peer involvement. In Figure 6–1, the three stages of engagement are pictured in a dynamic, synergistic way to reflect that the more engaged a community is and the earlier the intervention, the more recovery becomes possible. We recommend that early intervention for psychosis (EIP) programs use this diagram as a guiding principle in orienting EIP services toward engagement. More detailed information and specific strategies can be found in the Suggested Readings at the end of the chapter.

Stage 1: Engaging Communities Through Outreach Education

The earliest examples of first-episode psychosis programs engaging communities with comprehensive outreach education were English, Australian, Danish, and Norwegian initiatives, the most comprehensive being the Early Treatment and Intervention in Psychosis (TIPS) project in Norway (Joa et al. 2008). Within a comprehensive model of outreach, the TIPS project was able to show that by combining targeted outreach and an easy access referral system, the region's duration of untreated psychosis (DUP) was shortened from 114 weeks to 26 weeks, which equates to a more than 75% reduction in DUP (Johannessen et al. 2001). A follow-up study confirmed that the benefits of community education are maximized when outreach engages the community with consistent efforts over time, that is, dynamically reiterating the outreach messages to the targeted audiences (McFarlane et al. 2010).

Adding to the data to support the benefits of outreach education, the Portland Identification and Early Referral (PIER) program of Portland, Maine hosted a nationwide study in the United States and in 2016 published results that six distinct U.S. sites were able to both reduce stigma and improve early identification for individuals at risk for psychosis while adapting outreach efforts to the unique elements of their communities (Lynch et al. 2016). Furthermore, studies are now making it clear that outreach and community engagement do not, in fact, require significant funding but rather require creative use of current funding streams to maximize referrals (Baumann et al. 2013). In fact, community engagement can actually become the backbone of an EIP program's active referral network.

By developing a comprehensive outreach plan, the synergistic effect of multiple components of outreach education paves the way for EIP

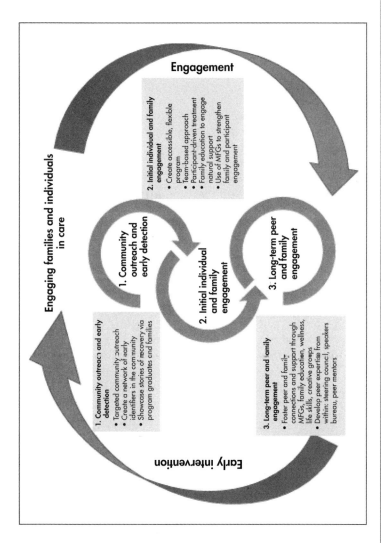

FIGURE 6–1. Engaging families and individuals in care.

Abbreviation. MFGs=multiple-family groups.

programs to operate within an engaged community—one that is aware and informed of the benefits of early intervention, one that is open and interested in accessing services across otherwise existing cultural and/ or economic divides, and one that is motivated and engaged to make a difference to end stigma against mental illness (McFarlane and Jaynes 2017). Within this framework, individuals who are in need of services are inherently more likely to engage in services. Likewise, their family members, friends, and professionals who interact with them most often (e.g., school staff, primary care providers) are more likely to refer (Ruff et al. 2012).

In 2017, McFarlane and Jaynes from the PIER program developed a technical assistance manual for the Substance Abuse and Mental Health Services Administration's Center for Mental Health Services, which outlines in greater detail what is defined as a "comprehensive outreach plan" to engage communities. This is the first manualized guide to walk program developers and clinicians through full implementation of an outreach plan, and it is available at the National Association of State Mental Health Program Directors (NASMHPD) website (McFarlane and Jaynes 2017). This guide provides an outline and step-by-step tools to support the seven primary components of a comprehensive outreach plan, including mapping community strengths and needs, establishing a steering council, developing and tailoring messages to specific targeted audiences, and other related efforts aimed at ensuring multifaceted, continuous community engagement (McFarlane and Jaynes 2017).

A crucial aspect of community engagement is the inclusion, on all levels, of peer experiences of successful, engaged treatment. Peer stories and voices illustrate the hope inherent in a successful outreach message and are the means to both promote early intervention and provide opportunities to showcase and engage young people and their families at all levels of recovery in mental health and wellness. With peer involvement, stories of people who have benefited from early intervention and are living well with good self-care and experiences of psychosis begin to go hand in hand with the message of early identification and reduced stigma. Maintaining these peer connections with program graduates in this nonclinical outreach/peer role provides incredible opportunities for wellness and relapse prevention for individuals, keeping them engaged in all phases of their mental health journey. Engagement then comes full circle—both helping individuals get to services sooner and helping them stay engaged and active longer in the realm of mental health and wellness. Young people in recovery benefit personally from the experience of directly helping others and give authentic voice to a misunderstood topic. Peer involvement will be discussed in more detail in stages 2 and 3, increasing and maintaining active engagement with participant and family members through all phases of recovery.

Stage 2: Increasing Engagement in Treatment for Individuals and Families

The next stage is engaging young people and family members in effective treatment. In this section, we outline important elements of early psychosis programming that contribute to strengthening engagement: a team-based program that is accessible, flexible, and culturally sensitive and offers individualized, person-centered, goal-driven treatment, with open involvement of family members and other supports identified by the individual. We also focus on the unique role that peer support plays with the team.

Creating Accessible, Flexible Programs for Engagement

Adolescents and young adults with early psychosis are at high risk of disengagement, with the most influential factors being duration of untreated psychosis, symptom severity at baseline, lack of insight, persistent substance abuse, and absence of family involvement and support (Doyle et al. 2014). Other influences are involvement with the criminal justice system and lack of youth-friendly services (Becker et al. 2016). It is understandable that individuals experiencing paranoid and disorganized thinking and fear about their safety may not readily engage in treatment. Therefore, offering a prolonged, individualized engagement period with involvement of family and other natural supports is critical to successful engagement.

Mental health systems and the rules that dictate treatment guidelines often unintentionally create barriers to access and engagement (Dixon et al. 2018). For example, outpatient treatment clinics often require multiple steps before engagement in treatment: the adult client must call a referral line; provide a lot of information, including history and insurance; attend an orientation appointment; and sometimes be put on a wait list for the next available intake appointment. If people do not show for appointments, they are often discharged without follow-up. Removing these practical barriers to engagement is a key component to engagement in EIPs (Dixon et al. 2018).

The timing of engagement is an important factor. A delay in help seeking can have long-term consequences in terms of the young person's insight about symptoms, willingness to engage with providers, treatment response, and outcomes. It can also increase family stress and negative family dynamics, which exacerbates symptoms (McFarlane 2016).

Stewart (2013) emphasizes that worsening of psychotic symptoms and hospitalization can be traumatic and act as a motivation toward recovery. Therefore, coordinated specialty care (CSC) team staff meeting young people in the hospital and assisting with their transition to community-based care can be a critical opening for engagement. At the PIER program, it is best practice to have both the clinician and peer support make a connection with the young person while he or she is in the hospital and offer the program as voluntary and flexible in meeting the individual's needs (Stewart 2013).

Ensuring That Services Are Person Centered and Goal Driven

Client narratives reveal an early disconnect between what the client thinks is happening and the actions of family, criminal justice, and health care systems that may lead to distrust (van Schalkwyk et al. 2015). Treatment providers may focus on symptom levels and behavioral changes, whereas the young person's goals may be related to relationships, housing, or school. It is important for the provider to listen to and validate the experiences and concerns of the young person and be responsive to his or her perceived concerns.

A literature review about common elements leading to engagement indicates the importance of comprehensive assessment of the client's values and beliefs, goals, race/ethnicity, sexual orientation, religion, and lifestyle choices (Becker et al. 2016). Cultural sensitivity to meaning and interpretation of experience are key to trust building. "Providers who are able to acknowledge cultural differences in how patients conceptualize symptoms, and address how such differences impact patients' decisions to follow providers' recommendations, may have greater success engaging patients of different cultures and ethnicities" (Kline and Thomas 2017, p. 75). Given local and cultural differences within communities, there needs to be some flexibility within evidence-based practices to individualize and adapt practices to meet the needs of diverse groups (Kline and Thomas 2017).

Recovery in mental health is broader than symptom reduction or removal. We need to ask service users more about what they value in terms of recovery. In one study's exploration of service users' views of recovery, four different recovery styles emerged: collaborative support and understanding, emotional change through social and medical support, regaining functional and occupational goals, and self-focused recovery (Wood et al. 2013). Collaborative support emphasizes positive thinking, openness to support, and understanding; emotional change through social and medical support highlights addressing emotional distress and depression as primary; and regaining functional goals illustrates the importance of reengaging in social and vocational roles. On the other hand, self-focused recovery is preferred by people with severe and enduring psychosis who may have had negative past experiences with treatment and who focus on the internal process of recovery (Wood et al. 2013).

EIP programs, such as CSC teams, offer a team-based approach in which engagement in treatment may occur through different pathways for different people on the basis of each person's identified goals. These pathways include cognitive-behavioral therapy for psychosis (CBTp), medication management, vocational or educational support, peer support and family psychoeducation, and group and recovery options. Individualized care driven by the participant's life goals and the convenience of "one-stop shopping" with services all on one team and easily accessible are important elements of engagement for young people (Lucksted et al. 2015). In one study, interviews with young people revealed that the combination of relationships with clinicians who are client centered and humanistic in addition to peers who have also experienced first-episode psychosis influenced their decision to stay in treatment (Stewart 2013). Key elements of individual engagement are "staff flexibility, mobility, patience, warmth, and stamina over time...to navigate ambivalence, illness and life changes" (Lucksted et al. 2015, p. 8).

Using Family Psychoeducation to Engage Family

Families coping with how to help a young person with untreated psychosis experience fear, isolation, and distress (Cairns et al. 2015). Without an understanding of psychosis, family members may misattribute changes to something other than psychosis, causing a delay in help seeking and leading to a crisis point where symptoms become unmanageable and dangerous (Chen et al. 2016; Connor et al. 2016). Additionally, family members' cultural beliefs can influence their interpretation of changes, leading them to seek help within their own community (Connor et al. 2016).

CSC teams providing early intervention in psychosis have a significant impact on engagement because they are able to offer education and proactive outreach not only to the client but to his or her support network as well (Dixon et al. 2018). Comprehensive monthly educational workshops enable families and community members alike to learn about psychosis as a spectrum of changes in thinking, perceptions, and mental processing. These workshops should be made available to any community member at no cost and include presentations by both peers with lived experience and professionals with specialized experience treating first-episode psychosis. The workshops emphasize the relationship between stressors, the environment, and symptoms and the important role of family and friends in partnering in treatment. The message of recovery and hope is key, with a combination of biological, psychological, and social interventions leading to the best outcomes (Addington et al. 2013). Offering educational workshops in a classroom format allows people to gather information before making a commitment to an EIP program.

Using Multiple-Family Groups to Strengthen Family and Participant Engagement

Family psychoeducation, which is delivered most effectively in a multiple-family group format (MFG-FPE), is considered an essential evidence-based component of early psychosis CSC treatment (Addington et al. 2013). The MFG-FPE model addresses the family's need for information, clinical guidance, and ongoing support during the recovery of their loved one. The model is based on a partnership between the family (broadly defined as the participant's trusted supports), the participant, and the CSC team. At EIP programs, groups are co-facilitated by a combination of disciplines (social worker, employment or education specialist, peer support, and case manager). The group is always inclusive of the young person but can benefit the family system with or without initial involvement from the client.

MFG-FPE is most effective when there is no delay in offering the group at the beginning of treatment, when the family most needs support (Fjell et al. 2007). Groups offer ongoing enrollment so newcomers can benefit from lessons learned by those at later stages of treatment and experience hope through those further along in recovery. Although psychoeducation can be provided in a single-family session, we have found that connecting families with other families is most powerful in deepening the family and individual's engagement with treatment. MFG-FPE addresses common feelings of isolation, stigma, family tension, and hopelessness in early psychosis by providing community, normalization, skill building, and hope. Clinicians will need supervision and coaching on how to present this resource to families because it is typical for people to refuse groups at the outset (Fjell et al. 2007).

Family Engagement Case Example

Laurence is a young man who describes that he has identified with ghosts and dark or evil creatures for as long as he can remember and that this has, in fact, fueled his creative style, identity, and art. At age 17, Laurence caught the attention of his high school counselor, who was concerned that he was "over-identifying" with ghosts in his often frightening graphic images and writing. She referred Laurence to the local EIP program; however, after the intake, his parents encouraged him to decline the program because they felt that early intervention for psychosis was not a fit. They felt that Laurence's creative side was being misrepresented and misunderstood, and they wanted to protect him from the stigma of "mental illness." Laurence's father was strongest in his reluctance to engage with EIP services and most protective of his son; his mother was uncertain and agreed to attend a community workshop to get more information "for future reference."

About a year later, in the stress of leaving home and transitioning to college, Laurence said, "I was really stressed and vulnerable...then something inside me just became bad or evil...and I was scared of it." Laurence was experiencing very distressing symptoms and was desperate for help. He called his mother, who immediately called the program to ask if it was "too late" to have Laurence start services. She then brought both Laurence and his father to another community workshop to learn more about psychosis. After the workshop, both Laurence and his parents immediately engaged fully in the program, and, as his father described, "I had no idea until I got here what this was or how to help him. I was just doing my best with all I knew as a dad." Laurence started learning words to describe his experiences in specific ways to ask for help from his family to support his recovery and wellness. Importantly, he also started learning how to let them know when *not* to worry and how to *not* hover too close. Laurence and his parents now regularly attend multiple-family problem-solving groups, which support this process openly, alongside other young people and their families who are having similar questions and struggles. His father jokes about his initial reluctance about services and how he's "come around" with the support of the group, the program, and, most importantly, Laurence.

Stage 3: Maintaining Active Engagement With the Participant and Family Members Through All Phases of Recovery With Peer Involvement

The last phase of engagement gives young people and families an opportunity to offer assistance to those in earlier phases of recovery through peer support, speaking opportunities, an advisory board, or mentorship, which in turn leads to earlier intervention and ultimately to social change and reduction of stigma. Similar to the model of peer-based recovery, we begin our discussion of the role of peer support with two narrative examples: first, a peer support's story of immersion into an EIP team and second, a participant's story of her experience being served by an EIP team with peer support.

Peer Narrative: Nyamuon

When I first started with the PIER program in the role of youth support partner, my goal was to use my own lived experience to help young people find a relatable person at the table and feel empowered by seeing that raw presence partnered alongside their clinical team. Through one-on-one work, I was able to form authentic connections with young people by being nonjudgmental, listening openly, and offering some of my own journey when relevant. Eventually, the young people learned how to trust and be honest about their experiences.

At the time of my own first treatment 10 years ago, I had already been dealing with symptoms and early warning signs of psychosis for some time. When my first suicide attempt landed me in an inpatient mental health facility, the stigma, shame, and fear of my mental illness being discovered by my family and community hindered me from being honest with the mental health professionals about my experience. Outside of the personal shame I had been feeling about the sexual abuse I believe sparked many of my struggles, I was also carrying the cultural responsibility to maintain normalcy and uphold my reputation and that of my family in our East African community. Service providers coming to the home or reaching out held a stigma in my community that assumed blame was being placed on the parents, finding them unfit to protect their children. These factors led to barriers in any real or effective attempts at treatment. I wasn't able to be honest and open about the number of symptoms I was having and how they were affecting me day to day.

As I became a peer support, through training in the components of CSC (early intervention, community outreach, CBTp, and MFG-FPE), I gained a deeper understanding of my own story and how long I had been impacted by trauma and psychosis. This led me to explore not only my experiences but also my interactions with the mental health system and providers. In my role as peer support these past 3 years, I have discovered possible engagement tactics that might have proven impactful for me and beneficial to building my confidence, voice, and ability to articulate what I was going through and what "better" would look like for me. Being able to draw from my story and openly talk about the journey from a place of strength and hope provides an example and motivation for others in the program to feel less isolated by their experience and hopefully be drawn or sparked to become a peer voice in supporting or encouraging others who follow.

Over time, I have fully integrated into the team and have become an equal and valued member. I have brought the youth peer support model training to the PIER team and given the team insight into a different, and more culturally informed, perspective. I have worked together with the team to incorporate the peer voice into community outreach presentations, family workshops, and initial meetings with clients and in co-facilitating a multiple-family group.

Working with many people in the immigrant community, one of the hurdles that prevents conversation around early detection or intervention is fear and lack of understanding or ability to relate to the information being shared about psychosis and other mental health terms. Peer support can and has acted as a bridge between communities and service providers in helping to normalize conversations about mental health. The peer support role offers "lived experience" examples of what clinicians and psychiatrists may discuss in more clinical terms. Peer involvement on a clinical team can offer a nonclinical, recovery-based perspective that incorporates personal wellness, building healthy natural supports in the community and opening opportunities for youth to establish their voice.

Peer Support Case Example: Helima

Helima, a 19-year-old young woman from an African country, did not have family involvement because she came to this country on her own. She was in a temporary living situation and attending high school sporadically. She had been hospitalized for suicidal ideation a year prior to her referral but did not reveal information about past trauma or the extent of her psychotic symptoms at the hospital. It was not until multiple emergency department visits with physical complaints that she was referred to an EIP program. Engaging her was challenging because she was afraid of being rehospitalized. She was open to EIP staff coming to her school to meet with her, especially after hearing that they might be able to support her with her goals of completing school and finding a job and more permanent housing. The team began to engage with the school social worker in order to meet Helima at school. There were multiple attempts because she sometimes did not show. The peer support and social worker finally were able to meet Helima at a school meeting. The peer support, Nyamuon, who was also from an African culture, shared parts of her own story in order to create a safe space and relatable language to break down barriers of shame. She established a cultural connection and shared experience with trauma and psychosis. Nyamuon was the liaison between Helima and the program, enabling Helima to begin to trust the team. Engagement was still a fluid process, and the initial focus was on getting Helima into a transitional housing program, which provided more structure and support. Eventually, she joined a multiple-family group, accompanied by Nyamuon, and began to feel more fully integrated with other peers and families in the program. She said, "What makes me feel hopeful is helping someone else and realizing I am not alone in my struggles."

EIP programs are beginning to incorporate peer and family support, leadership, and involvement in several aspects of their programs (Dixon et al. 2018), and a technical assistance manual, "Peer Involvement and Leadership in EIP Services," is available at the NASMHPD website (Jones 2016). The manual emphasizes involving peer and family members in advisory councils, community mapping of resources and strengths, and partnering with peer organizations in addition to using peer and family voices and stories of recovery whenever possible (Jones 2016). Since 2015, the PIER program has partnered with the youth-led peer support organization Youth Move Maine to include a positive peer presence at all outreach opportunities, clinical groups, family groups, and peer connections (as outlined in the section "Stage 2: Increasing Engagement in Treatment for Individuals and Families").

Since the late 1990s, the PIER program has been incorporating peer and family voice and engagement as people have come forth with an interest in giving back and supporting the early intervention movement. Videos and speakers bureaus allow peer and family voices to guide community education through hope, recovery, and resilience. In the PIER program, people tell their stories from the beginning in multiple-family groups, and over time, their stories emerge and expand as they make sense of their experiences and deepen their connection to a safe community. These stories are documented in a peer creative expression group through videos, stories, artwork, music, or poetry. Participants decide whether their stories are shared only with the group or more broadly.

One of our PIER graduates is now a psychiatric nurse practitioner and a regular speaker at conferences and in program videos, and she is influencing the field by providing treatment to others. Another graduate still comes back to speak to peers and families after 15 years because it is meaningful for her to offer her story of the ups and downs that ultimately shaped who she has become and made her stronger. Now that peer support has become a critical component of EIP programs, there is a lot of room for expanding how we involve peer and family voices to all aspects of engagement, creating social change and breaking down long-held stigmas and cultural divides.

Conclusion

Disengagement from mental health treatment occurs up to 50% of the time, with more than 70% of dropout occurring after the first or second visit (Lal and Malla 2015; Olfson et al. 2009). That said, treatment attendance is a limiting measure of meaningful engagement (Lal and Malla 2015), which we hope to have described in this chapter as a more multifaceted process. We recommend redefining engagement to include strengthening individual connections with participants through therapeutic alliance and program accessibility, as well as cultivating broader circles of support with well-engaged peers, families, and communities as a whole. These circles of engagement then become the cornerstone of stigma reduction, early intervention, and treatment models rooted in recovery, strength, and wellness.

KEY CONCEPTS

- Engagement is multifaceted and involves three primary stages: community outreach, individual and family engagement, and peer and family connections over time in recovery.

- Comprehensive community outreach with peer and family narratives reduces stigma and increases early detection.

- Communities, individuals, and families are strengthened when EIP programs are strongly rooted in engagement on multiple levels with treatment, recovery, and natural and peer connections.

Key Questions

1. How can EIP programs tailor evidence-based CSC models to individualized approaches with engagement as the primary premise?

2. How can CSC programs become more accessible to increase engagement in early stages?

3. How can we rethink agency policies and processes to incorporate engagement-influenced principles?

4. How can programs build in and manage outreach programming and recovery connections in addition to more traditional treatment models?

5. How can we engage youth as peers in nonclinical ways to maintain involvement over time?

Suggested Readings

Dixon LB, Holoshitz Y, Nossel I: Treatment engagement of individuals experiencing mental illness: review and update. World Psychiatry 15(1):13–20, 2016 26833597

Jones N: Peer Involvement and Leadership in Early Intervention in Psychosis Services: From Planning to Peer Support and Evaluation. Rockville, MD, Center for Mental Health Services, July 26, 2016. Available at: www.nasmhpd.org/sites/default/files/Peer-Involvement-Guidance_Manual_Final.pdf. Accessed September 28, 2018.

McFarlane WR, Jaynes R: Educating Communities to Identify and Engage Youth in the Early Phases of an Initial Psychosis: A Manual for Specialty Programs. Rockville, MD, Center for Mental Health Services, 2017. Available at: www.nasmhpd.org/sites/default/files/DH-Community_Outreach_Guidance_Manual__0.pdf. Accessed September 28, 2018.

McFarlane WR, Lynch S, Melton R: Family psychoeducation in clinical high risk and first-episode psychosis. Adolescent Psychiatry 2(2):182–194, 2012

National Alliance on Mental Illness: Engagement: A New Standard for Mental Health Care. Arlington, VA, National Alliance on Mental Illness, July 2016. Available at: www.nami.org/About-NAMI/Publications-Reports/Public-Policy-Reports/Engagement-A-New-Standard-for-Mental-Health-Care/NAMI_Engagement_Web.pdf. Accessed September 28, 2018.

References

Addington DE, McKenzie E, Norman R, et al: Essential evidence-based components of first-episode psychosis services. Psychiatr Serv 64(5):452–457, 2013 23370444

Baumann PS, Crespi S, Marion-Veyron R, et al: Treatment and early intervention in psychosis program (TIPP-Lausanne): implementation of an early intervention programme for psychosis in Switzerland. Early Interv Psychiatry 7(3):322–328, 2013 23445318

Becker KD, Buckingham SL, Rith-Najarian L, et al: The common elements of treatment engagement for clinically high-risk youth and youth with first-episode psychosis. Early Interv Psychiatry 10(6):455–467, 2016 26486257

Breitborde NJ, Moe AM, Ered A, et al: Optimizing psychosocial interventions in first-episode psychosis: current perspectives and future directions. Psychol Res Behav Manag 10:119–128, 2017 28490910

Cairns VA, Reid GS, Murray C: Family members' experience of seeking help for first-episode psychosis on behalf of a loved one: a meta-synthesis of qualitative research. Early Interv Psychiatry 9(3):185–199, 2015 24958353

Chen FP, Gearing RE, DeVylder JE, et al: Pathway model of parental help seeking for adolescents experiencing first-episode psychosis. Early Interv Psychiatry 10(2):122–128, 2016 24894667

Connor C, Greenfield S, Lester H, et al: Seeking help for first-episode psychosis: a family narrative. Early Interv Psychiatry 10(4):334–345, 2016 25303624

Dixon LB, Holoshitz Y, Nossel I: Treatment engagement of individuals experiencing mental illness: review and update. World Psychiatry 15(1):13–20, 2016 26833597

Dixon LB, Goldman HH, Srihari VH, et al: Transforming the treatment of schizophrenia in the United States: the RAISE initiative. Annu Rev Clin Psychol 14(1):237–258, 2018 29328779

Doyle R, Turner N, Fanning F, et al: First-episode psychosis and disengagement from treatment: a systematic review. Psychiatr Serv 65(5):603–611, 2014 24535333

Fjell A, Bloch Thorsen GR, Friis S, et al: Multifamily group treatment in a program for patients with first-episode psychosis: experiences from the TIPS project. Psychiatr Serv 58(2):171–173, 2007 17287370

Joa I, Johannessen JO, Auestad B, et al: The key to reducing duration of untreated first psychosis: information campaigns. Schizophr Bull 34(3):466–472, 2008 17905788

Johannessen JO, McGlashan TH, Larsen TK, et al: Early detection strategies for untreated first-episode psychosis. Schizophr Res 51(1):39–46, 2001 11479064

Jones N: Peer Involvement and Leadership in Early Intervention in Psychosis Services: From Planning to Peer Support and Evaluation. Rockville, MD, Center for Mental Health Services, July 26, 2016. Available at: https://www.nasmhpd.org/sites/default/files/Peer-Involvement-Guidance_Manual_Final.pdf. Accessed September 28, 2018.

Kline E, Thomas L: Cultural factors in first episode psychosis treatment engagement. Schizophr Res 195:74–75, 2017 28864280

Lal S, Malla A: Service engagement in first-episode psychosis: current issues and future directions. Can J Psychiatry 60(8):341–345, 2015 26454555

Lucksted A, Essock SM, Stevenson J, et al: Client views of engagement in the RAISE connection program for early psychosis recovery. Psychiatr Serv 66(7):699–704, 2015 25873029

Lynch S, McFarlane WR, Joly B, et al: Early detection, intervention and prevention of psychosis program: community outreach and early identification at six U.S. sites. Psychiatr Serv 67(5):510–516, 2016 26766751

McFarlane WR: Family interventions for schizophrenia and the psychoses: a review. Fam Process 55(3):460–482, 2016 27411376

McFarlane WR, Jaynes R: Educating Communities to Identify and Engage Youth in the Early Phases of an Initial Psychosis: A Manual for Specialty Programs. Rockville, MD, Center for Mental Health Services, 2017. Available at: www.nasmhpd.org/sites/default/files/DH-Community_Outreach_Guidance_Manual__0.pdf. Accessed September 28, 2018.

McFarlane WR, Cook WL, Downing D, et al: Portland identification and early referral: a community-based system for identifying and treating youths at high risk of psychosis. Psychiatr Serv 61(5):512–515, 2010 20439374

National Alliance on Mental Illness: Engagement: A New Standard for Mental Health Care. Arlington, VA, National Alliance on Mental Illness, July 2016. Available at: www.nami.org/About-NAMI/Publications-Reports/Public-Policy-Reports/Engagement-A-New-Standard-for-Mental-Health-Care/NAMI_Engagement_Web.pdf. Accessed September 28, 2018.

Olfson M, Mojtabai R, Sampson NA, et al: Dropout from outpatient mental health care in the United States. Psychiatr Serv 60(7):898–907, 2009 19564219

Ruff A, McFarlane WR, Downing D, et al: A community outreach and education model for early identification of mental illness in young people. Adolescent Psychiatry 2(2):140–145, 2012

Stewart KD: Factors contributing to engagement during the initial stages of treatment for psychosis. Qual Health Res 23(3):336–347, 2013 23196742

van Schalkwyk GI, Davidson L, Srihari V: Too late and too little: narratives of treatment disconnect in early psychosis. Psychiatr Q 86(4):521–532, 2015 25663602

Wood L, Price J, Morrision A, et al: Exploring service users perceptions of recovery from psychosis: a Q-methodological approach. Psychol Psychother 86(3):245–261, 2013 23184907

CHAPTER 7

Assessment of People in
the Early Stages of Psychosis

Barbara C. Walsh, Ph.D.

UNLIKE many medical illnesses and despite all the recent advances in the area of early psychosis research, we still do not have a gold standard laboratory test to mark the presence of psychosis (McGlashan et al. 2010). Diagnosis of the clinical high-risk phase and the recent-onset phase of psychosis relies on symptoms that can be observed by others or symptoms that can be reported by young people themselves, remembering that the young person may be suspicious or may be trying to hide his or her difficulties. Diagnosis requires a high level of sensitivity not only to existing symptoms but to the normal course of development of young people and to the gradual change in their psychosocial functioning. It is crucial for professionals to have an understanding of the array of presentations of psychotic disorders and the natural history of a psychotic episode, including the prodromal, active, and recovery phases, as well as proficiency in performing psychiatric assessment. Good assessment in early psychosis is an ongoing process, allowing for the fact that symptoms are fluid and change over time.

It is important to understand that when people seek an early psychosis evaluation, either they are distressed by their symptoms or others are noticing a change in their functioning due to these symptoms. For example, Alan experienced hearing the voice of the devil telling him to walk barefoot down the middle of the highway. He struggled against the commands of the devil, which left him distressed and drained of energy. Brenda experienced a cold wave over her body when she sat at the kitchen table. She reported that she thought this experience was the ghost of her dead grandmother coming to comfort her. This did not distress her at all, but she started spending more and more time sitting at the kitchen table waiting for Grandma rather than going to school and being with her friends. In Alan's case, the symptoms were causing distress, and in Brenda's case, the symptoms were interfering with functioning. In both examples, the person needed intervention and support.

The initial interview is a vital component of early identification and intervention work. It serves as the principal means for understanding the client's experiences and leads to a diagnosis and treatment plan. More than just taking a history to determine what condition the client struggles with and how he or she is affected by it, an effective assessment interview starts the therapeutic process. It has been stated that poor interviews and/or misinterpretation of a client's presentation can be critical to that person's future well-being and subsequent treatment (UK Essays 2013). For example, when young people present first with just the negative symptoms of psychosis, they are often misdiagnosed with other disorders such as major depressive disorder, attention-deficit/hyperactivity disorder, or even oppositional defiant disorder. They are started on a course of treatment that not only does not address their total clinical picture but actually may worsen their existing condition. An accurate assessment addressing the appropriate warning signs and symptoms can prevent this from happening.

A component of conducting an effective assessment interview is to have a framework to help explore potential problem areas and to recognize that the success of an assessment is based on establishing a relaxed, nonjudgmental atmosphere that promotes a trusting relationship, reduces tension, encourages engagement, and starts the therapeutic process. Being flexible in how the interview is conducted, respecting the client's needs, being empathetic, and engaging in active listening all contribute to successfully establishing a nonjudgmental atmosphere. Paranoia and perceptual distortions are often a part of the early phase of psychosis, and taking time to explain the interview process and what the client can expect helps to reduce concerns and anxiety associated with these symptoms. Being clear in defining expectations—what the young person can expect from the interviewer and what the interviewer can expect from him or her—reduces tension.

Many young people experiencing psychosis may be younger than 18 years or still living at home, so their parents or other family members may be attending the assessment with them. For older or more independent persons, the interviewer may want to encourage them to have a parent, spouse, or other relative accompany them to the interview. These involved family members may be able to provide details about the person's functioning and provide additional and/or collaborative information about his or her developmental, medical, and educational history and history of extended family mental health concerns.

With permission from the client, the interviewer works collaboratively with family members during the initial stage of the assessment to help define the family support system. The interviewer clearly defines the boundaries of confidentiality for everyone, emphasizing the type of information that cannot be kept private, especially around issues of self-harm or intent to harm others. Risk assessment, including issues of neglect, should be a part of every evaluation (Halpin 1995). With younger persons, these issues usually refer to physical or educational neglect from their parents, and with older persons, the issues may refer to neglect of dependents. Assessing for victimization by others applies to both younger and older persons. Risk assessment should include information about past episodes of abuse or neglect, history of self-injurious behavior, suicide attempts, and all relevant trauma history.

The interviewer should state that he or she will be meeting for a short time with everyone together and then will complete the majority of the interview with the client alone. The interviewer explains that he or she will be asking for information about things that the client might not be aware of, such as the status of the mother's pregnancy and delivery and attainment of developmental milestones. The interviewer helps the client understand that the interviewer is interested in the client's concerns as well as the concerns of family members, acknowledging that the client's perspective on things may differ from a family member's perspective and it is helpful for the interviewer to understand both perspectives. The interviewer works to balance rapport, assessment, psychoeducation, and assistance as he or she navigates through the interview. Family members are often distressed and anxious about the changes they see in their loved one, and they appreciate information and support. The family's distress, confusion, and denial, if present, need to be acknowledged. Dismissing presenting problems invalidates the family's experience and may impede diagnosis and future treatment for the client.

Family members also provide insight into the nature and culture of the family. For example, it is not uncommon in American Indian families for the entire family to accompany the young person to the assessment as a sign of support. Assessors must do their best to accommodate this practice, even if it differs from their usual approach. Traditional healers are often used in American Indian and other cultures, and assessors need to be familiar with indigenous beliefs and practices and to respect them even if they differ from their own. A sociocultural framework is needed during assessment so that diversity of values, interactional styles, and cultural expectations are all considered. The roles that culture and ethnicity or race play in the sociopsychological development of the client—

how they help the client form his or her own identification and how they impact the client's beliefs and behavior—are significant factors in understanding the psychological processes of the client. Asking open-ended follow-up questions allows clients to frame their experiences in their own way. This provides insight into the nature and context of the experiences for the individual and how they impact the client's perception of the intensity, frequency, distress, and interference from these experiences. In addition, the American Psychological Association recommends that all psychologists, regardless of their own ethnic or racial background, be aware of how their cultural background, experiences, attitudes, values, and biases influence psychological processes (American Psychological Association 1990).

A good place to start the assessment interview is with the reason for the referral. It is helpful to establish clients' understanding of the reason; obtain their insight into how their difficulties are impacting their day-to-day functioning; learn how they have attempted to cope with these difficulties; clarify their aspirations, hopes, and goals for the future; and evaluate their attitude toward the assessment interview and their level of cooperation. Understanding whether the client had any say in the decision to attend the interview can help or hinder how the interview progresses. It is possible that attendance was not presented as being optional, and the client may be angry and resentful about being there. He or she may not cooperate with the interview process. If this occurs, it can be helpful for the interviewer to acknowledge the situation before moving forward with the interview.

Case Example 1

Carter is a 16-year-old male adolescent who has been struggling in school, withdrawing socially, and becoming more and more irritable at home. His teacher recommended that his parents call the clinic to arrange an evaluation. Carter's parents, deeply concerned about their son, quickly acted on the suggestion and did not spend much time discussing the reason for the referral or the interview process with him. At the interview, Carter appeared sullen and withdrawn, and when he was alone with the interviewer he quickly answered "No" to all of the questions. The interviewer, without embarrassment or hesitation, acknowledged Carter's behavior and validated his right to refuse to answer the questions. The interviewer then explained to Carter that such a refusal would impede their understanding of his symptoms and the interviewer's ability to offer suggestions for improving things and would thus be a waste of time for both of them. Empowering Carter to make his own decision about participating in the interview allowed him to move forward with the assessment and obtain help.

Just like their family, young people may be confused and distressed by their symptoms. The assessment interview provides an opportunity to help them understand these symptoms and establish a framework for engagement and compliance with their future treatment. Interviewers should take the time to explain to clients that they ask everyone the same questions and that there are no right or wrong answers because everyone has different experiences. Many young people have not shared their symptoms with others, and they mistakenly believe they are the only ones who experience them. Knowing that others share these experiences, that there is a connection between psychotic-like experiences and more conventional ones, normalizes their experiences rather than identifying them as different, reassures the clients, and may encourage them to share more details of their symptoms and experiences.

Case Example 2

Daniela, a 17-year-old female adolescent, was referred for assessment because school staff noticed she could no longer pay attention and attend to her schoolwork. She had always been an excellent student, so this was quite a departure from her normal presentation. Daniela did not offer any explanation to her teachers or family for this change. When she arrived at the clinic, the interviewer took the time to show her the assessment form and to explain to her that the questions they would be asking were not designed specifically for her experiences but were the same questions asked of everyone. Halfway through the interview, Daniela looked at the interviewer with tears in her eyes and asked, "You mean there are enough kids who experience these things that you have the questions written out?" The interviewer replied yes. Daniela visibly relaxed and began to share more details about the voices and intrusive thoughts that she was experiencing in school on a daily basis. This additional information helped the interviewer to understand and communicate about the change in Daniela's academic performance. It might also be helpful to recognize that when discussing a person's internal experiences, a softer approach provokes less reactivity than a more direct approach. Statements such as "I'm guessing it might be scary for you when you hear voices" tend to be accepted more easily than a statement such as "You get scared when you hear voices."

The interviewer should also take the time to explain that the purpose of the interview is to increase the client's understanding of what he or she is experiencing and to determine what might help the client feel and do better in his or her daily life. The interviewer should help the client understand that the interview is not intended to label or judge him or her but rather to reduce his or her level of stress. The Personal Assessment and Crisis Evaluation (PACE) Clinic in Melbourne, Australia acknowledges that young people can be difficult to engage because of the nature of their symptoms, their lack of familiarity with or stigma about mental health services, and their ambivalence about their need for treatment (Thompson 2012). Staff at the PACE Clinic recommend using excellent communication skills, including active listening and empathy; providing information and education about symptoms; and working collaboratively with family members with the knowledge and consent of the young person to help foster engagement. They also recommend offering the client a choice in where the assessment interview should take place, which may require the use of mobile outreach teams to conduct assessments outside the office and outside normal office hours. Assessments should take place at a location and time that are suitable and that accommodate the needs and preferences of the client and his or her family to allow for school and work commitments.

The early identification and intervention model stresses the importance of assessing the entire spectrum of the client's well-being (Goldner-Vukov et al. 2007). This helps to establish the framework for evaluating potential problem areas and for making an accurate diagnosis regarding prodromal and psychotic symptoms. In addition to the reason for referral and presenting problems and concerns, the framework should include many other elements that are based on both interviewing and observation skills.

Good observation skills allow the interviewer to collect information that might not be in the client's awareness. It is important to pay close attention to the client's presentation during the entire assessment, taking note of anything unusual in his or her appearance in terms of self-care, dress, and makeup. Observing abnormal motor activity, eye contact, mannerisms, and posture as well as abnormalities in rate, tone, or ability to express and comprehend language adds important clinical details to the assessment. The interviewer should also observe whether the client attends to the questions and whether his or her thoughts are connected and logical. The interviewer should take notice of untimely or excessive affect, lack of affect, or affect that does not match thought content. All of these observations provide information that is vital in making a valid assessment and diagnosis.

Other elements of the framework for the assessment are obtained by directly interviewing the client. The interviewer should keep the client talking with as little intrusion as possible. This is why open-ended questions are so valuable. "How so?" or "Can you tell me more about that?" serve as requests that keep the person talking. "To what extent" can change any question to an open-ended one. For example, when inquiring about the impact of depressive symptoms on a client's sleep, the interviewer can ask "To what extent did your sleep change?" instead of "Did your sleep change?" Phrasing makes a big difference in how questions are perceived. Instead of "How often have you been hospitalized?" the interviewer can say, "Please tell me about your other hospitalizations." The interviewer should avoid phrasing questions in the negative, which implies an expected answer. For example, "You haven't been smoking pot regularly, have you?" demands the answer "No." Double questions, such as "Have you had problems with your sleep or appetite?" may be efficient, but they are often confusing, and the client may respond to one part of the question and ignore the other.

There are also some other techniques that might be helpful with this process. Experienced interviewers rely on nonverbal encouragements to keep the client talking. Maintaining continuous eye contact, smiling or nodding for appropriate responses, and leaning in a little closer all indicate interest in what the person is saying. This technique increases rapport and the person's sense of well-being. Reassurance is a technique an interviewer uses to increase the client's level of comfort during the interview. To be effective, reassurance needs to be sincere, factual, and specific to the situation. It should not appear forced or fake. The interviewer should avoid generalizations. Because the interviewer cannot predict the future, stating "I'm sure it will be fine" can seem hollow or can reduce the interviewer's credibility with the client.

A technique that encourages continued disclosure is to repeat the client's last word. For example, if the client endorses that he or she has been feeling paranoid recently, the interviewer can respond with "Paranoid?" to encourage the client to continue along that same line of thought. It also helps to briefly summarize what has been said so that the interviewer and client are on the same page. For example, "As I understand it, you have been feeling paranoid recently." There are times when the client does not need encouragement to give information and, in fact, may need encouragement to be brief. In this situation, the interviewer must encourage brevity without impairing rapport. It is effective to state "I really want to hear more about that, but I am aware that our time today is limited, so I am going to ask you to focus on this specific question." The interviewer can nod or smile approval when he or she gets the brief answer that provides the needed information.

Capturing the client's medical and psychiatric history is another piece of the framework addressed through the direct interviewing process. It is important to learn about general medical symptoms, previous diagnoses, previous hospitalizations and medical procedures, and all prescribed medications or supplements. Medication side effects can produce a variety of mood symptoms. You may occasionally encounter a client whose depression was caused by cancer or a psychosis that was the result of an endocrine disorder. The interviewer should explore all past psychiatric symptoms and treatment, including hospitalizations, and treatment compliance for both prescribed medications and therapies. Blood work, physical examinations, and perhaps even a neurological consultation may be warranted. Often, a mental status examination is included in this part of the assessment interview.

Once the interviewer has captured the client's major areas of difficulty, he or she can explore all the details of the current episode of illness. This establishes a timeline for how and when the illness began, its symptoms, the consequences, and possible stressors. The interviewer should learn as much as possible about the symptoms: Are they constant or intermittent? Are they changing in intensity or frequency? Are they connected to certain places, situations, or time of day? After first obtaining a complete educational, occupational, and social history, the interviewer can query for the changes that have occurred because of these symptoms. The interviewer should explore for changes in sleep pattern, weight, energy level, and mood variation. He or she should also query for the impact the symptoms are having on marital or love relationships, sexuality and sexual activity, and friendships. The interviewer should explore for any difficulties with impulsivity and any involvement with the police or legal issues, including past arrests or incarcerations, probation status, and pending court appearances. A history of past domestic or legal issues can help assess for future risk of violence and help the interviewer ensure his or her own personal safety. The interviewer should watch for indicators of potential violence in the client such as the use of threats or insults, rising pitch in the person's voice, aggressive behavior, or significant body language such as agitation or clenched fists. The interview should be conducted in a room that provides easy access to the exit for both interviewer and interviewee and that is equipped with an alarm or is within earshot of other professionals who can provide help if needed.

The interviewer also should probe for information regarding drug and alcohol experimentation and misuse. Orygen Youth Health approximates that 60%–70% of young people with early psychosis report some misuse of substances (Crlenjak et al. 2014). This makes screening for misuse essential in early psychosis programs. The wording of the questions is important for obtaining honest information. Asking "How often do you smoke pot in an average week?" as opposed to "Do you smoke pot?" encourages clients to be open about their use. Further, it is helpful to let clients know that this question is asked without judgment or prejudice and that the information is necessary in order to best understand the nature of their condition and how to appropriately work with them in pursuit of their goals. Clients should know that admitting to misuse of substances is not grounds for termination from treatment so they can feel comfortable with being more forthcoming. It is important to include synthetic, over-the-counter, and prescription drugs in the queries. In addition to identifying the types of substances and the length and frequency of use, the interviewer should query for the impact the use has on the person's day-to-day life and functioning. Substance use can impact job attendance and performance, family and marital relationships, friendships and social activity, financial status, medical health, and legal status. Inquiring about the success or failure of any prior substance misuse treatment is very important in understanding the severity of the issue for this particular client and its relationship to the symptoms he or she is experiencing.

Many tools are available to help with the evaluation and diagnosis of early psychosis. You will find that these tools all share certain interview techniques. Questions are worded in a softer manner that allows clients to endorse their experiences freely: "Does it seem like your mind (ears/eyes) is playing tricks on you?" "Do you become confused between what is real and what is imaginary?" "Do you find yourself feeling mistrustful or suspicious of others?" "Do you feel like you have special powers or abilities?" "Do you behave without regard to painful consequences?" Following up these questions with "How so?" "Can you tell me more about that?" or "What did you make of that when it happened?" helps the interviewer understand the client's internal experiences. It is then crucial to inquire whether the experience was captivating or distressing to the client and whether it had an impact on his or her behavior or functioning. These are all components of making an accurate assessment of experiences and of developing the most appropriate treatment plan. Some of the assessments, such as the Structured Interview for Psychosis-Risk Syndromes (SIPS; Miller et al. 2003), are effective in diagnosing the at-risk phase as well as documenting the onset of transition to full psychosis, capturing the affective comorbidities and substance use issues. Professionals should take the time to become familiar with the most commonly used assessment tools and how they are suited to meet the needs of the population they serve (Fulford et al. 2014). Familiarity with these tools also helps identify the gaps in proper assessment in early psychosis and aids in the improvement of existing tools or the development of new tools. State-of-the-art assessment can play a pivotal role in ensuring early identification and intervention in psychosis.

Termination of assessment involves a summary of the client's participation in the process and the outcome of the assessment. Setting a tone that is optimistic and avoids a deterministic viewpoint of psychosis and emphasizes hope for recovery is crucial. The amount of information shared depends on the nature of the outcomes, the state of the client's condition, and his or her ability to understand the information and the recommendations for proposed treatment, further evaluation, or referral. Brain imaging or neurocognitive testing for memory, attention, executive functioning, language, and visuospatial and motor skills might be part of the recommendations for future assessment.

It is important to remember that assessment in early psychosis is an ongoing process and allows for the possibility that the diagnosis may change over time. If no diagnosis is determined at the time of the initial assessment, the recommendation might be to have the client return if symptoms worsen or new symptoms emerge. Persons coming for evaluation are experiencing some level of distress from their experiences, and even if they do not meet criteria for the at-risk or early-onset phase or another comorbid diagnosis, they are in need of support. Establishing an open discussion regarding the future course of action is important for the client being assessed. For professionals working in early psychosis programs, it is important that they continue to enhance their core skills in assessment and interviewing with additional training and supervision so they can successfully provide beneficial evaluations.

KEY CONCEPTS

- Making an early psychosis diagnosis is a key component in determining eligibility for coordinated specialty care services.

- Effective assessment skills of youth presenting with psychotic symptoms are essential in mental health evaluation.

- Structured interviews are used to support valid and reliable diagnostic evaluation.

Discussion Questions

1. How can your team support accurate diagnosis early in the course of psychosis and how might this effect prognosis?

2. How would you ensure that assessment is culturally informed?

3. What systems are in place, or what might need to be developed, in your agency to conduct a structured interview reliably?

Suggested Readings

Comas-Diaz L, Griffith EH: Clinical Guidelines in Cross-Cultural Mental Health. New York, Wiley, 1988

Garlikov R: The Socratic method: teaching by asking instead of by telling, 2012. Available at: http://www.garlikov.com/Soc_Meth.html. Accessed February 13, 2019.

Miller TJ, McGlashan T, Woods SW, et al: Symptom assessment in schizophrenia prodromal states. Psychiatr Q 70:273-287, 1991

References

American Psychological Association: Guidelines for Providers of Psychological Services to Ethnic, Linguistic, and Culturally Diverse Populations. Washington, DC, American Psychological Association, August 1990. Available at: www.apa.org/pi/oema/resources/policy/provider-guidelines.aspx. Accessed October 1, 2018.

Crlenjak C, Ratheesh A, Blaikie S, et al: Let Me Understand: Assessment in Early Psychosis. Melbourne, Australia, Orygen Youth Health Research Centre, 2014

Fulford D, Pearson R, Stuart BK, et al: Symptom assessment in early psychosis: the use of well-established rating scales in clinical high-risk and recent-onset populations. Psychiatry Res 220(3):1077–1083, 2014 25278477

Goldner-Vukov M, Duska-Cupina D, Moore L, et al: Early intervention in first episode psychosis: hope for a better future. Srp Arh Celok Lek 135:11–12, 2007 18368910

Halpin S: Assessment in Early Psychosis. New Lambton, NSW, Australia, Hunter New England Health, 1995. Available at: http://sydney.edu.au/medicine/psychiatry/workshops/presentations/assess_early_psychosis (workshop).pdf. Accessed October 1, 2018.

McGlashan TH, Walsh BC, Woods SW: The Psychosis-Risk Syndrome: Handbook for Diagnosis and Follow-up. New York, Oxford University Press, 2010

Miller TJ, McGlashan TH, Rosen JL, et al: Prodromal assessment with the structured interview for prodromal syndromes and the scale of prodromal symptoms: predictive validity, interrater reliability, and training to reliability. Schizophr Bull 29(4):703–715, 2003 14989408

Thompson AD: The Pace Clinical Manual: A Treatment Approach for Young People at Ultra High Risk of Psychosis. Melbourne, Australia, Orygen Youth Health, 2012

UK Essays: Ensuring Effective Assessment in Psychiatry and Mental Health Nursing Essay. Nottingham, UK, UKEssays, November 2013. Available at: www.ukessays.com/essays/nursing/ensuring-effective-assessment-in-psychiatry-and-mental-health-nursing-essay.php?cref=1. Accessed October 1, 2018.

CHAPTER 8

Assessment and Targeted Intervention in Individuals at Clinical High Risk for Psychosis

Skylar Kelsven, M.S.
Kristin Cadenhead, M.D.

Case Example

Jane is a 21-year-old Latina college student in the fourth year of a 5-year structural engineering degree at a top university. She was referred by her therapist to a local early psychosis treatment center for evaluation of symptoms indicative of possible prodromal psychosis. She experienced a number of subsyndromal psychotic-like symptoms over the past 2 years, but these symptoms had increased in intensity within the last 7 months. Her psychiatric history was significant for anxiety and mood symptoms in the context of childhood sexual abuse and neglect. Jane reported experiencing dissociative reactions, hypervigilance, avoidance, and feelings of alienation in response to trauma-related stimuli that had occurred in childhood. In addition, she reported experiencing periods of elevated and expansive mood that persisted for 2–3 days, followed by periods of distinct low mood that lasted for weeks to months. She reported smoking marijuana consistently since age 16 but using no other drugs. She reported receiving psychotherapy and psychopharmacological intervention (sertraline) for posttraumatic stress disorder (PTSD). She has a family history of PTSD in both parents and bipolar disorder in her father.

Jane was interviewed with the Structured Clinical Interview for DSM-IV Axis I Disorders, Clinician Version (SCID-CV; First et al. 1997) and the Structured Interview for Psychosis-Risk Syndromes (SIPS; Miller et al. 1999). Jane stated that the presenting concerns had been present for the past 2 years but had worsened significantly within the past year. She reported multiple unusual, delusional-like beliefs such as sensing that something was present around her and that she was being observed. When queried further, Jane shared that the unexplained presence could be demons or ghosts and revealed that she avoided being alone for fear of possibly being possessed. She noted that although these experiences were distressing, she recognized that her ideas were unlikely. Jane described herself as superstitious and admitted to putting salt in her windows and hanging crosses. She reported believing she has some psychic tendencies but was able to spontaneously generate insight around the reality of this belief.

Jane disclosed that she has started to disassociate more over the past year, daydreaming often and subsequently losing track of time. Jane shared that she finds it increasingly difficult to determine reality from daydreams and that she engages in a lot of "second-guessing" as to whether or not these experiences are real. She indicated that she has had these experiences for as long as she can remember. In the past year, Jane reported that these symptoms could no longer be ignored, caused her to avoid being around other people, and impacted her concentration in class. Jane reported feeling hypervigilant of her surroundings and even mistrustful of her close friends and boyfriend, suggesting suspiciousness and emerging paranoia. She explained feeling that others were thinking about and talking about her negatively but denied being convinced these thoughts were real. Further, Jane reported a number of perceptual changes, including seeing shadows out of the corner of her eye, accompanied by worries that these shadows might be a demon. Jane reported feeling as though something touched her, which frightened her and caused her to change locations. Jane also reported hearing a high-pitched ringing noise and music, with no apparent source, approximately three times per week.

When asked about possible disorganization of speech, Jane recounted having trouble expressing herself to others, indicating that she mumbled more than she had in the past and that her friends expressed having difficulty understanding her. Jane stated that she had experienced an increased incidence of losing her train of thought. During the evaluation, the evaluator had to steer Jane back to the question at hand and repeat questions. Jane disclosed that prior to the interview, she had just completed her worst school year to date, with grades dropping from As and Bs to Cs and Ds. Despite her reported dysfunction and decline in school achievement, Jane reported that she believed herself to be very intelligent and indicated that with "hard work" she could potentially become a senator or accomplish something that would greatly impact humanity. Jane reported that these grandiose beliefs were present intermittently.

Jane met criteria for psychosis-risk syndrome (subtype attenuated positive symptom syndrome) per the Scale of Prodromal Symptoms (SOPS; Miller et al. 1999) (see Table 8–3 for a scoring summary). SCID diagnoses included PTSD and bipolar II disorder. Jane also underwent brief neuropsychological assessment during her initial clinical visit. Tests administered included the Hopkins Verbal Learning Test–Revised (HVLT-R; Benedict et al. 1998) and the Brief Assessment of Cognition in Schizophrenia–Symbol Coding (BACS-SC; Keefe et al. 2004). Jane's performance on the HVLT-R was below average (HVLT-R Total Recall raw score=20), whereas her performance on the BACS-SC was within normal limits (BACS-SC raw score=61). Comprehensive neuropsychological assessment and magnetic resonance imaging were conducted several days after the clinical interview and did not reveal any abnormalities or gross impairments.

Jane's story is not atypical. If the clinician is unfamiliar with the criteria for psychosis-risk syndrome, it is not uncommon for him or her to incorrectly assume that this may be an example of acute psychosis or conceptualize the experiences as better explained by PTSD. Unfortunately, this quandary is far too common, leaving youth at clinical high risk for psychosis without appropriate diagnosis or intervention. In this chapter we broadly review the definition and diagnosis of psychosis-risk syndrome, validated assessment tools for identifying individuals at clinical high risk for psychosis, and targeted interventions for use in this population. Jane's story will be carried throughout this chapter as a means to illustrate the nuances of assessment and intervention in individuals at clinical high risk for psychosis.

Definition and Diagnosis

Definition

The term *prodrome* is derived from the Greek words *pro* (before) and *dromos* (running), with prodromos meaning "precursor." In contemporary medicine, the term prodrome is used to describe an early symptom indicating the onset of a disease or illness. Formal diagnosis of a prodromal state is made retrospectively. This means that before a period of prodrome can be accurately identified, disease onset must occur. Subsequently, the period of respective changes during the time leading up to disease onset is labeled the *prodromal state* or prodrome.

The psychosis prodrome has been objectively defined in a number of ways. In 2013, the *Diagnostic and Statistical Manual of Mental Disorders*, 5th Edition (DSM-5) included *attenuated psychosis syndrome* in a list of conditions for future study (American Psychiatric Association 2013). The Structured Interview for Psychosis-Risk Syndromes (SIPS) defines it as "prodromal-risk syndrome for psychosis." The Comprehensive Assessment of At-Risk Mental States (CAARMS; Yung et al. 2005) terms it "ultra-high risk for onset of first psychotic disorder." All iterations of the term refer to the same set of defined symptoms that we will hereinafter refer to as *psychosis-risk syndrome*, of which there are three subtypes: 1) genetic risk and deterioration syndrome, also known as the vulnerability group; 2) attenuated positive symptom syndrome, also known as the attenuated psychosis group; and 3) brief intermittent psychotic syndrome, also known as the brief limited intermittent psychotic symptoms group (Table 8–1). Individuals who meet criteria for one of the psychosis-risk syndromes are referred to as being at clinical high risk (CHR) for psychosis or in the prodrome of the first episode of psychosis.

Nomenclature aside, medical treatment intervention and practice have shifted from an emphasis on curative to preventive care. As a result, mental health care providers are forced to conceptualize and assess for pathology in a different way. Such is the case with psychotic disorders, in which the opportunity for intervention and possible prevention occurs during a nonspecific phase of functional decline and emerging psychotic-like experiences (i.e., psychosis-risk syndrome).

Diagnostic Features

Compared with psychotic disorders, the symptoms of psychosis-risk syndrome are less severe and more transient. Diagnosis requires that symptoms are associated with functional impairment and/or distress that is of recent onset or worsening. Symptoms are not long-standing trait pathology; rather, individuals present with marked changes in their mental state, evidenced through reports from self and concerned others. Further, insight remains largely intact (Table 8–2). Affected individuals maintain reasonable cognitive flexibility regarding psychotic-like experiences and generally appreciate that altered perceptions and/or unusual thought content are not real. Insight may be expressed spontaneously, or the interviewing clinician may need to probe overtly for insight. Although establishing the presence of insight is not emphasized in proposed DSM-5 diagnostic criteria for attenuated psychosis syndrome, it appreciably discriminates between psychosis risk and frank psychosis (Box 8–1). For further reading on attenuated psychosis syndrome, see DSM-5 (American Psychiatric Association 2013, pp. 783–786).

Box 8–1. DSM-5 proposed diagnostic criteria for attenuated psychosis syndrome

---

A. At least one of the following symptoms is present in attenuated form, with relatively intact reality testing, and is of sufficient severity or frequency to warrant clinical attention:

1. Delusions.
2. Hallucinations.
3. Disorganized speech.

B. Symptom(s) must have been present at least once per week for the past month.
C. Symptom(s) must have begun or worsened in the past year.
D. Symptom(s) is sufficiently distressing and disabling to the individual to warrant clinical attention.
E. Symptom(s) is not better explained by another mental disorder, including a depressive or bipolar disorder with psychotic features, and is not attributable to the physiological effects of a substance or another medical condition.
F. Criteria for any psychotic disorder have never been met.

Source. Reprinted from American Psychiatric Association: *Diagnostic and Statistical Manual of Mental Disorders*, 5th Edition, Arlington, VA, American Psychiatric Association, 2013. Copyright © 2013 American Psychiatric Association. Used with permission.

Risk and Prognostic Factors

Psychosis-risk syndrome typically emerges in mid to late adolescence or early adulthood. Preceding development can be normal, or the presence of impaired cognition, impaired social development, and negative symptoms may be observed. Specific subtypes of psychosis-risk syndrome are identified through a formal structured clinical interview and are differentiated through individual risk factors, as discussed in the next section. Broadly, risk factors for psychosis-risk syndrome include presence of attenuated positive symptoms, negative symptoms, cognitive impairment or cognitive decline, decline in social and/or role functioning, and family history of psychosis.

Assessment

A number of structured interviews have been developed for evaluation of psychosis-risk syndrome. The selected assessment tools for identification of CHR individuals reviewed in this section show excellent overall prognostic accuracy and interrater reliability in trained raters (Fusar-Poli et al. 2015; Miller et al. 2003). The use of these tools in non-help-seeking individuals from the general population is not recommended because these instruments were developed for and validated in help-seeking populations.

Structured Interview for Psychosis-Risk Syndromes

SIPS is a diagnostic semistructured interview designed to be used with an accompanying severity scale, the Scale of Prodromal Symptoms

TABLE 8–1.   Psychosis-risk syndrome diagnostic subtypes

CHR subtypes

SIPS	CAARMS	SIPS diagnostic features	CAARMS diagnostic features
Genetic risk and deterioration syndrome	Vulnerability group	1. The person has met criteria for schizotypal personality disorder, now or in the past, *and/or* the person has a first-degree relative with a psychotic disorder. 2. The person has experienced at least a 30% drop in GAF score compared with 1 year ago, sustained over the past month.	1. The person has met criteria for schizotypal personality disorder, now or in the past, *and/or* the person has a first-degree relative with a psychotic disorder. 2. The person has experienced a 30% drop in SOFAS (Goldman et al. 1992; Yung et al. 2005) within the past year, occurring within the past month and sustained for at least a month, *or* SOFAS score is ≤50 over the past 12 months or longer.

TABLE 8–1. Psychosis-risk syndrome diagnostic subtypes *(continued)*

CHR subtypes

SIPS	CAARMS	SIPS diagnostic features	CAARMS diagnostic features
Attenuated positive symptom syndrome	Attenuated psychosis group	1. The person scored 3–5 on one or more of SOPS items P1, P2, P3, P4, or P5. 2. The symptoms are *not* better accounted for by a DSM-5 disorder. 3. The symptoms occurred at an average frequency of at least once per week in the past month.	Subthreshold intensity 1. Global score: unusual thought content 3–5, nonbizarre ideas 3–5, perceptual abnormalities 3–4, and/or disorganized speech 4–5 2. Frequency score: unusual thought content, nonbizarre ideas, perceptual abnormalities, and/or disorganized speech 3–6 for at least a week or 2 on more than two occasions, with symptoms occurring during the last year Subthreshold frequency 1. Global score: unusual thought content 6, nonbizarre ideas 6, perceptual abnormalities 5–6, and/or disorganized speech 6 2. Frequency score: unusual thought content, nonbizarre ideas, perceptual abnormalities, and/or disorganized speech 3, with symptoms occurring during the past year 3. The person has experienced a 30% drop in SOFAS within the past year, occurring within the past month and sustained for at least a month, *or* SOFAS score is ≤50 over the past 12 months or longer.

TABLE 8–1.   Psychosis-risk syndrome diagnostic subtypes *(continued)*

CHR subtypes

SIPS	CAARMS	SIPS diagnostic features	CAARMS diagnostic features
Brief intermittent psychotic syndrome	Brief limited intermittent psychotic symptoms group	1. The person scored 6 on one or more of SOPS items P1, P2, P3, P4, or P5. 2. Symptoms are not better explained by a DSM-5 disorder. 3. Symptoms are not seriously dangerous or disorganizing. 4. The person does not meet DSM-5 criteria for a psychotic disorder. 5. The symptoms currently are present for at least several minutes per day (not more than 1 hour) at least one time per month, up to an average frequency of several minutes per day 4 days per week over 1 month.	1. Global score: unusual thought content 6, nonbizarre ideas 6, perceptual abnormalities 5–6, and/or disorganized speech 6 2. Frequency score: unusual thought content, nonbizarre ideas, perceptual abnormalities, and/or disorganized speech 4–6, with symptoms occurring during the past year 3. For each episode, symptoms are present for less than 1 week, and symptoms spontaneously remit on every occasion. 4. The person has experienced a 30% drop in SOFAS within the past year, occurring within the past month and sustained for at least a month, *or* SOFAS score is ≤50 over the past 12 months or longer.

Note.   P1–P5 refer to positive symptom domains.
Abbreviations.   CAARMS= Comprehensive Assessment of At-Risk Mental States; CHR= clinical high risk; GAF=Global Assessment of Functioning; SIPS=Structured Interview for Psychosis-Risk Syndromes; SOFAS=Social and Occupational Functioning Assessment Scale; SOPS=Scale of Prodromal Symptoms.

TABLE 8–2.   Determining the presence of insight in psychosis

Definition of insight	Clinical considerations
Awareness of or acknowledgment that one's thoughts and behaviors are the result of mental illness, with recognition of the need for treatment and/or questioning of the reality of one's beliefs or experiences	• Does the individual spontaneously report awareness that his or her experiences or beliefs are not real or are the product of his or her own mind? If yes: insight intact. • Can doubt about the reality of delusional thinking or hallucinatory experiences be induced by others or by contrary evidence? If yes: insight intact. • Despite contrary evidence, does the individual remain fully convicted that his or her beliefs or experiences are real? If yes: loss of insight.

(SOPS), as well as the Criteria of Prodromal Syndromes (COPS) to operationalize the definition of psychosis-risk onset (Miller et al. 1999). The goal of these integrated tools is to 1) systematically identify the presence or absence of a prodromal-risk state (SIPS interview), 2) measure the severity of prodromal symptoms cross-sectionally and longitudinally (SOPS ratings), and 3) operationalize the threshold of psychosis (COPS diagnosis). For further reading on symptom assessment, see Miller et al. (1999).

The SOPS includes four symptom constructs measured through 19 specific items and subscales: 1) positive symptoms, 2) negative symptoms, 3) disorganization symptoms, and 4) general symptoms. The positive symptom construct is measured through five subscales (see Table 8–3).

Two different severity scales are used for quantifying symptoms on the SOPS. The positive symptom items are rated on the following scale: 0=absent, 1=questionably present, 2=mild, 3=moderate, 4=moderately severe, 5=severe but not psychotic, and 6=severe and psychotic. A score of 6 indicates the presence of a positive symptom that is at a psychotic level of intensity, whereas a score of 3–5 is considered to be not psychotic but subsyndromal. Further, positive symptoms rated as a 3 denote that symptoms reoccur meaningfully but the individual functions mostly as usual despite this increase in symptom frequency. Positive symptoms rated a 4 denote that some degree of distress, confusion, bewilderment, or unease occurs in conjunction with symptom presentation. Positive symptoms rated a 5 denote that the symptoms have become so distressing that behavioral changes occur in the individual

TABLE 8–3.   COPS scoring summary for Jane

| | SOPS positive symptom domain | | | | |
	P1: Unusual thought content and delusional ideas	P2: Suspicious and persecutory ideas	P3: Grandiosity	P4: Perceptual abnormalities and hallucinations	P5: Disorganized communication
Severity rating	4	3	4	4	4
Description of symptom domain	Sense that ideas, experiences, or beliefs may be coming from outside oneself or that they may be real but doubt remains intact Distracting and bothersome May affect functioning	Concerns that people are untrustworthy and/or may harbor ill will Sense of unease and need for vigilance (often unfocused). Mistrustful Recurrent (yet unfounded) sense that people might be thinking or saying negative things about him or her	Notions of being unusually gifted, powerful, or special; has exaggerated expectations Person may be expansive but can redirect to the everyday on own	Illusions or momentary formed hallucinations that are ultimately recognized as unreal but can be distracting, curious, and unsettling May affect functioning.	Circumstantial speech (i.e., eventually getting to the point) Difficulty directing sentences toward a goal Sudden pauses Can be redirected with occasional questions and structuring
Onset	"For as long as I can remember"	1 year ago	"For as long as I can remember"	"For as long as I can remember"	1 year ago
Increase	1 year ago	NA	1 year ago	1 year ago	NA

TABLE 8–3. COPS scoring summary for Jane (*continued*)

	SOPS positive symptom domain				
	P1: Unusual thought content and delusional ideas	**P2: Suspicious and persecutory ideas**	**P3: Grandiosity**	**P4: Perceptual abnormalities and hallucinations**	**P5: Disorganized communication**
Better explained by another DSM disorder?	Not likely	Not likely	Rule out bipolar disorder (manic episode)	Not likely	Not likely

Diagnosis achieved using above criteria: attenuated positive symptom syndrome.

Note. P1–P5 refer to positive symptom domains.
Abbreviations. COPS= Criteria of Prodromal Syndromes; NA=Not applicable; SOPS=Scale of Prodromal Symptoms.

in response to the symptom occurrence. Positive symptoms rated as a 6 imply that insight is completely lost and that the symptoms are experienced with full conviction, potentially affect the person's behavior, and are experienced as bothersome or distressing. The fundamental difference between ratings of 3–5 versus 6 is insight. Insight into the reality of symptoms remains intact for severity ratings of 3–5. Rating an item at the level of 6 marks that the symptom is experienced with full conviction and there has been a total loss of insight.

For positive symptom items rated at a severity level of 3 or higher, symptom onset, symptom worsening, symptom frequency, and whether or not the symptom is "better explained by another DSM disorder" are also recorded. Symptom onset refers to the date at which the positive symptom rating achieved a score of between 3 and 6 for the *first* time. This could be a retrospective rating and requires careful probing by the interviewer to elicit information from the individual regarding when he or she first noticed the symptom meaningfully occur. Finally, the likelihood that positive symptoms rated as 3 or higher are "better explained by another DSM disorder" is indicated. If the co-occurring disorder has been present continuously throughout positive symptom presentation, then it must be differentiated whether or not the symptoms are more characteristic of a psychosis-risk syndrome or of the co-occurring disorder. In the example of Jane, her feelings of frank superiority occur only in the context of mania and are therefore "likely" better explained by mania rather than psychosis-risk syndrome.

Negative, disorganized, and general symptoms items are rated on a similar SOPS scale ranging from 0 (absent) to 6 (extreme); however, these symptom ratings are not used for making a psychosis-risk diagnosis on the COPS. Instead, these ratings are useful in providing both descriptive and quantitative estimates of the diversity and severity of accompanying negative, disorganized, and general symptoms.

The COPS operationalizes three psychosis-risk syndromes: 1) genetic risk and deterioration syndrome, 2) attenuated positive symptom syndrome, and 3) brief intermittent psychotic syndrome. Genetic risk and deterioration syndrome is defined by a combined genetic risk for a psychosis spectrum disorder and a recent history of functional decline. Attenuated positive symptom syndrome is defined by the presence of attenuated positive symptoms of sufficient severity and frequency. Brief intermittent psychotic syndrome is defined by the presence of frank psychotic symptoms that are brief or intermittent when current psychotic syndrome can be ruled out because sufficient frequency, duration, and urgency criteria have not been met. Positive symptoms experienced at a level of psychotic intensity (i.e., unusual thought content, suspiciousness, or grandiosity with delusional conviction; perceptual abnormalities of hallucinatory intensity; and/or speech that is incoherent or unintelligible) that occur for at least 1 hour per day at a minimum average of at least 4 days per week and/or are seriously disorganizing or dangerous are considered to be indicative of a psychotic syndrome, *not* psychosis-risk syndrome. For specific scoring criteria, refer to Table 8–1. Figure 8–1 models onset of psychosis-risk symptoms using associated assessment criterion from the SIPS and CAARMS.

Using the information from the case example, Jane meets the criteria for attenuated positive symptom syndrome. Her symptoms are described as recurrent and distressing. Over the past year, the symptoms became more frequent, started to affect her behaviors, and impacted her social functioning, as well as her academic achievement. Insight into the reality of these symptoms remained intact, as evidenced by either spontaneously divulged doubt or doubt induced by further questioning. Table 8–3 breaks down the scoring of Jane's symptoms using the SIPS-associated COPS criteria.

Comprehensive Assessment of At-Risk Mental States-Brief

The Comprehensive Assessment of At-Risk Mental States-Brief (CAARMS-B) is a semistructured interview designed for use by mental health professionals in Australia to identify the prodrome of a first psychotic episode using validated criteria and reliable methodology (Yung et al. 2005). Its function is to assess psychosis-like pathology and determine whether an individual meets criteria for being at ultra-high risk for onset of first psychotic disorder. CAARMS-B is designed for repeated use over time, from monthly to biyearly. CAARMS-B aims to 1) determine if an individual meets the criteria for an at-risk mental state, 2) rule out or confirm acute psychosis, and 3) map a range of psychopathology and functioning factors over time in young people at ultra-high risk of psychosis. CAARMS-B ratings are completed on a range of subscales that target different areas of psychopathology and functioning. From these ratings it is then possible to extract information relating to these aims.

The following constructs are used to evaluate presence and severity of psychopathology and functional impairment: 1) disorders of thought content, 2) perceptual abnormalities, 3) conceptual disorganization, 4) motor changes, 5) problems with concentration and attention, 6) problems with emotion and affect, and 7) subjectively impaired energy and impaired tolerance to normal stress. The severity of each of these constructs is rated using a global rating scale score as follows: 0=never/absent, 1=questionable, 2=mild, 3=moderate, 4=moderately severe, 5=severe, and 6=psychotic and severe. Ratings for each of the CAARMS-B subscales are anchored with content-specific benchmarks (as with the SIPS); however, several severity rating themes exist throughout the scale. A severity level rating of 2 indicates that the person is "not concerned/ worried about the experience." A severity level rating of 4 indicates that the symptom "does

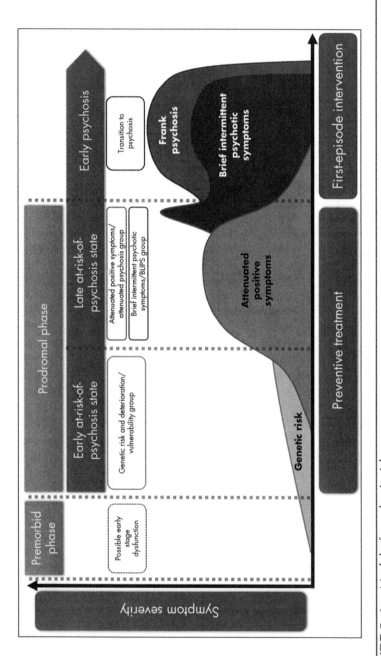

FIGURE 8–1. Model of psychosis risk onset.

Abbreviation.   BLIPS=brief limited intermittent psychotic symptoms.
Source.   Adapted from Fusar-Poli et al. (2013).

not result in a change in behavior but may be associated with mild distress." A severity level rating of 5 indicates that the symptom "may result in some minor change in behavior and may be frightening or associated with some distress." A severity level rating of 6 indicates that the symptom "may have marked impact on behavior and may be very distressing" (Yung et al. 2005). As previously discussed with the SIPS, a rating of 6 on the CAARMS-B subscales distinguishes frank psychotic symptoms (full conviction with no insight) from the psychosis-like experiences (doubt remains intact and insight is either spontaneously divulged or can be induced given contrary evidence from others) that are indicated in the 1–5 range.

Onset and offset dates, frequency and duration of occurrence, pattern, and level of distress are also recorded. Symptoms rated as a 6 that last for more than a week at a time are considered to be above the psychosis-risk threshold and should instead be considered evidence for presence of frank psychosis. Frequency and duration are rated through a frequency scale score ranging from 0 (absent) to 6 (continuous). Pattern of symptoms is used to determine whether or not the presenting symptoms are accounted for by the use of alcohol or illicit substances in order to denote whether there is a relation between symptoms and substance use. Finally, level of distress experienced by the symptom is rated on a scale of 0=not at all distressed to 100=extremely distressed.

CAARMS-B operationalizes three groups of ultra-high-risk individuals: 1) the vulnerability group, 2) the attenuated psychosis group, and 3) the brief limited intermittent psychotic symptoms group. The vulnerability group is defined as young people at risk of psychosis due to the combination of a trait risk factor and a significant deterioration in mental states and/or functioning. The attenuated psychosis group is defined as young people at risk for psychosis due to a subthreshold psychotic syndrome, in which the experienced symptoms do not reach a threshold level for psychosis because of either subthreshold intensity (not severe enough) or subthreshold frequency (occurrence not often enough). The brief limited intermittent psychotic symptoms group is defined as young people at risk of psychosis due to a recent history of frank psychotic symptoms that resolved spontaneously (without antipsychotic intervention) within 1 week. For specific scoring criteria, refer to Table 8–1 and Figure 8–1. For further reading on this assessment measure, see Yung et al. (2005).

Again, using the information from the case example, Jane would meet CAARMS-B criteria for attenuated psychosis group: subthreshold intensity. Her symptoms are recurrent and have increased in intensity over the past year. However, insight remains intact and Jane is able to generate insight into the reality of these experiences. Table 8–4 breaks down the scoring of Jane's symptoms using the CAARMS-B-associated criteria.

TABLE 8–4. CAARMS-B scoring summary for Jane

	CAARMS-B symptom domains			
	Unusual thought content	**Nonbizarre ideas**	**Perceptual abnormalities**	**Disorganized speech**
Global rating	5	4	4	4
Description of symptom domain	Unusual thoughts that contain completely original and highly improbable material Person can doubt these thoughts (i.e., thoughts not held with delusional conviction) or does not believe them all the time May result in some minor change in behavior, but this change is minor May be frightening or associated with some distress	Clearly idiosyncratic beliefs that, although possible, have arisen without logical evidence (*more severe than a rating of 3, in which belief may be supported by some logical evidence and is not entirely implausible*) May include thoughts that others wish the person harm (without logical evidence) or thoughts of having special powers Beliefs may be easily dismissed by individual but associated with mild degree of distress	Much clearer hallucinatory experiences that are more external to self (*more severe than a rating of 3, in which they are described as "distortions," "illusions," or "indistinct murmurs"*) Examples: hear name being called, phone ringing May be fleeting or transient Person is able to give plausible explanation for experiences, but they may be associated with mild degree of distress	Clear evidence of mild disconnected speech and thought patterns Links between ideas are tangential; person experiences an increased feeling of frustration in conversations
Frequency score	3	2	3	2

Diagnosis achieved using above criteria: attenuated psychosis group

Abbreviations. CAARMS= Comprehensive Assessment of At-Risk Mental States.

Risk Calculator

Using data from more than 500 individuals determined to be at clinical high risk for psychosis, the North American Prodrome Longitudinal Study (NAPLS) Consortium developed a diagnostic algorithm that can ascertain the probability of conversion to psychosis in CHR youth (Cannon et al. 2016). This risk calculator combines a unique set of demographic (age, family history of psychosis), clinical (unusual thought content and suspiciousness), neurocognitive (verbal learning and memory, speed of processing), and psychosocial (traumas, stressful life events, decline in social functioning) predictor variables to generate a specific number representing an individual's probability of transitioning to psychosis within 1–2 years. The calculator is available online at http://riskcalc.org/napls.

The risk calculator performs well, with a concordance index (C-index) of 0.71. This index score is comparable to that of established calculators used for the identification of recurrence risk in cardiovascular disease and cancer (C-index values ranging from 0.58 to 0.81). The calculator assumes that the ratings and scores input into the algorithm are obtained by a clinician or health professional. In addition, a SIPS-based diagnosis of a prodromal risk syndrome must be established because the calculator is not operational without this information. Use of this calculator in non-help-seeking, nondistressed individuals from the general population is not recommended. For further reading, see Cannon et al. (2016).

If the above criteria are satisfied, the following information is then input into the calculator: 1) age in years (range of 12–35), 2) Brief Assessment of Cognition in Schizophrenia (BACS) symbol coding total raw score, 3) Hopkins Verbal Learning Test–Revised (HVLT-R) total raw score, 4) undesirable life events raw score (obtained through the Research Interview Life Events Scale), 5) number of types of trauma observed (obtained through the Childhood Trauma and Abuse Scale), 6) sum of rescaled SIPS ratings for positive symptom domains P1 and P2 (unusual beliefs and suspiciousness subscales), 7) change in global social role functioning over the past year (measured using the Global Functioning: Social Scale and calculated by subtracting the individual's lowest score in the past year from the highest score in the past year), and 8) family history of psychosis in first-degree relative (yes or no) (Cannon et al. 2016). SIPS scores on P1 and P2 are rescaled such that scores 0–2 on the original scale are redefined as 0, scores 3–5 on the original scale are redefined as 1–3, respectively, and score 6 on the original scale is redefined as 4.

As an example, the following information was input into the calculator for Jane (Figure 8–2): 1) age=21 years, 2) BACS symbol coding total raw score=61, 3) HVLT-R total raw score=20, 4) undesirable life events raw score=21, 5) number of types of trauma observed=6, 6) sum of rescaled SIPS ratings for P1 and P2=3, 7) change in global social functioning over the past year=3, and 8) family history of psychosis=no.

This profile yielded a 1-year probability of conversion to psychosis of 26.5% and 2-year probability of conversion to psychosis of 33.9% (Figure 8–3).

Prodromal Questionnaire-Brief

The previously discussed semistructured interviews have established validity and reliability for identifying individuals who are at the highest risk for developing psychosis. However, these interviews are time consuming, typically requiring 1–2 hours to administer and score by a trained clinician. Because of the cumbersome nature of these structured interviews, screening tools have been developed for the purpose of distinguishing between individuals who might benefit from further psychosis-risk assessment and those who would not. One such screening tool is the Prodromal Questionnaire-Brief (PQ-B; Loewy et al. 2011). Use of the PQ-B can limit the costs associated with unnecessarily administering lengthy interviews in clinical settings where time is a limited resource. The PQ-B is a 21-item self-report scale. It has established concurrent validity in differentiating between individuals who will qualify for a psychosis-risk diagnosis from those who do not meet criteria. The PQ-B consists of 21 yes or no questions; questions receiving a yes answer are followed by distress ratings on a scale of 1 (strongly disagree) to 5 (strongly agree). This yields two composite scores: total score (range 0–21) and distress score (range 0–105). For total score, a cut-off ≥3 has 89% sensitivity and 58% specificity, and for distress score, a cut-off ≥6 has 88% sensitivity and 68% specificity. Using these cut-offs, the PQ-B has been established as a reliable and valid way of differentiating individuals who may qualify as having psychosis-risk syndrome and/ or psychotic syndrome from individuals with no diagnosis, thereby reducing costs associated with administering lengthy structured interviews to individuals who will likely not meet criteria for psychosis-risk syndrome.

It is important to emphasize that the PQ-B is not meant to replace traditional structured interviews for diagnosing a psychosis-risk syndrome. It is not a diagnostic tool. The PQ-B is meant to serve as the first step in a two-step process of identifying help-seeking individuals who may benefit from further in-depth assessment in the form of a structured interview (i.e., SIPS or CAARMS).

Cultural Considerations in Assessment and Diagnosis

In assessment and diagnosis of mental disorders, it is critical that providers consider the complexity of culture in presenting symptoms.

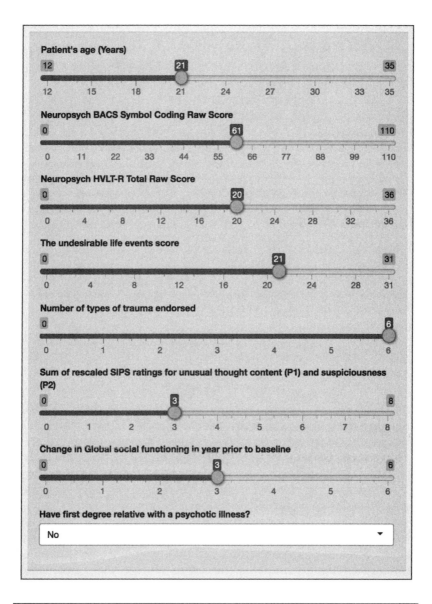

FIGURE 8–2. Risk calculator input.

There have been attempts to look at the impact of culture on experience and development of psychosis-risk syndrome, but more research is needed to provide definitive recommendations regarding the impact of culture on the diagnosis and treatment of psychosis risk. Despite this,

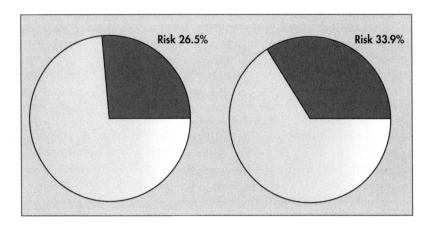

FIGURE 8–3.   Risk calculator output: Jane's 1-year and 2-year probabilities of conversion to psychosis.

This calculator was based on a Cox proportional hazards regression model that was developed from a cohort consisting of 596 clinical high-risk participants from the second phase of the North American Prodrome Longitudinal Study.

we can refer to several particularly robust cultural considerations revealed through research on the impact of culture in early psychosis.

During assessment, clinicians must differentiate between culturally sanctioned response patterns and persistent abnormal experiences. For example, an individual may report hearing voices during a religious ceremony, but if these voices are not experienced as persistent or distressing and are not considered abnormal by other members of that religious community, then the symptom should not be considered pathological. Religious background must be taken into account, especially when assessing for delusional beliefs or perceptual abnormalities. Other considerations include socioeconomic status, narrative expression and language, emotional expression and posturing, race, and ethnicity. Clinicians need to rule out linguistic variation and language barriers when assessing for disorganized speech and alogia. Differences in style of emotional expression, eye contact, and body language should not be mistaken for negative or disorganized symptoms.

Ideas that might be considered delusional in one culture, such as witchcraft, voodoo, or nonmedical healing, may be commonly accepted in another culture; therefore, the etiology of beliefs must be assessed. Several specific cultural concepts of distress should be considered in assessment of psychotic-like symptoms. *Ataque de nervios, nervios, maladi moun*, and *taijin kyofusho* are all examples of culture-bound syndromes that may better account for symptoms such as depersonalization, perceptual abnormalities, or overvalued beliefs (see "DSM-5 Glossary of

Cultural Concepts of Distress," American Psychiatric Association 2013, pp. 833–837).

Stigma associated with the diagnostic label of psychosis-risk syndrome is another domain of cultural consideration. The interpretation of this diagnostic label may vary between cultures or languages for individuals and their families. Research in the area of stigma and diagnostic labeling of psychosis-risk syndrome is ongoing. Of note, studies involving Chinese individuals with psychosis-risk syndrome and Latino CHR individuals indicate that current diagnostic labeling may be stigmatizing and associated with reduced help-seeking behaviors (Lee et al. 2017; Tsai et al. 2015). For some individuals, the assignment of a diagnosis may be experienced as relieving, reducing confusion and uncertainty regarding the meaning of symptoms, as well as increasing hope through recommendations for treatment. For others, the understanding of this label may result in feelings of hopelessness, loss of independence, or increased isolation. When the cultural interpretation of diagnostic labeling is of concern for individuals, it may be appropriate to disclose diagnostic information in terms of symptoms rather than diagnostic labeling (Mittal et al. 2015). Guiding individuals through the meaning of and treatment recommendations for psychosis-risk syndrome may be particularly important. *Risk for* does not equate to *certainty of* a psychotic disorder developing. Clients should be well informed of the limits to diagnostic accuracy of psychosis-risk syndrome, as well as the benefits of intervening early to prevent further impairments.

Treatment

As will be discussed in later chapters, there are many targeted interventions shown to be effective in reducing or improving social, cognitive, and functional impairments in first-episode or early psychosis. The search for effective treatment interventions for psychosis-risk populations is ongoing. Research that focuses explicitly on vulnerability for psychosis risk not only brings the field closer to understanding the causal processes and mechanisms that need to be therapeutically addressed once psychosis occurs but also aids in preventing the onset of psychosis or, at least, attenuating the duration and intensity of symptoms and accompanying functional impairments.

Cognitive-behavioral therapy, social skills training (CBSST), cognitive therapy, family-focused therapy, and supportive contact have all shown low to moderate effect sizes for reducing risk of a psychotic disorder and improving symptoms as well as overall functioning. Additional randomized controlled trials are under way to evaluate the effectiveness of these psychosocial interventions and characterize long-term outcomes of such treatments in psychosis-risk syndrome (CBSST trial in CHR youth ongoing; Cadenhead et al. 2018). Current treatment guidelines of attenuated psychosis syndrome proposed by the American Psychiatric Association recommend "careful assessment and frequent monitoring" (Woods et al. 2010). Low-risk, nonpharmacological interventions are recommended over the use of drug treatment for psychosis-risk syndromes, and treatment recommendations are based largely on presenting symptoms and co-occurring disorders. Comorbid disorders should be treated simultaneously while psychotic-like symptoms are being monitored. If frank psychotic symptoms emerge, the use of antipsychotic medication should be considered.

Receiving psychosis-risk-specific treatment is correlated with lower risk of psychosis at 1-, 2-, and 3-year follow-up (Fusar-Poli et al. 2013). Preventive interventions in psychosis-risk youth are feasible and valuable to improving prognosis. Early intervention is associated with decreased duration of untreated psychosis (DUP). Longer DUP has been associated with poor prognostic outcomes, high costs, and reduced functioning (Allott et al. 2018; Fusar-Poli et al. 2017).

In the case example, Jane received treatment for symptoms of PTSD but chose not to engage in treatment specific to psychosis-risk syndrome.

Case Example *(continued)*

One year after the initial interview, Jane presented at a university-based psychosis evaluation clinic to complete a follow-up SIPS assessment. Her symptoms had increased to include stable persecutory and grandiose delusions and fully formed auditory and visual hallucinations, as well as disorganized appearance and behavior. These symptoms had reportedly increased during the preceding month and were experienced at a level of full conviction; insight into these symptoms was no longer intact and could not be induced. Jane was ultimately diagnosed with schizoaffective disorder, bipolar type. Careful monitoring of Jane's symptoms allowed for immediate detection of psychosis, intervention with psychotherapy, and initiation of mood stabilizer and antipsychotic medication. Ultimately, repeated psychosis-risk assessment and careful monitoring facilitated early detection and intervention, thereby reducing Jane's DUP.

KEY CONCEPTS

- The concept of preserved insight is one of the key features in differential diagnosis of psychosis-risk syndrome versus full psychotic disorders and refers to the awareness or acknowledgment that one's thoughts and behaviors are the result of mental illness, with recognition of the need for treatment, and/or questioning of the reality of one's beliefs or experiences.

- One of the Conditions for Further Study in DSM-5, attenuated psychosis syndrome involves the presence of psychosis-like experiences that are below the threshold for a full psychotic disorder. As compared with the symptom criteria for full psychotic disorders, symptoms of attenuated psychosis syndrome are more transient and less severe and involve greater preservation of insight.

- Duration of untreated psychosis (DUP) is the period of time from onset of frank psychosis to initiation of adequate treatment. Longer DUP is associated with poorer prognosis in individuals with psychosis.

- Criteria of Prodromal Syndromes identifies three psychosis-risk syndrome subtypes:

  1. Genetic risk and deterioration syndrome (GRDS)—Criteria are met if an individual 1) has a first-degree relative with a psychotic disorder and/or has ever met DSM-5 schizotypal personality disorder criteria and 2) demonstrates a 30% or greater drop in Global Assessment of Functioning within the past year. GRDS is similar to the vulnerability group from the Comprehensive Assessment of At-Risk Mental States-Brief (CAARMS-B).

  2. Attenuated positive symptom syndrome (APSS)—Symptoms are experienced as unwilled, not easily ignored, confusing, bothersome, or distressing to affected individuals and may affect an individual's daily functioning. APSS is similar to the attenuated psychosis group from CAARMS-B.

  3. Brief intermittent psychotic syndrome (BIPS)—Criteria are met if frank psychotic symptoms occur for at least several minutes a day at a frequency of at least once per month; preservation of insight is typically lost during symptom occurrence. BIPS is similar to the brief limited intermittent psychotic symptoms group from CAARMS-B.

Discussion Questions

1. In what way is insight a clinically relevant diagnostic feature in psychosis-risk syndrome?

2. Structured assessments classify three distinct subtypes of psychosis-risk syndrome. What are these subtypes? How do the criteria for each subtype differ?

3. In assessment of psychosis-risk syndrome, clinicians must differentiate between culturally sanctioned response patterns and persistent abnormal experiences. Additionally, culture must be considered when assigning diagnostic labels. Why is this of particular importance for psychosis-risk syndrome?

4. Even though research on effective intervention in psychosis risk is ongoing, what treatment options should be considered after identifying psychosis-risk syndrome? Why is early intervention important in psychosis risk?

Suggested Readings

American Psychiatric Association: Conditions for Further Study: Attenuated psychosis syndrome, in Diagnostic and Statistical Manual of Mental Disorders, 5th Edition. Arlington, VA, American Psychiatric Association, 2013, pp 783–86

American Psychiatric Association: Glossary of cultural concepts of distress, in Diagnostic and Statistical Manual of Mental Disorders, 5th Edition. Arlington, VA, American Psychiatric Association, 2013, pp 833–837

Cannon TD, Yu C, Addington J, et al: An individualized risk calculator for research in prodromal psychosis. Am J Psychiatry 173(10):980–988, 2016 27363508

Fusar-Poli P, Borgwardt S, Bechdolf A, et al: The psychosis high-risk state: a comprehensive state-of-the-art review. JAMA Psychiatry 70(1):107–120, 2013 23165428

Loewy RL, Pearson R, Vinogradov S, et al: Psychosis risk screening with the Prodromal Questionnaire–Brief version (PQ-B). Schizophr Res 129(1):42–46, 2011 21511440

Marshall M, Lewis S, Lockwood A, et al: Association between duration of untreated psychosis and outcome in cohorts of first-episode patients: a systematic review. Arch Gen Psychiatry 62(9):975–983, 2005 16143729

Miller TJ, McGlashan TH, Woods SW, et al: Symptom assessment in schizophrenic prodromal states. Psychiatr Q 70(4):273–287, 1999 10587984

Yung AR, Yuen HP, McGorry PD, et al: Mapping the onset of psychosis: the Comprehensive Assessment of At-Risk Mental States. Aust N Z J Psychiatry 39(11–12):964–971, 2005 16343296

References

Allott K, Fraguas D, Bartholomeusz CF, et al: Duration of untreated psychosis and neurocognitive functioning in first-episode psychosis: a systematic review and meta-analysis. Psychol Med 48(10):1592–1607, 2018 29173201

American Psychiatric Association: Diagnostic and Statistical Manual of Mental Disorders, 5th Edition. Arlington, VA, American Psychiatric Association, 2013

Benedict RHB, Schretlen D, Groninger L, Brandt J: The Hopkins Verbal Learning Test-Revised: normative data and analysis of interform and test–retest reliability. Clin Neuropsychol 12:43–55, 1998

Cadenhead K, Addington J, Cornblatt B: Cognitive behavioral social skills training for youth at clinical high risk for psychosis: Recovery Through Group (ReGroup). Presented at International Conference on Early Intervention in Mental Health, Boston, MA, October 2018

Cannon TD, Yu C, Addington J, et al: An individualized risk calculator for research in prodromal psychosis. Am J Psychiatry 173(10):980–988, 2016 27363508

First MB, Spitzer RL, Gibbon M, Williams JBW: Structured Clinical Interview for DSM-IV Axis I Disorders, Clinician Version (SCID-CV). Washington, DC, American Psychiatric Press, 1997

Fusar-Poli P, Borgwardt S, Bechdolf A, et al: The psychosis high-risk state: a comprehensive state-of-the-art review. JAMA Psychiatry 70(1):107–120, 2013 23165428

Fusar-Poli P, Cappucciati M, Rutigliano G, et al: At risk or not at risk? A meta-analysis of the prognostic accuracy of psychometric interviews for psychosis prediction. World Psychiatry 14(3):322–332, 2015 26407788

Fusar-Poli P, McGorry PD, Kane JM: Improving outcomes of first-episode psychosis: an overview. World Psychiatry 16(3):251–265, 2017 28941089

Goldman HH, Skodol AE, Lave TR: Revising Axis V for DSM-IV: a review of measures of social functioning. Am J Psychiatry 149(9):1148–1156, 1992 1386964

Keefe RS, Goldberg TE, Harvey PD, et al: The Brief Assessment of Cognition in Schizophrenia: reliability, sensitivity, and comparison with a standard neurocognitive battery. Schizophrenia research, 68(2-3):283–297, 2004 15099610

Lee EHM, Ching EYN, Hui CLM, et al: Chinese label for people at risk for psychosis. Early Interv Psychiatry 11(3):224–228, 2017 25721613

Loewy RL, Pearson R, Vinogradov S, et al: Psychosis risk screening with the Prodromal Questionnaire–Brief version (PQ-B). Schizophr Res 129(1):42–46, 2011 21511440

Miller TJ, McGlashan TH, Woods SW, et al: Symptom assessment in schizophrenic prodromal states. Psychiatr Q 70(4):273–287, 1999 10587984

Miller TJ, McGlashan TH, Rosen JL, et al: Prodromal assessment with the structured interview for prodromal syndromes and the scale of prodromal symptoms: predictive validity, interrater reliability, and training to reliability. Schizophr Bull 29(4):703–715, 2003 14989408

Mittal VA, Dean DJ, Mittal J, et al: Ethical, legal, and clinical considerations when disclosing a high-risk syndrome for psychosis. Bioethics 29(8):543–556, 2015 25689542

Tsai KH, López S, Marvin S, et al: Perceptions of family criticism and warmth and their link to symptom expression in racially/ethnically diverse adolescents and young adults at clinical high risk for psychosis. Early Interv Psychiatry 9(6):476–486, 2015 24576106

Woods SW, Walsh BC, Saksa JR, McGlashan TH: The case for including attenuated psychotic symptoms syndrome in DSM-5 as a psychosis risk syndrome. Schizophr Res 123(2–3):199–207, 2010 20832249

Yung AR, Yuen HP, McGorry PD, et al: Mapping the onset of psychosis: the Comprehensive Assessment of At-Risk Mental States. Aust N Z J Psychiatry 39(11–12):964–971, 2005 16343296

Medical Workup for First-Episode Psychosis

Agnieszka Kalinowski, M.D., Ph.D.
Jacob S. Ballon, M.D., M.P.H.

PSYCHIATRY is in the midst of an explosion in scientific and technical advances that are beginning to explain complex behavioral phenomena in ways never before possible. With these advances, we are better able to understand the core pathophysiology that links disparate symptoms and better explain complex syndromes throughout medicine. Schizophrenia is, and has been, a diagnosis of exclusion, yet patients with psychosis are often given only cursory medical evaluation. Psychiatrists then bear the burden of not missing a reversible condition, especially early in the disease course when families may be perplexed and seeking explanations for the sudden change in their loved one's behavior.

Given the wide range in presentations of early psychosis, psychiatrists are often called on to lead a medical workup. Consider the following vignette:

Case Example 1

Abraham is a 19-year-old former honors student who has experienced a significant loss of functioning, including needing nearly full assistance with activities of daily living, over the past 3 years and is nearly unable to talk. At the time of his initial presentation, he reported hearing voices telling him that he was stupid and had a new-onset germ phobia requiring him to wash his hands frequently. He developed many other rituals as well that he had not demonstrated previously. Abraham started taking an antipsychotic medication but showed minimal response, and his functional decline continued. After several antipsychotic trials, Abraham started taking clozapine, but it was also ineffective for his symptoms. Electroconvulsive therapy and benzodiazepine treatments were tried to help with catatonia, but there was no change in Abraham's level of cognition or other symptoms despite high doses. Ultimately, he was admitted to a psychiatric unit for closer observation and consideration of a medical washout. A panoply of specialty consults and tests were performed, yet there were no notable findings. At the suggestion of rheumatology staff, an empirical trial of steroids was considered. After 3 days of taking high doses of methylprednisolone, Abraham began to speak in partial sentences and was able to start performing activities of daily living for the first time in 2 years. Although an ultimate diagnosis is elusive for Abraham, steroid-responsive autoimmune encephalitis is most likely. However, there was never a seropositive test to confirm the focus of an autoimmune condition. Abraham continues to receive potent anti-inflammatory treatment and continues to slowly regain the abilities that were lost over the course of his illness.

Although Abraham's case includes an unusual presentation and a dramatic outcome, with media streaming with information about new possible causes of psychosis, psychiatrists and other mental health professionals may often feel compelled to do more extensive medical workups. These more comprehensive workups are discussed in the literature (Coleman and Gillberg 1997; Freudenreich et al. 2009; Golomb 2002), and the list of possible etiologies (e.g., autoimmune, postinfectious, paraneoplastic) keeps growing. Disagreement exists as to what extent these workups are able to identify a potentially reversible cause of psychosis, but a study from 1987 showed that up to 3% of cases have identifiable causes other than a primary psychiatric disorder, many of which are reversible if identified in a timely manner (Johnstone et al. 1987).

Extensive medical workups are typically not pursued when the patient's age and duration of onset of symptoms, types of symptoms (predominantly paranoia and auditory hallucinations), and level of social and occupational functioning match a generally understood canonical pattern that most medical professionals would agree is likely to be due to a primary psychiatric condition (Freudenreich et al. 2009). On the other hand, there can be substantial variability in symptom presentation, and finding a reversible cause early in the disease course is clearly worthwhile. Delineating a prudent balance between testing for all possible causes of psychosis, including the long list of rare disorders, compared with minimal testing focused on finding the most common disorders, is often unclear. Furthermore, although an argument can be made for an extensive workup for a person in the first episode of psychosis, the feasibility may be challenging in many practice settings because of cost and unavailability of resources.

The American Psychiatric Association (APA) guidelines for initial medical workup of first-episode psychosis were published in 2004 (Lehman et al. 2004), with an update provided in 2009 (Dixon et al. 2009; see also Freudenreich et al. 2009); these suggested baseline tests are presented in Table 9–1. The updated guidelines added routine testing for HIV, even without risk factors and urine toxicology, as recommended by the Centers for Disease Control and Prevention. Current guidelines for a medical workup for people with onset of psychosis are grounded in the idea that if there is an alternative medical explanation, then the foundational history and/or physical examination should provide an initial clue to guide further workup (Table 9–2). Often, this may be the case—seizures in a young woman suggesting limbic encephalitis, an abnormal neurological examination suggesting stroke, or tachycardia occurring in a patient with thyrotoxicosis.

TABLE 9–1. Baseline medical evaluation of patients with first-episode psychosis

Type of test	Test
Physical examination	• Vital signs • Complete physical examination, including detailed neurological examination • Weight, height, and body mass index • Clinical assessment of extrapyramidal symptoms and abnormal movements
Laboratory and ancillary tests	• Fasting blood glucose and/or hemoglobin A1c • Lipid panel • Prolactin level • Electrocardiogram for QTc monitoring and cardiac status • Pregnancy test (for women of child-bearing age)

However, what may be unsettling is the idea that there may be instances when psychosis is truly the only indication of illness, yet a medical cause can still be present. A study published in 2011 in which lumbar punctures were performed on 155 consecutive people who presented with new-onset psychosis found an alternative medical cause that changed the clinical management in 5 (3%) of the patients (Kranaster et al. 2011). These alternative diagnoses included herpes simplex encephalitis, neuroborreliosis, multiple sclerosis, and two cases of chronic inflammation of the central nervous system of uncertain origin. Hauntingly, the authors stated that the patients in these 5 cases did not differ in their clinical presentation from the other patients with psychosis, and their history and physical examination were unremarkable.

TABLE 9–2.	Suggested workup for medical causes of psychosis
Type of test	**Test**
Tests for common, treatable causes	• Complete blood count
	• Basic metabolic panel
	• Liver function tests
	• Urine toxicology screen
	• Thyroid function tests
	• HIV screen
	• Urine heavy metals
	• Vitamin B_{12}
	• Antinuclear antibodies test
	• Test for syphilis (fluorescent treponemal antibody absorption preferred)
Tests for conditions that should be considered if history or the physical point to a possible positive finding	• Magnetic resonance imaging of the brain with and without contrast
	• Electroencephalogram
	• Hepatitis B and C screen
	• Lumbar puncture (or peripheral blood) for infectious and paraneoplastic antibodies
	• Ceruloplasmin, serum copper
	• Quantiferon and/or chest X-ray
	• Erythrocyte sedimentation rate and C-reactive protein
	• Neuropsychological and/or cognitive testing
Specialty consultations	• Genetics workup (e.g., karyotype, fluorescence in situ hybridization, sequencing)
	• Neurology for workup of demyelinating disorders, seizure, or encephalitis
	• Neurosurgery if potential tumor or other structural brain abnormalities are seen
	• Immunology for workup of autoimmune or postinfectious disorders
	• Endocrinology if consideration for significant hormonal abnormalities
	• Rheumatology for workup of autoimmune concerns or vasculitis

Because of the burgeoning delineation of paraneoplastic syndromes, pediatric acute-onset neuropsychiatric syndrome (PANS), and other postinfectious syndromes, along with increased access to genetic testing, psychiatrists are in the uncomfortable position of wading through an onslaught of complex information in hopes of finding an identifiable, reversible etiology that can be treated and saving their patient with new-onset psychosis the concerning future of chronic schizophrenia. Navigating this information is challenging, even for clinicians in well-resourced medical centers and teaching hospitals. Clear guidelines, epidemiology, and even "typical" clinical phenotypes do not yet exist. At the same time, glimpses of hope are on the horizon with each new discovery and successful treatment. Table 9–3 is an assembly of the medical causes that are known to be related to or to cause psychosis. It is based on Freudenreich and Golomb's lists (Freudenreich et al. 2009; Golomb 2002), with more recent additions, particularly in the autoimmune encephalitis category. The same principle of starting with a thorough history and physical examination applies in approaching this comprehensive differential diagnosis.

Questions often arise about what sorts of tests should be included in a standard or expanded workup. For example, should a lumbar puncture (LP) be a part of the standard medical workup? We propose that consideration be made for the likelihood of a positive finding and whether or not there will be a likely change in clinical management based on the outcome of the test. If those standards are sufficiently met, LP should be offered to patients and their family as an option, and if the procedure is desired but not feasible within the practice where the patient is being seen, a referral should be considered. This is also how we would suggest approaching other invasive or expensive diagnostic testing such as magnetic resonance imaging, electroencephalography, neuropsychological testing, and send-out blood tests. Although it is generally unlikely that any one test will uncover a consequential finding, there can be a rationale for obtaining these tests if there is an increased index of suspicion for a positive finding and the tests are available. More easily, common conditions that are potentially reversible should be routinely evaluated through screening for thyroid function, HIV, vitamin B_{12} deficiency, and presence of heavy metals. In the following subsections, we review and suggest updates to the available guidelines for working up the first presentation within the heterogeneous category of early psychosis, while providing a logical and accessible framework for psychiatrists and other personnel working with patients to follow.

Where to Start

The most current guidelines from the APA regarding the initial workup of first-episode psychosis were published in 2004 and updated in 2009

TABLE 9–3.	Medical causes of psychosis

Neurological disorders

- Epilepsy

- Head trauma

- Neuropsychiatric diseases: Huntington's disease, Wilson's disease, Parkinson's disease, familial basal ganglia calcification, Friedreich's ataxia

- Dementias: Alzheimer's disease, frontotemporal dementia, Lewy body disease

- Space-occupying lesions and structural brain abnormalities: primary brain tumors (e.g., meningiomas), secondary brain metastases, brain abscesses and cysts, tuberous sclerosis, midline abnormalities (e.g., corpus callosum agenesis, cavum septi pellucidi), cerebrovascular malformations (e.g., involving the temporal lobe), hydrocephalus

- Demyelinating diseases: multiple sclerosis, leukodystrophies (e.g., metachromatic leukodystrophy, X-linked adrenoleukodystrophy, Marchiafava-Bignami disease), Schilder's disease

- Narcolepsy

- Stroke

Autoimmune diseases

- Rheumatological diseases: systemic lupus erythematosus, rheumatic arthritis, myasthenia gravis, Hashimoto's thyroiditis, steroid-responsive nonvasculitis autoimmune inflammatory meningoencephalitic syndrome

- Paraneoplastic diseases: Morvan's syndrome; limbic encephalitis, including but not limited to antibodies against Hu, Ma2, CV2/CRMP5, amphiphysin, anti-AMPAR, NMDAR, NR1, NR2, voltage-gated potassium channel antibody syndrome, GlyR, D2RA, GABAR, metabotropic glutamate receptor antibody, or IgLON5

- Postinfectious disease: pediatric acute-onset neuropsychiatric syndrome

Infections

- Viral: HIV, viral encephalitis (e.g., herpes simplex, measles, cytomegalovirus, rubella, Epstein-Barr, varicella)

- Bacterial/fungal: neurosyphilis, neuroborreliosis (Lyme), tuberculosis, *Cryptococcus* infection

- Other: prion disease (e.g., Creutzfeldt-Jakob disease), central nervous system–invasive parasitic infections (e.g., cerebral malaria, toxoplasmosis, neurocysticercosis), sarcoidosis

Endocrinopathies

- Hypoglycemia, Addison's disease, Cushing's syndrome, hyperthyroidism and hypothyroidism, hyperparathyroidism and hypoparathyroidism, hypopituitarism

---

TABLE 9–3. Medical causes of psychosis *(continued)*

Nutritional deficiencies

- Magnesium deficiency, vitamin A deficiency, vitamin D deficiency, zinc deficiency, niacin deficiency, vitamin B_{12} deficiency

Toxic and metabolic diseases

- Amino acid metabolism: Hartnup disease, homocystinuria, phenylketonuria, urea cycle disorders, hyperornithinemia-hyperammonemia-homocitrullinuria syndrome, isovaleric acidemia

- Storage disorders: GM2 gangliosidosis, Fabry's disease, Niemann-Pick disease type C, Gaucher's disease–adult type

- Porphyrias (acute intermittent porphyria, porphyria variegate, hereditary coproporphyria)

- Heavy metals: lead, mercury, Wilson's disease

Chromosomal abnormalities

- Fragile X syndrome, 22q11 deletion syndrome (velocardiofacial syndrome, DiGeorge syndrome), Klinefelter's syndrome, XXX syndrome, metachromatic leukodystrophy

---

(Dixon et al. 2009; Lehman et al. 2004). The APA clearly suggests a complete medical history; physical examination; and basic blood tests, such as complete blood count, electrolyte and liver function tests, and thyroid testing (thyroid-stimulating hormone [TSH]). Questions regarding travel history, developmental history, and infectious and environmental exposures are particularly important in the initial history taking. Further, if the patient's medical history includes a history of neurological or infectious illnesses, then the workup may prompt further testing in those directions. Family history of immigration (especially from underdeveloped nations), infections, developmental disorders, cancers, or endocrine disorders should be evaluated. Although many metabolic disorders are screened for during routine prenatal screening, this may not always be done in underdeveloped countries. The history should include a clear time course for the development of the index episode of psychosis, including a search for a clearly identifiable prodromal period.

In this initial stage it is also crucial to include a primary care physician on the team of people working with the individual experiencing symptoms. Although many people with the first episode of psychosis will be referred by pediatricians or adult primary care providers, teaming up to work in concert on the workup is essential. Obtaining a more thorough history and physical, or a second look at the existing history and examination results, may help to pick up subtle clues that could change the index of suspicion for different potentially affected systems or disorders. Typical mimickers of schizophrenia such as amphetamine abuse, hyperthyroidism, and pituitary tumor should be considered as a part of the initial differential diagnosis and ruled out by standard laboratory testing and examination.

High-Yield Conditions for Consideration in Initial Workup

The most common possible conditions other than schizophrenia spectrum disorders that need to be ruled out in all individuals at the first episode of psychosis include infectious diseases, paraneoplastic and autoimmune disorders, toxic-metabolic disorders, endocrine disorders, neurological disorders, and genetic disorders. Although not an exhaustive list of potential causes (see Table 9–3), these high-yield conditions should be considered in all initial workups.

Infectious Diseases

Psychosis can be the initial presentation in patients with HIV, and all patients should be considered for an HIV test as part of their initial evaluation. In a recent study out of South Africa, where HIV is highly prevalent, researchers looked at 159 consecutive individuals who presented to an academic emergency department with a first episode of psychosis (Laher et al. 2018). Of these, 40% had HIV as at least a comorbidity. Beyond the contribution of HIV to the likelihood for developing psychosis, 84% of HIV-positive subjects had further underlying medical conditions considered to be potentially causative in the development of the psychotic symptoms. These other conditions included infections, such as meningitis, tuberculosis, or fungal pneumonia; renal or hepatic dysfunction; or stroke. In those first-episode patients who were HIV negative, 35% were found to have an underlying medical condition, such as epilepsy, ischemic stroke, or meningitis, that was considered most likely responsible for the psychotic symptoms.

Rates of infectious agents and availability of treatment vary throughout the world and are an important factor in history taking. Country of origin and/or history of immigration from underdeveloped countries should also lead to consideration of potential causes of psychosis that are less common in more developed countries. For example, many providers may not be accustomed to seeing psychosis as a manifestation of malaria, which should be considered in patients who have immigrated from or traveled to malaria-infected areas. Similarly, tertiary syphilis, neurocysticercosis, and other infectious complications may give risk to psychosis in someone from an underdeveloped or under-resourced area.

Along with the manifestations of acute infections, our understanding of the impact of previous infectious exposures is evolving at a rapid rate. PANS refers to a panoply of symptoms that are often associated with prior streptococcus or other infections. Although PANS is a rare condition, it can be striking to see a precipitous and rapid decline in function, often over only several days, occur in a previously healthy young person. In people experiencing these syndromes, there is typically a sudden onset of symptoms, often with an initial presentation of psychosis in conjunction with obsessive-compulsive behaviors, change in intellectual function, and tics (Chang et al. 2015). Testing for PANS is challenging, and referral to an institution with specific expertise in this area is important when symptoms match this pattern and time course (Frankovich et al. 2015).

Paraneoplastic and Autoimmune Disorders

Paraneoplastic syndromes have received more attention since journalist Susannah Cahalan wrote about her experience of anti-*N*-methyl-D-aspartate (anti-NMDA) receptor encephalitis in the book *Brain on Fire* (Cahalan 2012). Under the general category of autoimmune encephalopathies, the first symptoms tend to be psychiatric, describing a process by which an autoantibody targets the brain and disrupts function or causes inflammation. Delirium, catatonic features, anterograde amnesia, personality change, rapid progression of symptoms, fluctuating symptoms, and seizures may occur in conjunction with elevated inflammatory markers such as erythrocyte sedimentation rate and C-reactive protein (Oldham 2017). Recent viral illnesses are seen in more than half of patients with anti-NMDA receptor encephalitis and often co-occur with gonadal tumors. Similarly, smokers with small cell lung cancer can manifest with paraneoplastic encephalomyelitis.

Autoimmune encephalitis can occur in the context of systemic autoimmune disorders such as antiphospholipid antibody syndrome; Sjögren's syndrome; polymyositis; vasculitis syndrome; and large, medium, or small vessel vasculitis. Unusual accompanying symptoms, such as arthralgias or unexplained hypoventilation, could also be helpful in tipping the clinician toward evaluation of the patient for autoimmune encephalopathy. Unfortunately, peripheral blood antibodies do not seem to be sufficient to rule out the disorder, and false positives occur in the normal population, so only antibody testing from cerebrospinal fluid is conclusive (Gaughran et al. 2018).

Numerous autoimmune disorders are associated with psychosis, and many times, psychosis is the first presenting symptom. A patient with systemic lupus erythematosus may present with psychosis up to 2%–3% of the time (Kosmidis et al. 2010; Patten et al. 2005); thus, a test looking for the antinuclear antibody is recommended in people with a first episode of psychosis. There are increasing numbers of autoantibodies associated with psychosis to varying degrees, as well as other neuropsychiatric manifestations (Ho et al. 2016). In addition, comorbid rheumatological and autoimmune disorders occur at increased rates in patients with schizophrenia (Chen et al. 2012).

Toxic-Metabolic Disorders

Many potential environmental or toxic exposures, such as heavy metal toxicity, can contribute to the risk for psychosis. When taking an initial history, it is important to survey for potential lead exposure. Lead may contribute to numerous neuropsychiatric symptoms, including poor concentration and low IQ, but at sufficient levels can also contribute to psychosis (Vorvolakos et al. 2016). Although lead exposure is less common now because of the reduction of lead-containing pipes, paints, and gasoline, there is still potential for exposure in old buildings and/or for people with a prior exposure in an underdeveloped country.

In addition to environmental exposures, there can also be issues with the metabolism or storage of heavy metals in the body. Wilson's disease is a copper storage disorder manifested most commonly by tremors; hepatic dysfunction; and psychiatric symptoms, including depression or psychosis (Zimbrean and Schilsky 2014). Elevated liver enzymes or unusual tremor, especially if the patient is particularly sensitive to extrapyramidal symptoms from antipsychotic medication, should prompt an investigation into Wilson's disease.

B_{12} and folate deficiencies can manifest with fatigue, personality changes, or psychosis. Historical clues to such deficiencies include a vegetarian diet, alcohol abuse, or oral contraceptive use. In the case of B_{12} deficiency, patients may also complain of parasthesias or fatigue. Similarly, pellagra or B_3 (niacin) deficiency can lead to psychosis, typically in patients with chronic alcoholism.

Endocrine Disorders

Derangements in cortisol have well-known psychiatric manifestations. For example, elevated cortisol levels can manifest with lability, irritability, mania, or psychosis with associated cognitive slowing and poor short-term memory, which may overlap with clinicians' expectations for schizophrenia. Cushingnoid features such as upper-body obesity with thin arms and legs, bruising, purple striae, menstrual irregularities, vertigo, hyperglycemia, "moon" facies, fluid retention, thin skin, and high blood pressure are other clues that may prompt testing. However, an estimated 50% of patients will present with psychiatric symptoms prior to physical signs or symptoms (Rasmussen et al. 2015). Low cortisol levels, on the other hand, typically result in fatigue, weight loss, malaise, memory impairment, and confusion.

Assessing for changes in thyroid function is typically part of routine testing on initial medical evaluations because it is well known that individuals with thyroid disease can present with psychiatric complaints. Classically, hyperthyroidism manifests with elevated heart rate, diaphoresis, and anxiety, but at especially high levels of circulating thyroid hormone, people may present with psychotic symptoms (Brownlie et al. 2000). Often referred to as a thyroid storm, this extreme form of thyrotoxicosis is a life-threatening emergency and requires urgent hospitalization if evident.

In contrast to the thyroid storm, people with hypothyroidism may also present with psychosis. At extremely low levels of circulating thyroid hormone, and consequently significantly elevated TSH, patients may develop myxedema and can present with psychotic symptoms. The psychotic symptoms correlate with a significant slowing of metabolism, and fatigue, depression, weight gain, and confusion often precede the psychotic symptoms (Heinrich and Grahm 2003).

Neurological Disorders

People with structural abnormalities such as chronic subdural hematomas, cerebral contusions, glial cell tumors, and meningiomas that compress underlying cortex and impair processing may present with psychotic symptoms (Kar et al. 2015). Similarly, ischemic strokes or brain metastases have been documented in people who present with psychosis. Associated neurological signs and/or symptoms that suggest structural brain abnormalities require follow-up with brain imaging (Khandanpour et al. 2013). Notably, a typical brain imaging pattern for a person with schizophrenia includes reduction in gray matter; paucity of axons and dendrites in the cortex; compensatory enlargement of the lateral and third ventricles; and volumetric loss, especially in the temporal lobes. On positron emission tomography, there is often decreased activity in the frontal lobe. Suspicion for a structural neurological condition would increase if the onset of psychosis is acute or subacute, if there are other neurological symptoms such as weakness or change in coordination, if there are concurrent or historical comorbid cancer diagnosis and treatment, or if the psychosis has atypical features such as nonauditory hallucinations.

Seizures, specifically temporal lobe epilepsy (TLE), may manifest initially with depression and behavioral changes that may be confused with schizophrenia (Kandratavicius et al. 2014). Classically, people with TLE may experience delusions that they are dead that occur paroxysmal with the ictal activity. Additionally, patients with a history of seizures have an increased risk for developing a psychotic illness. This is particularly true for patients with TLE (7%), which may lead to scarring of the hippocampus, a structure implicated in the pathophysiology of schizophrenia (Kandratavicius et al. 2014). A clear time course for the seizures, including periods of confusion and urinary incontinence, should be assessed in the history. Because latency in response is a common manifestation of a psychotic process, psychosis can be confused with potential partial-complex seizure activity. Long-term electroencephalogram monitoring may be required to identify seizure activity. Identifying a seizure disorder is important not only for assessment; it may also guide antipsychotic selection because antipsychotic medications variably lower the seizure threshold.

Genetic Disorders

Velocardiofacial syndrome, or 22q11 deletion syndrome, has an incidence of 1:2,000–4,000 in the population, has wide variability in presentation, and can often be missed. Identification is important because it may suggest alternative treatment approaches (Carandang and Scholten 2007) and provide the patient and family with another community for potential engagement and support. Typical co-occurring symptoms include a submucosal cleft palate, learning disorder in childhood, and short stature (McDonald-McGinn et al. 2015). Seizures, renal agenesis, and cardiac and immune abnormalities may also be present. Testing is best done in consultation with medical geneticists.

Conclusion

Expanded workup should be pursued when there is indication after the basic workup that an underlying reversible condition may exist. In these cases, one must consider the index of suspicion for various causes and target the workup in the direction that seems most likely. Not all of the testing reviewed here would be indicated in most patients, and, in fact, many cases will warrant investigation in only one of these categories, if any. However, when history, physical, family history, and/or other telltale signs point in the direction of another potential cause or contributor to onset of psychosis, a targeted workup should be commenced.

A word of caution about pursuing medical workups is warranted. The following vignette illustrates a common story within our clinic.

Case Example 2

Tyler is a 19-year-old who presented with 2–3 months of delusions and obsessive-compulsive symptoms. He was previously a high school honor student and had been accepted by an elite university but had to drop out of school after one quarter because of the onset and worsening of his psychiatric symptoms. He had numerous physical complaints, and initial laboratory workup showed unexpected levels of inflammation and insulin resistance. This prompted further workup with endocrinology to understand whether there was a hormonal connection to the insulin resistance and with immunology and rheumatology to ascertain potential causes of the inflammation. Despite a thorough workup from these services, including several visits and numerous tests, a decision was made by an outside consultant to try empirical treatment with intravenous immunoglobulin (IVIg). Although Tyler's parents initially felt that he improved from the IVIg, the effect was short lived. Discussion of options for further pursuit of a medical cause of his psychosis continued, and his parents often focused much of the clinical sessions on asking about further consultations throughout the medical center. Tyler's treatment team recognized that pursuit of alternative explanations was interfering with effective treatment of his ongoing psychosis. After several months, his parents agreed to a referral for Tyler to see one of the team's psychologists to begin cognitive-behavioral therapy for psychosis. At this point, despite seeking further medical workup, Tyler and his family began to understand the nature of his experience, and Tyler achieved tremendous symptomatic improvement. He was able to join a book club and participate in regular volunteer work in a capacity beyond what he had been capable of for the previous 2 years.

In Tyler's case, when looking at how the process unfolded, it is clear that time was lost in pursuit of the medical workup at the expense of engaging in effective psychiatric treatment. This example demonstrates the importance of setting reasonable expectations at the onset of a detailed medical workup for psychosis, as well as a plan for initiating care to achieve relief and begin healing as the workup proceeds. In some cases, as the psychiatric diagnosis becomes clearer and/or the search for medical causes becomes more remote, patients and families may become desperate to deepen the search. This understandable reaction can shift attention away from initiation of evidence-based therapies for psychosis. For example, when there is concern for infectious causes such as Lyme disease, there may not be objective markers to guide treatment. It is helpful to delineate with patients and families what tests you agree to run to rule out a suspected condition and what you will do with the results, as well as the limits of those tests. To continue to pursue a lengthy medical workup when the likelihood of a primary psychotic disorder is becoming clear can be a disservice to both patients and families.

On the other hand, mental health providers must also be fierce advocates for patients as they enter the general medical system. Too often, elements of the physical examination or history are overlooked, written off as psychiatric, and not given the attention they deserve. Further, people with psychotic disorders may misattribute somatic sensations, leading to further misunderstanding. For example, a patient might describe feeling unusual body sensations and suggest that they may be a result of body control due to hallucinations, when in fact he or she may be experiencing the onset of a neurological condition. Mental health professionals must insist on the appropriate workup and testing when the circumstances dictate and not settle for simple explanations in complex situations without careful consideration of what is being excluded.

KEY CONCEPTS

- Approach workup of psychosis methodically, starting with the basics: history, physical examination, and routine laboratory tests.

- Consider additional testing as your index of suspicion increases in a particular direction. There should be a rationale for ordering more invasive tests.

- Assemble a team. The workup may be complex and often requires outside consultation from specialty providers. Make sure to include primary care in the earliest stage of the workup if not already involved.

- Remember the patient and family in the process while pursuing medical workup. Work with families to set expectations for the workup and remember to focus on providing treatment while a workup is pending.

Discussion Questions

1. What resources in your area can you use to provide a complete workup for a person who comes to you in a first episode of psychosis?

2. How will you work with families to understand the road map and limitations of the medical workup? What can you do to manage expectations?

3. How might you respond to a family who asks for more extensive workup than you judge to be warranted? How can you maintain a therapeutic connection with the patient and family while setting appropriate limits on the medical workup?

Suggested Readings

Chang K, Frankovich J, Cooperstock M, et al: Clinical evaluation of youth with pediatric acute-onset neuropsychiatric syndrome (PANS): recommendations from the 2013 PANS Consensus Conference. J Child Adolesc Psychopharmacol 25(1):3–13, 2015 25325534

Freudenreich O, Schulz SC, Goff DC: Initial medical work-up of first-episode psychosis: a conceptual review. Early Interv Psychiatry 3(1):10–18, 200921352170

Kandratavicius L, Hallak JE, Leite JP: What are the similarities and differences between schizophrenia and schizophrenia-like psychosis of epilepsy? A neuropathological approach to the understanding of schizophrenia spectrum and epilepsy. Epilepsy Behav 38:143–147, 201424508393

Khandanpour N, Hoggard N, Connolly DJA: The role of MRI and CT of the brain in first episodes of psychosis. Clin Radiol 68(3):245–250, 201322959259

Oldham M: Autoimmune encephalopathy for psychiatrists: when to suspect autoimmunity and what to do next. Psychosomatics 58(3):228–244, 201728545782

References

Brownlie BE, Rae AM, Walshe JW, et al: Psychoses associated with thyrotoxicosis—"thyrotoxic psychosis": a report of 18 cases, with statistical analysis of incidence. Eur J Endocrinol 142(5):438–444, 2000 10802519

Cahalan S: Brain on Fire: My Month of Madness. New York, Free Press, 2012

Carandang CG, Scholten MC: Metyrosine in psychosis associated with 22q11.2 deletion syndrome: case report. J Child Adolesc Psychopharmacol 17(1):115–120, 2007 17343559

Chang K, Frankovich J, Cooperstock M, et al: Clinical evaluation of youth with pediatric acute-onset neuropsychiatric syndrome (PANS): recommendations from the 2013 PANS Consensus Conference. J Child Adolesc Psychopharmacol 25(1):3–13, 2015 25325534

Chen S-J, Chao Y-L, Chen C-Y, et al: Prevalence of autoimmune diseases in inpatients with schizophrenia: nationwide population-based study. Br J Psychiatry 200(5):374–380, 2012 22442099

Coleman M, Gillberg C: A biological approach to the schizophrenia spectrum disorders. J Neuropsychiatry Clin Neurosci 9(4):601–605, 1997 9447505

Dixon L, Perkins D, Calmes C: Guideline Watch (September 2009): Practice Guideline for the Treatment of Patients With Schizophrenia. Arlington, VA, American Psychiatric Association, 2009

Frankovich J, Thienemann M, Pearlstein J, et al: Multidisciplinary clinic dedicated to treating youth with pediatric acute-onset neuropsychiatric syndrome: presenting characteristics of the first 47 consecutive patients. J Child Adolesc Psychopharmacol 25(1):38–47, 2015 25695943

Freudenreich O, Schulz SC, Goff DC: Initial medical work-up of first-episode psychosis: a conceptual review. Early Interv Psychiatry 3(1):10–18, 2009 21352170

Gaughran F, Lally J, Beck K, et al: Brain-relevant antibodies in first-episode psychosis: a matched case-control study. Psychol Med 48(8):1257–1263, 2018 28920570

Golomb M: Psychiatric symptoms in metabolic and other genetic disorders: is our "organic" workup complete? Harv Rev Psychiatry 10(4):242–248, 2002 12119310

Heinrich TW, Grahm G: Hypothyroidism presenting as psychosis: myxedema madness revisited. Prim Care Companion J Clin Psychiatry 5(6):260–266, 2003 15213796

Ho RC, Thiaghu C, Ong H, et al: A meta-analysis of serum and cerebrospinal fluid autoantibodies in neuropsychiatric systemic lupus erythematosus. Autoimmun Rev 15(2):124–138, 2016 26497108

Johnstone EC, Macmillan JF, Crow TJ: The occurrence of organic disease of possible or probable aetiological significance in a population of 268 cases of first episode schizophrenia. Psychol Med 17(2):371–379, 1987 3602229

Kandratavicius L, Hallak JE, Leite JP: What are the similarities and differences between schizophrenia and schizophrenia-like psychosis of epilepsy? A neuropathological approach to the understanding of schizophrenia spectrum and epilepsy. Epilepsy Behav 38:143–147, 2014 24508393

Kar SK, Kumar D, Singh P, et al: Psychiatric manifestation of chronic subdural hematoma: the unfolding of mystery in a homeless patient. Indian J Psychol Med 37(2):239–242, 2015 25969617

Khandanpour N, Hoggard N, Connolly DJA: The role of MRI and CT of the brain in first episodes of psychosis. Clin Radiol 68(3):245–250, 2013 22959259

Kosmidis MH, Giannakou M, Messinis L, Papathanasopoulos P: Psychotic features associated with multiple sclerosis. Int Rev Psychiatry 22(7):55–66, 2010 20233114

Kranaster L, Koethe D, Hoyer C, et al: Cerebrospinal fluid diagnostics in first-episode schizophrenia. Eur Arch Psychiatry Clin Neurosci 261(7):529–530, 2011 21298501

Laher A, Ariefdien N, Etlouba Y: HIV prevalence among first-presentation psychotic patients. HIV Med 19(4):271–279, 2018 29282832

Lehman AF, Lieberman JA, Dixon LB, et al: Practice guideline for the treatment of patients with schizophrenia, second edition. Am J Psychiatry 161(2 suppl):1–56, 2004 15000267

McDonald-McGinn DM, Sullivan KE, Marino B, et al: 22q11.2 deletion syndrome. Nat Rev Dis Primers 1:15071, 2015 27189754

Oldham M: Autoimmune encephalopathy for psychiatrists: when to suspect autoimmunity and what to do next. Psychosomatics 58(3):228–244, 2017 28545782

Patten SB, Svenson LW, Metz LM: Psychotic disorders in MS: population-based evidence of an association. Neurology 65(7):1123–1125, 2005 16217073

Rasmussen SA, Rosebush PI, Smyth HS, Mazurek MF: Cushing disease presenting as primary psychiatric illness: a case report and literature review. J Psychiatr Pract 21(6):449–457, 2015 26554329

Vorvolakos T, Arseniou S, Samakouri M: There is no safe threshold for lead exposure: a literature review. Psychiatriki 27(3):204–214, 2016 27837574

Zimbrean PC, Schilsky ML: Psychiatric aspects of Wilson disease: a review. Gen Hosp Psychiatry 36(1):53–62, 2014 24120023

▮▮▮▮▮▮

CHAPTER
10

Assessing and Treating Trauma in Team-Based Early Psychosis Care

Rachel L. Loewy, Ph.D.
Tara Niendam, Ph.D.
Paula Wadell, M.D.

IN this chapter, we address the assessment and treatment of posttraumatic stress within the framework of team-based treatment of early psychosis. First, we discuss the prevalence of trauma exposure in psychosis, highlighting different types of trauma that are particularly relevant to first-episode psychosis (FEP) and briefly discuss models of the relationship between trauma and psychosis. Next, we propose universal screening for trauma exposure and posttraumatic stress symptoms in early psychosis services and describe assessment tools and best practices for assessment procedures. Then we explain how trauma-informed care (TIC) can be applied to early psychosis programs. Finally, we review evidence-based trauma-specific interventions that can be used by early psychosis teams, including cognitive-behavioral therapy (CBT), family interventions, and medication management. We also provide a case example to illustrate how each component of care can apply to an individual presenting with trauma and psychosis. Given the relative lack of attention to trauma in early psychosis work and the hesitation that many providers express regarding addressing trauma with their clients, we hope that this chapter gives both novice and experienced early psychosis team members more confidence that they can safely and effectively treat traumatic experiences and symptoms to promote resilience and recovery.

Case Example

Maria, a 25-year-old woman, was referred to the FEP program by her older sister, Sarah, who was concerned about Maria's recent hospitalization after a 3-month period of homelessness. Sarah reported that Maria experienced periods of depression, anxiety, strange thoughts, and unusual behaviors. Maria presented to the clinic for the clinical intake with her sister. Maria reported periods of chronic depression since childhood that worsened after high school graduation. She reported that she worked odd jobs after graduation, but nothing ever seemed to stick. In the fall of the previous year, Maria reported that she began to hear whispers coming from the vents in her apartment. At first, she wondered if they were the voices of angels or demons. Sarah reported that the family lost touch with Maria at this time until they received a call from the local psychiatric hospital. Maria had been evicted from her apartment after she smashed the walls looking for "the demons" and trying to release "the angels." She had painted her walls with crosses and said that she had been chosen by God to save the world. After being evicted, Maria was homeless and lived in her car. Police brought her to the hospital because she was yelling at people in a parking lot and threatening to hurt them. Maria reported that she felt others were noticing her "brown skin" and that they had hostile intentions toward her, including wanting to hurt her. In the past month, Maria reported that her new medications had helped to quiet the whispers, but she still felt unsafe when walking in public. She also reported periods of suicidal ideation, wondering if death would be better than burdening her family. When asked about their early history, Maria and Sarah reported they were adopted as children from Guatemala, noting that their biological parents died in 1992 during the civil war. Maria was 9 and Sarah was 12 at the time of their adoption. Sarah reported that their biological father had a history of drinking too much and would often get angry and hit his family to "get them in line."

Trauma Types and Prevalence

Trauma in Early Psychosis

Exposure to traumatic events is, unfortunately, quite common in psychosis, occurring at much higher rates than in the general population (Varese et al. 2012). History of trauma exposure is related to a variety of poorer outcomes, including more severe symptoms, worse social functioning, substance use, homelessness, and risk for suicide. The relationship of trauma and psychosis is likely reciprocal; early trauma may contribute to later risk for psychosis, and young people with psychosis are at increased risk for bullying and interpersonal victimization (see Figure 10–1). Traumatic experiences can shape the form of psychotic symptoms, such as suspiciousness, and many people experience psychotic symptoms, such as auditory hallucinations, in the context of posttraumatic stress disorder (PTSD). Finally, psychotic symptoms can themselves be frightening and experienced as traumatic, as can hospitalizations and involuntary restraint. Furthermore, compared with the general population, people with psychotic disorders are at higher risk for revictimization.

Childhood Trauma

A meta-analysis of psychosis and adverse childhood events (sexual abuse, physical abuse, emotional/psychological abuse, neglect, parental death, and bullying) reviewed 36 studies in three categories of research: 1) case-control studies that compared individuals with psychosis to those without psychosis and those with childhood trauma exposure to those without a childhood trauma history; 2) prospective cohort studies that followed people with and without childhood trauma over time, and 3) cross-sectional cohort studies that examined the relationship of trauma to psychotic-like experiences in the general population (Varese et al. 2012). Varese and colleagues found significant relationships between childhood trauma and psychosis across all three types of studies and concluded that childhood adversity is strongly associated with increased risk for psychosis.

Bullying and Interpersonal Victimization

People with psychosis may have experienced bullying by peers in childhood during the *prodrome* or pre-psychotic phase of their disorder or after onset of their first psychotic episode. In some cases, these experiences meet narrow definitions of trauma, such as interpersonal violence or verbal threat of harm, and in others, they represent a painful pattern of verbal abuse and rejection that can nonetheless be stressful and psychologically traumatizing, especially in childhood and adolescence. These kinds of experiences can often affect mood and social functioning and influence the form of psychotic symptoms through mistrust, paranoid delusions, and hallucinations.

Community, Intergenerational, and Identity-Based Trauma

In addition to direct experiences of trauma, individuals with FEP may be exposed to violence in their families and communities that must be

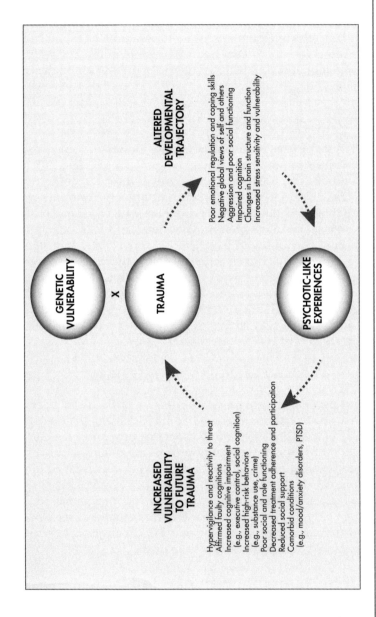

FIGURE 10–1. Cycle of trauma, psychotic-like experiences, and vulnerability.

Abbreviation. PTSD=posttraumatic stress disorder.

Source. Reprinted from Mayo D, Corey S, Kelly LH, et al.: The role of trauma and stressful life events among individuals at clinical high risk for psychosis: a review. *Frontiers in Psychiatry* 8:55, 2017. Used with permission.

accounted for in treatment of their psychosis. This can impact treatment when family members, seen as important sources of support in FEP care, are either perpetrators or themselves victims of assault, abuse, and/or neglect. In communities with high levels of ongoing violence, perceived threat must be examined in the context of reality-based threats. Furthermore, discrimination based on personal identity or characteristics (e.g., sex, race, ethnicity, sexuality, religion, intersectionality) and historical or institutionalized discrimination must be thoughtfully included in conceptualization and treatment of trauma and psychosis. Careful discussion in assessment and treatment from a cultural humility approach can differentiate these elements rather than assuming that symptoms are psychotic or, alternatively, assuming that they are nonpsychotic responses to discrimination.

Temporal Characteristics of Trauma

Trauma may be a single event, or it may be chronic abuse and victimization. It also can be experienced in multiple domains. This can affect the severity of posttraumatic stress (PTS) as well as the presentation of symptoms in response to a single time-limited event or complex PTSD as a result of prolonged periods of victimization. Complex PTSD can carry higher levels of risky behaviors and self-harm, as well as additional symptoms of changes in perceptions of self, others, and relationships that may be misdiagnosed as personality disorders. Additionally, past traumatic experiences are treated differently from ongoing abuse or victimization, which requires establishing current safety first and foremost. FEP programs should have established policies on reporting abuse communicated clearly to clients and families at the outset of program participation, with every effort made to deal with reporting as collaboratively as is legally allowed.

Assessment

Case Example *(continued)*

During the initial evaluation, the examiner asked Maria to complete the Posttraumatic Stress Disorder Checklist for DSM-5 (PCL-5), a brief self-report screening questionnaire for trauma experiences and symptoms (Weathers et al. 2013a). On this measure, Maria endorsed experiencing physical abuse by her father, observing the physical abuse of other family members, experiencing the sudden death of a family member, and being around war. She also reported that she had quickly left a neighborhood when a number of U.S. Immigration and Customs Enforcement trucks appeared in the street, noting that she was terrified that she could be deported because of her undocumented status. She reported that the experience of abuse by her father was the most distressing of these experiences. In response to this abuse, she endorsed multiple trauma symptoms, including hypervigilance, re-experiencing, blaming herself, and feelings of low self-worth and avoidance. The examiner also completed a semistructured interview about Maria's trauma experiences and symptoms. Maria met criteria for PTSD, according to the *Diagnostic and Statistical Manual of Mental Disorders,* 5th Edition (DSM-5; American Psychiatric Association 2013).

Trauma Screening

Universal screening for both exposure to traumatic events and related PTS symptoms should be part of every initial evaluation for FEP services. Although we appreciate that an extensive intake process can be burdensome to clients, families, and clinicians, attention to trauma is critical for 1) differential diagnosis and 2) collaborative treatment planning. Because of feelings of shame and avoidance, many people will not report trauma unless specifically asked about it. Compassionate trauma screening can make someone feel understood and "seen" as a whole person, with a full life history, rather than a constellation of psychotic symptoms. However, repeated screening may be necessary because some people will be more comfortable reporting trauma after the therapeutic relationship develops over time. High levels of distress related to PTS can interfere with engagement and must be addressed. In fact, many individuals with FEP may identify relief from PTS as a primary treatment target that is more important to them than first targeting hallucinations or delusions.

Trauma Measures

Several validated measures for assessing trauma and PTS that can be used in FEP programs are discussed in this subsection and are listed on the website for the National Center for PTSD (www.ptsd.va.gov/professional/index.asp). In some cases, programs may be required by their operating agency, municipality (city, state, or county) or funding organization (e.g., Substance Abuse and Mental Health Services Administration [SAMHSA]) to use a specific measure. If the measure recommended for general mental health programs is insufficient for the FEP service, we encourage programs to negotiate with the relevant parties. The FEP service should consider whether it is important to have one measure that can be used across a wide age span, such as from adolescence to adulthood. Some measures are self-report, whereas others are semistructured interviews. Some options can offer client self-report and caregiver or provider versions to allow multiple informants to contribute to the assessment.

Although the gold standard for diagnosis of PTSD is a semistructured interview such as the Clinician-Administered PTSD Scale (CAPS-5; Weathers et al. 2013b) or the Structured Clinical Interview for DSM-5® Disorders—Clinician Version (SCID-5-CV; First et al. 2016), the choice of the correct tool may be based on the population served by the FEP program as well as the resources available. For example, the Life Events Checklist (LEC; Gray et al. 2004, Weathers et al. 2013c) can be used to evaluate the presence of traumatic events. The PTSD Checklist for DSM-5 (PCL-5) is a 20-item self-report screen that can be combined with the LEC to assess associated PTS. This combination can be used to determine whether additional assessment is warranted and to monitor change in symptoms in response to treatment. In children, the Child and Adolescent Trauma Screen (CATS; Sachser et al. 2017) provides the ability to examine traumatic events and associated symptoms in a manner that is parallel to the PCL-5 with LEC. The Traumatic Events Screening Inventory for Children (TESI-C; Ippen et al. 2002; Ribbe 1996) is a semistructured interview that includes child and caregiver self-report versions to screen for traumatic events and assesses PTS related to each event. The National Center for PTSD provides excellent free resources for assessment of trauma experiences and symptoms for children and adults (see Recommended Resources).

Differential Diagnosis

A very common referring question posed to early psychosis (EP) services who provide diagnostic evaluations is differential diagnosis of PTSD versus a primary psychotic disorder. In many cases this is a false dichotomy because the same individual can present with both PTS and psychotic symptoms. Although prevalence rates vary, one large study estimated that 16% of people with schizophrenia spectrum disorders meet formal diagnostic criteria for PTSD (de Bont et al. 2015). Subthreshold PTS symptoms are measured less often but occur at even higher rates, and psychotic-like symptoms are common enough in PTSD that there has been debate about whether there is actually a psychotic subtype of PTSD.

In terms of clinical presentation, hallucinations must be distinguished from vivid memories, flashbacks, and dreams that occur as reexperiencing of traumatic events. Details of the symptoms and their explanation are important. Both types of symptoms can be upsetting, but one has a known source, whereas the other may be experienced as unrelated to the trauma or being of unknown origin (e.g., the perpetrator's voice vs. an unidentified voice). Paranoia must be differentiated from exaggerated suspiciousness and mistrust that does not reach delusional severity. Here, the level of conviction may be helpful (e.g., "I am sure he wanted to hurt me" vs. "I think he wanted to hurt me, but it's possible that was my imagination"). Dissociation must be differentiated from delusional experiences (e.g., "I felt as if I was not present in my body" vs. "Another being took over control of my body"). These cases can be complex and often require consultation, supervision, or group discussion to reach a consensus regarding the differential diagnosis. Further complicating factors include the triggering effect of stress in exacerbating both types of symptoms and the high rates of substance use to cope with PTS, which can trigger or induce psychosis. Finally, some EP services may not accept PTSD with psychotic features as an eligible diagnosis for services, whereas others do accept it.

Cultural Factors

A variety of cultural factors can influence an individual's exposure to trauma, as well as that person's ability to access appropriate care. The DSM-5 Cultural Formulation Interview (American Psychiatric Association 2013) could be useful as the clinician works to understand how an individual's cultural experience impacts his or her experience of symptoms related to psychosis, trauma, or other domains. In the case of Maria, her lived experience as a survivor of a civil war was not seen by her as the most significant traumatic experience in her life. Additionally, her identification as Latina was associated with increased fear of deportation and a perception of others as being hostile toward her. These fears and concerns are not wholly inaccurate, and it is important for the clinician to consider these factors when attempting to determine which experiences are treatment targets. Language, religion, racial and ethnic identity, gender and sexual identity, and acculturation represent some of the cultural areas that must be explored with clients as part of the treatment planning process to ensure accurate identification of treatment targets for both psychosis and trauma symptoms.

Treatment Approaches to Trauma in Early Psychosis

Case Example *(continued)*

During the first meeting with her clinician, Maria was provided with feedback about the results of her intake evaluation. The clinician discussed Maria's experiences of depression, auditory hallucinations, and delusions as well as her experiences of trauma and the associated symptoms. At first, Maria was surprised at being asked to discuss her painful childhood memories when she was seeking care for her psychosis. The clinician took time providing education about the relationship between stress and symptoms, noting that traumatic experiences are one form of stress that can impact recovery. The clinician then laid out a plan for care, in which education about psychosis, depression, and trauma would be provided along with skills to improve Maria's ability to cope with stress and reduce her symptoms. The clinician asked Maria's permission to share this information with Sarah and their adoptive parents, who wanted to be active participants in Maria's care because she was now living at home with them. Maria reported that she was primarily concerned about her depression and hearing the voices, so the clinician agreed to target those symptoms first. As those experiences improved, the clinician stated that they would re-evaluate Maria's depression, psychosis, and trauma symptoms to determine which direction to take next.

Trauma-Informed Care

Although there are different models of TIC, their primary aim is to help survivors resolve trauma rather than be retraumatized by their interactions with services and systems. These approaches promote awareness of the signs and effects of trauma and support trauma-sensitive interactions by educating staff at all system levels—from the phone or front desk administrative staff who first interact with clients, through frontline providers, to the financial billing staff and upper management. Trauma-sensitive policies and procedures are integrated throughout the organization. SAMHSA has developed a number of TIC resources based on six core principles:

1. *Safety*: making physical and psychological safety of all clients and staff a priority
2. *Trustworthiness and transparency*: conducting all operations and making decisions with transparency and the goal of building and keeping trust with those served
3. *Peer support*: promoting trauma recovery through use of peers
4. *Collaboration and mutuality*: sharing power and decision making between clients and staff and also between all staff members in different roles
5. *Empowerment, voice, and choice*: promoting empowerment and resiliency for clients and staff through respectful, shared decision-making
6. *Cultural, historical, and gender issues:* moving past stereotypes and biases to offer culturally sensitive and responsive services

Although we are unaware of a formalized approach to integrating TIC into EP services in the published literature, many organizations that receive SAMHSA funding or provide an array of services have used a trauma-informed approach, as have some stand-alone EP clinics. The TIC principles defined above overlap substantially with many aspects of coordinated specialty care models, although TIC may also have particular challenges that require attention in integration, as summarized in Table 10–1. For example, all programs working with this population should have clear procedures in place to ensure the physical safety of all clients and staff, communicated with transparency to all. Sensitivity to suspiciousness and paranoia, much like trauma, means checking in with clients frequently to gauge their sense of psychological safety.

Collaborative decision making is a hallmark of many EP programs, which offer a variety of services tailored to the needs and goals of individuals. Peer staff in EP programs are often individuals with lived experience of psychosis, who, given the high rates of trauma experienced by individuals with psychosis, are often also trauma survivors. Training and supervision of peers should focus on experiences of trauma and how they may interact with psychosis. Prioritizing self-care for staff in EP clinics can reduce workforce turnover by addressing vicarious trauma and burnout. Shifting the power balance between staff and clients and between different staff members may be more of a challenge for EP programs embedded in medical models and systems. As we have discussed previously, ensuring staff members' knowledge of and sensitivity to identity-related trauma and discrimination, as well as historical trauma, is necessary to understand clients' experiences and promote recovery from both psychosis and trauma.

Case Example *(continued)*

Maria felt very unsafe in public and, at times, felt very uncomfortable in the clinic waiting room. To help with this fear, she checked in with the clinic coordinators on arriving at the clinic, and the peer case manager, Kevin, went out to the lobby to sit with her. Maria liked Kevin, so this helped her feel safer and more relaxed while she waited. Consistent with TIC, the team prioritized Maria's sense of safety, and Kevin helped level the balance of power by interacting with her as a supportive peer with his own recovery experience rather than as a doctor in a position of authority.

Cognitive-Behavioral Therapy

The use of cognitive-behavioral approaches to treating psychosis allows for easy integration of specific trauma approaches based in CBT in order to address both trauma and psychosis. Evidence-based treatments for trauma, such as trauma-focused cognitive-behavioral therapy (TF-CBT) for youth and prolonged exposure (PE) or eye movement desensitization therapy (EMDR) for adults, have a foundation in cognitive-behavioral theory. In a recent review, Cragin et al. (2017) found studies that demonstrated the effectiveness of these trauma treatments in individuals with established psychosis and PTSD; however, the authors' survey of EP

TABLE 10–1. Elements of trauma-informed care and coordinated specialty care for first-episode psychosis

TIC principle	CSC compatibility	Potential integration challenges
1. Safety	• Clear guidelines should be communicated to clients, family members, and staff for assessing and ensuring physical safety of clients, family, and staff, including abuse, SI/ HI reporting, and evaluations for hospitalization. • Attention should be paid to the client's perceived threat in the moment in clinic and other situations. • Flexibility is key in offering services in clinic, at the client's home, or in neutral community spaces.	All staff, not just individual providers, require training in assessing fearfulness and safety.
2. Trustworthiness and transparency	• A team-based approach that honors contributions of all team members is required. • Patience and flexibility are needed in establishing trust when clients feel suspicious.	Organizational transparency requires particular attention in busy, complex team-based programs.
3. Peer support	• Peers and family partners often work in CSC programs.	Additional training in disclosure and support of trauma may be required for peers and family partners.

TABLE 10–1.   Elements of trauma-informed care and coordinated specialty care for first-episode psychosis (*continued*)

TIC principle	CSC compatibility	Potential integration challenges
4. Collaboration and mutuality	• Treatment planning is characterized by shared decision making, including defining specific treatment goals and selecting CSC elements with particular clients and families.	Organizations need to be thoughtful in leveling power differences between staff in programs with a medical model orientation.
5. Empowerment, voice, and choice	• There should be a focus on strengths-based perspectives, resilience, and recovery orientation.	Programs should be responsive to varying levels of goals for achievement, particularly in supported education or employment models that may have traditionally focused on lowered expectations.
6. Cultural, historical, and gender issues	• Cultural or contextual sensitivity is often built into clinical assessment and conceptualization of psychosis. • Identity issues often are important for transitional-age youth.	Attention to these issues can lapse when training and supervising staff in multiple evidence-based approaches.

Abbreviations.   CSC=coordinated specialty care; SI/HI=suicidal ideation/homicidal ideation; TIC=trauma-informed care.

program providers indicated uncertainty regarding how to address trauma symptoms in early psychosis.

Within an integrated trauma-psychosis cognitive-behavioral framework, the clinician and client collaboratively develop a conceptualization of how the trauma experiences and psychosis symptoms are being maintained and contribute to current distress. The clinician provides psychoeducation around both psychosis and trauma, such as information on how stress can lead to the exacerbation of both psychosis and trauma symptoms. Information about the rates of certain traumatic events or types of trauma symptoms can also be provided. The clinician and client work to develop a set of coping skills to manage symptoms and distress. Measuring distress regularly through subjective distress ratings and addressing it directly and early in the therapy with coping skills are critical to giving clients an early positive experience of the treatment and to providing them coping skills to support later exposure practices. Coping skills can address relaxation, awareness of affect, and regulation as well as cognitive coping skills.

Relapse and safety planning are essential for maintaining stability in an outpatient setting. At this point, it would be important to reassess the severity of trauma and psychosis symptoms to determine the focus of subsequent treatment. If psychosis is stable, trauma treatment would suggest that exposure—through creation of a trauma narrative—would be the next step. Such a narrative would be shared with a caregiver in the case of a TF-CBT approach or the clinician in the case of PE or EMDR. As noted by Cragin and colleagues (2017), exposure is an essential component in the treatment of trauma symptoms in individuals with psychosis and should not be avoided in cases where psychosis symptoms are stable. If psychosis symptoms are not stable, ongoing psychoeducation around trauma and enhancement of coping skills to manage trauma-related symptoms would be appropriate in the context of treatment that focuses on psychosis symptom reduction. Regardless of whether the client's level of trauma symptoms warrant exposure to trauma history, CBT for psychosis would use exposure as one method for addressing psychosis symptoms. For example, a client and provider may walk around public places, identify times when the client feels strangers are looking at him or her (or not), and use cognitive skills (e.g., "Catch it, check it, change it") to evaluate the client's belief that people are out to get him or her.

Case Example *(continued)*

As Maria engaged in EP services, her depression and auditory hallucinations improved; however, she continued to feel very unsafe in public. As part of the treatment conceptualization, Maria had learned that part of her anxiety was related to experiences of trauma and realistic concerns about her immigration status, whereas another piece was associated with potentially unrealistic beliefs that other people judged or persecuted her because of the darker color of her skin. As part of her treatment, Maria and her clinician developed a hierarchy of anxiety-provoking experiences so that they could analyze and examine her thoughts in real time. Maria realized that she often felt afraid when walking in her neighborhood, worrying that someone might assault her because of her skin color. To address this fear, as part of her treatment, Kevin took walks with Maria in her neighborhood, allowing them to actively record her thoughts and try alternative thoughts (cognitive coping) while measuring her emotional response (assessing distress).

Family Involvement

CSC for early psychosis sees family involvement as a core component in supporting understanding and recovery. Family members who actively support the client should also receive psychoeducation on psychosis and trauma. Family can support use of effective coping skills when the client is in the community and provide feedback to the clinician about their effectiveness in reducing distress in the real world. TF-CBT incorporates sharing of the trauma narrative with a nonoffending caregiver as part of the exposure process. If this is appropriate for the EP client, it could also be included in the integrated trauma-psychosis treatment approach. However, this may or may not be appropriate for adult clients. In general, sharing the trauma narrative with someone other than the clinician should be discussed with the client to determine the best approach. Overall, family members or other loved ones should be seen as natural and ongoing supports for youth and adults with psychosis, and EP care should strive to enhance these supports through education and collaboration, regardless of the symptoms that are being targeted.

Case Example *(continued)*

Maria actively participated in individual and group treatment. Biweekly family sessions included her biological sister, Sarah, and their adoptive parents. Maria was encouraged to share information on psychosis and trauma symptoms with her family, with the support of her clinician. She also shared her favorite coping skills, which included deep breathing and meditation, and asked her family to prompt her to use her skills when she is upset. Maria was able to identify family arguments and large crowds as triggers for her anxiety. Specifically, she reported that she was often overwhelmed by Sarah's critical comments and tendency to yell when upset. The clinician reflected that both Maria and Sarah had experienced verbal and physical abuse by their biological parents and noted that both of them could benefit from improved coping and communication skills. Sarah and Maria agreed. Maria asked her family to participate in an upcoming communication skills group for families so they could improve their communication as a family. They expressed appreciation for the help with understanding more about Maria's experiences and how they could be more supportive. They were also impressed by how much knowledge Maria had gained. Sarah reported that she was pleased to have Maria participate in a recent family barbecue, noting that it was nice to see her enjoy being with family again.

Medication Management

There are currently no guidelines for the psychopharmacological treatment of comorbid trauma and psychosis. Generally, the treatment of comorbidity should be modeled on the evidence for each disorder. Antipsychotic medications are the appropriate treatment for psychosis and have all been shown to be more effective than placebo (Schatzberg et al. 2010). Antipsychotic medications have also been studied in the treatment of PTSD. Studies of risperidone, olanzapine, and quetiapine demonstrated some efficacy, with the greatest impact seen on reduction of intrusive traumatic ideation and hypervigilance (Ahearn et al. 2011; Carey et al. 2012). The most widely studied medications for the treatment of PTSD are the selective serotonin reuptake inhibitors, with paroxetine and sertraline both having specific U.S. Food and Drug Administration approval.

All other medications used in PTSD are off label. Randomized placebo-controlled treatment studies have shown some efficacy in the reduction of symptom severity with a range of other antidepressants, including fluoxetine, amitriptyline, imipramine, mirtazapine, nefazodone, phenelzine, and venlafaxine (Ipser and Stein 2012). There are data regarding the use of antidepressants in schizophrenia because of the frequent presence of depressive symptoms in first-episode clients (Koreen et al. 1993; Tapp et al. 2001), but studies have suggested that depressive symptoms may resolve with antipsychotic medication, and therefore initial treatment with an antipsychotic alone is generally recommended to minimize medications and potential side effects (Robinson et al. 2014). Data supporting the use of other medication classes in PTSD are limited and show conflicting evidence (Raskind et al. 2018). The only class considered relatively contraindicated is the benzodiazepines, which can worsen symptoms in PTSD (Guina et al. 2015).

Training and Consultation

As with all evidence-based interventions, implementing trauma-informed care and trauma-specific interventions requires allocated resources from finances, administrative planning, and staff time for training and ongoing supervision and consultation. Although these approaches are compatible in many ways with team-based early psychosis programs and can build on skills and elements already in place, they do require a long-term commitment from program leadership for successful integration. There are a number of resources available for training and consultation, starting with online resources and toolkits and including expert consultation on both the organizational changes required and specific clinical supervision. Many care systems are asking all organizations to include trauma-informed approaches and may offer free trainings, workshops, and technical support. The resource list provided at the end of this chapter includes several organizations that can respond to requests for training and technical assistance.

Conclusion and Future Directions

Given the very high rates of trauma seen in EP populations, team-based EP care must include assessment and treatment of trauma. Treatment should include both trauma-informed practices throughout the service and evidence-based psychotherapy for trauma; neither is a sufficient approach on its own. Staff providing medication management should also be familiar with treating both psychosis and PTS, with particular attention to how benzodiazepines are used. Clinicians are often concerned that addressing trauma with clients with EP may exacerbate psychotic symptoms, similar to the long-held but erroneous view that talk therapy is contraindicated for psychosis. Without training in evidence-based assessment and treatment of trauma, many clinicians hesitate to address the trauma, inadvertently contributing to retraumatization or client disengagement and withholding chances for full recovery. Identifying when a client has sufficient coping skills to tolerate exposures and when PTS is a priority for treatment is a decision to be made in collaboration with the client and with good clinical supervision and consultation. Although EP care already requires intensive training in evidence-based practices and additional training may initially feel burdensome to teams, a focus on trauma will actually help clinicians be more effective with some of their most distressed clients and will help staff understand their own reactions to working with this population, with a focus on self-care to address vicarious trauma. The relative lack of attention to trauma in psychosis until more recently leaves many avenues in need of further research to help guide EP teams. However, we hope we have made a sufficient argument for attention to trauma in EP care, with the ultimate goal of supporting the whole person and promoting recovery from both psychosis and trauma.

KEY CONCEPTS

- Trauma occurs at high rates in the first-episode psychosis population, including childhood trauma, bullying and victimization, intergenerational trauma, and traumatic hospitalization experiences.

- Assessment of both trauma exposure and posttraumatic stress symptoms is important for every client and may need to be repeated over time as the therapeutic relationship develops.

- Trauma treatment can be safe and effective for individuals with psychosis.

Discussion Questions

1. How do you assess trauma exposure and symptoms in your program?

2. How might a trauma history affect a client's perceptions and expectations of treatment for psychosis?

3. How could a trauma-informed perspective inform the operation of your program, from the first contact to the last?

4. How should each member of the treatment team approach trauma issues with clients and their families?

5. How can therapists integrate trauma-specific interventions into their treatments for clients with psychosis?

Recommended Resources

Frontiers: Trauma, Psychosis, and Posttraumatic Stress Disorder. Available at www.frontiersin.org/research-topics/4761/trauma-psychosis-and-posttraumatic-stress-disorder. Accessed December 4, 2018.

National Association of State Mental Health Program Directors Center for Trauma-Informed Care: www.nasmhpd.org/content/national-center-trauma-informed-care-nctic-0

National Center for PTSD: www.ptsd.va.gov/professional/index.asp

National Child Traumatic Stress Network: www.nctsn.org

Substance Abuse and Mental Health Services Administration: SAMHSA's Concept of Trauma and Guidance for a Trauma-Informed Approach. Pub ID SMA14-4884. Rockville, MD, Substance Abuse and Mental Health Services Administration, 2014. Available at: https://store.samhsa.gov/product/SAMHSA-s-Concept-of-Trauma-and-Guidance-for-a-Trauma-Informed-Approach/SMA14-4884.html. Accessed December 4, 2018.
TF-CBT Therapist Certification Program: https://tfcbt.org

References

Ahearn EP, Juergens T, Cordes T, et al: A review of atypical antipsychotic medications for posttraumatic stress disorder. Int Clin Psychopharmacol 26(4):193–200, 2011 21597381

American Psychiatric Association: Diagnostic and Statistical Manual of Mental Disorders, 5th Edition. Arlington, VA, American Psychiatric Association, 2013

Carey P, Suliman S, Ganesan K, et al: Olanzapine monotherapy in posttraumatic stress disorder: efficacy in a randomized, double-blind, placebo-controlled study. Hum Psychopharmacol 27(4):386–391, 2012 22730105

Cragin CA, Straus MB, Blacker D, et al: Early psychosis and trauma-related disorders: clinical practice guidelines and future directions. Front Psychiatry 8:33, 2017 28321193

de Bont PA, van den Berg DP, van der Vleugel BM, et al: Predictive validity of the Trauma Screening Questionnaire in detecting post-traumatic stress disorder in patients with psychotic disorders. Br J Psychiatry 206(5):408–416, 2015 25792693

First MB, Williams JBW, Karg RS, et al: Structured Clinical Interview for DSM-5® Disorders—Clinician Version. Arlington, VA, American Psychiatric Association, 2016

Gray M, Litz B, Hsu J, Lombardo T: Psychometric properties of the Life Events Checklist. Assessment 11(4):330–341, 2004 15486169

Guina J, Rossetter SR, DeRhodes BJ, et al: Benzodiazepines for PTSD: a systematic review and meta-analysis. J Psychiatr Pract 21(4):281–303, 2015 26164054

Ippen CG, Ford J, Racusin R, et al: Traumatic Events Screening Inventory-Parent Report Revised. Washington, DC, National Center for PTSD, 2002

Ipser JC, Stein DJ: Evidence-based pharmacotherapy of post-traumatic stress disorder (PTSD). Int J Neuropsychopharmacol 15(6):825–840, 2012 21798109

Koreen AR, Siris SG, Chakos M, et al: Depression in first-episode schizophrenia. Am J Psychiatry 150(11):1643–1648, 1993 8105706

Mayo D, Corey S, Kelly LH, et al: The role of trauma and stressful life events among individuals at clinical high risk for psychosis: a review. Front Psychiatry 8:55, 2017 28473776

Raskind MA, Peskind ER, Chow B, et al: Trial of prazosin for post-traumatic stress disorder in military veterans. N Engl J Med 378(6):507–517, 2018 29414272

Ribbe D: Psychometric review of Traumatic Event Screening Instrument for Children (TESI-C), in Measurement of stress, trauma, and adaptation. Edited by Stamm BH. Lutherville, MD, Sidran Press, 1996, pp 386–387

Robinson DG, Correll C, Kurian B, et al: NAVIGATE psychopharmacological treatment manual. Bethesda, MD, National Institute of Mental Health, April 1, 2014. Available at: www.navigateconsultants.org/wp-content/uploads/2017/05/Prescribers-Manual.pdf. Accessed October 5, 2018.

Sachser C, Berliner L, Holt T, et al: International development and psychometric properties of the Child and Adolescent Trauma Screen (CATS). J Affect Disord 210:189–195, 2017 28049104

Schatzberg AF, Cole JO, DeBattista C: Antipsychotic drugs, in Manual of Clinical Psychopharmacology. Arlington, VA: American Psychiatric Publishing, 2010, pp 169–279

Tapp A, Kilzieh N, Wood AE, et al: Depression in patients with schizophrenia during an acute psychotic episode. Compr Psychiatry 42(4):314–318, 2001 11458306

Varese F, Smeets F, Drukker M, et al: Childhood adversities increase the risk of psychosis: a meta-analysis of patient-control, prospective- and cross-sectional cohort studies. Schizophr Bull 38(4):661–671, 2012 22461484

Weathers FW, Litz BT, Keane TM, et al: The PTSD checklist for DSM-5 (PCL-5). Washington, DC, National Center for PTSD, 2013a

Weathers FW, Blake DD, Schnurr PP, et al: The Clinician-Administered PTSD Scale for DSM-5 (CAPS-5). Washington, DC, National Center for PTSD, 2013b

Weathers FW, Blake DD, Schnurr PP, et al: The Life Events Checklist for DSM-5 (LEC-5). Washington, DC, National Center for PTSD, 2013c

Intervening Early

A TEAM-BASED APPROACH

Iruma Bello, Ph.D.
Debra R. Hrouda, Ph.D.
Lisa Dixon, M.D., M.P.H.

SPECIALIZED multi-element early intervention services for the treatment of first-episode psychosis (FEP) have been in existence for at least two decades in both Australia and parts of Europe and Canada. Research studies have consistently found that individuals who receive these services early in their illness trajectory demonstrate short-term positive outcomes (Gafoor et al. 2010; Grawe et al. 2006). More recently, studies in the United States have obtained similar positive results (Dixon et al. 2015; Kane et al. 2015; Srihari et al. 2015). A recent meta-analysis by Correll and colleagues (2018) also found that individuals receiving early intervention services had better outcomes than those receiving treatment as usual. These research findings have led to a broad implementation effort of specialized early intervention services across the United States that have come to be known as coordinated specialty care (CSC) services.

Coordinated Specialty Care

CSC is an early intervention treatment approach for young people experiencing a first episode of nonaffective psychosis. It consists of a multidisciplinary team with specialized training to deliver assertive care management, individual or group psychotherapy, supported employment and education services, family education and support, appropriate pharmacotherapy, and primary care coordination. The program philosophy emphasizes the delivery of person-centered, recovery-oriented, culturally competent care using shared decision making (Heinssen et al. 2014). The National Institute of Mental Health defined CSC on the basis of the national and international body of research focused on early psychosis; the positive findings of the Recovery After an Initial Schizophrenia Episode (RAISE) studies conducted in the United States provided further support for CSC (Azrin et al. 2016).

There are several types of CSC programs that are being implemented throughout the United States, including Navigate, OnTrackNY, the Early Assessment and Support Alliance (EASA), FIRST Coordinated Specialty Care, and Specialized Treatment Early in Psychosis (STEP). Although all of these programs have comparable key elements, there are some differences in the way the teams are structured or the way in which the services are provided and the level of manualization associated with each approach. Nonetheless, they all share the philosophy that the nonspecifics related to delivery of CSC services (including team members' attitudes, youth orientation, flexibility, team collaboration, and recovery orientation), which can convey to participants and families a sense of compassion, warmth, and hope for the future, are paramount for ensuring the successful implementation of CSC and helping young people attain good outcomes.

The ability to connect with young people experiencing FEP in a collaborative and productive way that respects their personal values and keeps them at the center of the team's efforts is fundamental for being able to deliver the CSC interventions. Therefore, in most of this chapter we focus on describing 1) the specific interventions delivered across CSC teams, using a time-limited framework for service delivery, 2) the important factors associated with working within a multidisciplinary treatment team, and 3) the underlying clinical concepts that drive all of the evidence-based practices delivered under CSC. A vignette is used throughout to illustrate the implementation of each of these components. In the final section of this chapter, we provide guidance on adaptations that should be considered when implementing CSC services in rural settings.

Case Example

Jasmin is a 19-year-old Latina living with her mother, aunt, uncle, and two younger siblings. Jasmin's father lives in the Dominican Republic, and she visits him regularly. When Jasmin was 10 years old, her mother brought her and her siblings to live in the United States with Jasmin's maternal uncle and his wife to provide them with better educational opportunities. Jasmin's mother works at a bank, and the aunt and uncle have their own small business selling jewelry. Jasmin's relationship with her family is close but marked by discord related to their differing views on religion.

Throughout her childhood, Jasmin was a good student interested in the sciences. She was accepted to an out-of-state college with a scholarship. During the first semester of her sophomore year, Jasmin began taking courses related to her engineering major and began experiencing school as increasingly stressful. Her GPA declined, which further increased her stress level because she feared she might lose her scholarship. She also started spending more time drinking with friends during the weekends as a way to cope. She was arrested for public intoxication once. By the end of the semester, Jasmin became increasingly distressed. She stopped sleeping and ate very little, spending most days at the library studying for finals. She also started experiencing auditory and visual hallucinations and started believing that her teachers were plotting to get her expelled from school. Jasmin's friends noticed the change in her demeanor, hygiene, and thinking and decided to take her to the school's counseling center. This resulted in her first hospitalization, where she was prescribed antipsychotic medication.

On discharge from the hospital, Jasmin returned to live with her family and took a medical leave from school. Although she was experiencing fewer voices and visual hallucinations and no longer believed that her professors were plotting against her, Jasmin felt apathetic, refused to meet with friends, barely interacted with her siblings, and spent a lot of time alone in her room watching television. Jasmin's mother searched for appropriate mental health services online and contacted a local CSC program. Once evaluated by the team, Jasmin was found to be eligible and was offered services, and she agreed to enroll in the program.

Coordinated Specialty Care Interventions

CSC programs provide a suite of evidence-based practices that have been shown to be effective in treating individuals diagnosed with schizophrenia. At a minimum, services offered include care management, individual and family therapy, supported employment and education services, medication management, and coordination with primary health care. Some teams offer enhanced services such as peer support services for participants and for family members, treatments for cognitive health, cognitive-behavioral therapy for psychosis (CBTp), occupational therapy, and supported housing. Interventions are delivered using a phased, time-limited framework that typically lasts 2–3 years. Within the CSC model, participants are not required to engage in any of the interventions in order to maintain enrollment, although everyone is connected to a primary provider who serves as the point person for the participant and family members. It is the participant's and family's ability to engage with the team in a flexible way that allows the interventions to be tailored specifically to each individual and his or her set of circumstances to promote achievement of school, work, and relationship goals.

At the outset of treatment, teams focus on forging highly collaborative and engaging alliances with participants and family members through the use of specific assertive outreach and engagement strategies (Bennett et al. 2017). For instance, successful teams are able to remain proactive in connecting with participants and family members throughout all phases of treatment, which might include the use of various forms of communication (phone, texting, e-mail, and in-person meetings). The time and location of sessions are flexible and responsive to the needs of the participants and family members (e.g., in the home, community, or clinic, with increased or decreased frequency as needed). Considerations of transportation, work schedules, and other caregiving are critical, especially in areas that are geographically spread out where public transportation may not be readily available. The flexibility of team members to be creative in communication and scheduling is essential in developing a solid working alliance.

Teams provide important information for participants to consider all relevant treatment choices rather than dictating treatment recommendations, which helps ensure that treatment decisions are guided by pressing concerns expressed by participants and family members—not the priorities of the team. Providers maintain a flexible and consistent stance toward treatment, which allows them to respond sensitively and practically to the range of situations that might arise on an as-needed basis. At the same time, they focus on demonstrating to the participant and family members that the team will remain a consistent presence by behaving in a reliable manner and offering support, empathy, and trustworthiness (Bennett et al. 2017). This therapeutic alliance usually serves to ensure that treatment engagement remains across time and serves as the foundation for introducing and delivering the pharmacological, psychosocial, and other treatments offered. Teams typically have the flexibility to keep the participant's file open in the program for longer periods of time than in traditional clinical settings, even when there is little contact with the participant.

Once rapport has been established and the team is able to gain a more in-depth understanding of the individual and his or her natural supports, preferences, values, and worldview, interventions can be tailored accordingly and delivered as intensely as necessary to promote recovery. The final phase of treatment is focused on transitioning the individual from the team on the basis of his or her continued needs and preferences. Some options might include a CSC step-down program if available, regular outpatient clinic care, or other less traditional supports offered through school or the community.

Case Example *(continued)*

When Jasmin arrived at the CSC clinic, she was surprised at how youth-friendly and nontraditional the environment felt. She noticed that there were other younger individuals like herself in the waiting room, the decor was warm and appealed to her, and there was even a computer room where several young people were congregating and seemed to be discussing a computer game. Jasmin and her mother met with Martha, her assigned primary therapist. Unlike other providers Jasmin had encountered at the hospital, Martha did not start by asking Jasmin about her diagnosis or whether she was taking her medications as prescribed. The meeting did not feel rushed, and Jasmin felt heard and involved in the process. Jasmin quickly got the impression that Martha wanted to really get to know her as a person and understand her point of view.

Initially, Martha spent time discussing with Jasmin and her mother the services the team could provide and how these services would be focused on helping Jasmin achieve her personal goals, which included finishing her engineering degree. Martha described the various ways in which the team had worked with other participants and introduced Jasmin and her mother to the various team members. Martha maintained a curious stance, which conveyed support, reassurance, and hope. She offered to communicate with Jasmin via text and to visit her at home to get to know the rest of the family who were unable to make it to the clinic. Martha spent several meetings both at the clinic and at the family's home learning about Jasmin's needs and concerns as well as those of her family members.

At first, Jasmin conveyed that she did not want to meet with any other team members. However, over time, as Martha got to know Jasmin and her family and the things they found to be important, she was able to make individualized recommendations about how working more closely with other team members might be beneficial. Together, they settled on the plan that Jasmin would benefit from receiving CBTp in their sessions to help cope with the symptoms she continued to experience and would also start meeting with the team psychiatrist to discuss medication side effects.

Because Jasmin continued to express the goal of completing her engineering degree, she and Martha decided that Jasmin would meet with the supported employment and education specialist, Scott, to start to figure out how to get back on track. Martha recommended that Jasmin also meet with the peer support specialist for added support and perspective. At first, Jasmin was hesitant, but after one meeting with Paul, the peer specialist, she agreed that it was helpful to interact with and get the perspective of someone who had experienced similar symptoms and shared how he pursued his goals with the support of mental health services. Throughout her treatment with the team, Jasmin at times would meet with specific team members more frequently, particularly when she needed more support or when she was struggling with an increase in symptoms. However, she appreciated being able to decrease the frequency of these meetings and meet with fewer team members during those times when she was feeling more stable and was busy pursuing her educational goals. The fact that she did not feel pressured to follow a regimented treatment schedule allowed her to remain working with the team for 2 years.

Working Within a Multidisciplinary Treatment Team

One of the central elements of providing CSC services is the effective use of a multidisciplinary treatment team. CSC teams are composed of a variety of providers. Most commonly, these include a team leader, who provides administrative and supervisory oversight, and licensed therapists (e.g., psychologists, social workers, mental health counselors, occupational therapists) able to provide therapeutic interventions. These interventions might include individual and group evidence-based psychosocial treatments such as CBTp, social skills training, motivational interviewing, harm reduction, and family education and support. The team also includes medical providers (e.g., prescriber, nurse) able to deliver medication management, health and wellness interventions, and primary care coordination and trained employment or education support specialists who provide community-based support for attaining school and work goals based on the individualized placement and support model. Some teams may also include additional care managers, peer specialists for participants, and peer specialists for family members.

The number of providers necessary to fulfill all of these roles sometimes depends on the configuration of the specific CSC model being followed (e.g., OnTrackNY vs. Navigate vs. EASA), the available resources within a specific agency, and the size of the cohort being served. It is common for team members to hold multiple roles. For example, in addition to having administrative and supervisory responsibilities, the team leader might also deliver individual psychotherapy to a group of participants. The roles of primary therapist and care manager might be combined, with the primary therapist also in charge of managing referrals and performing eligibility evaluations, or the primary therapist might work primarily to provide family education and support. Although most teams have four to six providers (some part time and some full time) serving 30–35 participants, the number of team members is less important than the amount of effort devoted by each provider to working on the CSC team and ensuring that all the roles are covered.

Team collaboration is another essential element for delivering effective CSC treatment. This is accomplished by having weekly team meeting attended by all team members where providers have an opportunity to at least briefly discuss each individual with whom they are working, provide feedback, and review progress toward treatment goals. These meetings can also serve as a platform for team members to strategize about how they might work together to help each participant achieve his or her goals, process and troubleshoot challenges they might be encountering with specific participants and family members, and ensure that the team's culture remains recovery oriented and person centered.

Case Example *(continued)*

During a particular team meeting, Martha noted that she noticed Jasmin decompensating during the past month after she stopped taking her medication, which was leading Martha to believe that Jasmin was not ready to take a course at her local college next semester. Paul reminded Martha that the term *decompensating* is not recovery oriented and encouraged Martha to instead describe in detail the behavioral changes she has noticed and how these changes are affecting Jasmin and her family so that the team could strategize together. Additionally, Paul said that he would share aspects of his recovery story during his next meeting with Jasmin to see if he could provide her with added support.

Scott shared that there is a zero exclusion principle for engaging in work and school, which means that the team should support individuals in their work and school goals without presuming readiness or their ability to succeed. He shared how he has worked with many participants whose symptoms seem to decrease when they are able to actively work on their goals, and taking a class might be just what Jasmin needs at this moment to help her feel better. He offered to work with Jasmin on her preferences to determine good next steps.

This discussion allowed Martha to feel supported by her team on several levels. Jasmin's care was now based on multiple perspectives, which provided a more optimistic outlook and helped relieve some of Martha's concerns. On a practical level, other team members with expertise in their respective areas developed a plan to help support Jasmin and her family.

Clinical Concepts That Drive Coordinated Specialty Care Treatment

Four clinical concepts and practices lie at the core of all services provided by CSC teams: health, home, purpose, and community. Providers within CSC teams are expected to deliver recovery-oriented, person-centered, culturally competent services that are guided by a framework of shared decision making regarding treatment options. Teams that are recovery oriented ascribe to the definition of recovery promoted by the Substance Abuse and Mental Health Services Administration: "A process of change through which individuals improve their health and wellness, live a self-directed life, and strive to reach their full potential"

(Substance Abuse and Mental Health Services Administration 2011). A CSC team might implement the four dimensions of recovery as follows:

1. *Health*: The team works with service participants and their families to make informed decisions to assist individuals in managing symptoms and to support physical and mental health.
2. *Home*: The team helps individuals and their families with concrete case management services, including assistance with insurance, entitlements, and a stable and safe place to live.
3. *Purpose*: All members of the team work with the service participant in order to clarify and meet personal goals around work and/or school.
4. *Community*: The team is responsive to participants' preferences regarding their desired level of interaction with family and friends. Simultaneously, the team also encourages the development of such relationships, including involvement in community groups that may foster support, friendship, and hope.

When working from a recovery perspective, providers convey a sense of hope and focus on individual strengths and resiliency rather than symptoms and impairment. Participants view the process of recovery as one that is nonlinear and progresses over time, allowing them to achieve important life goals (Bennett et al. 2017).

Person-centered care works alongside a recovery philosophy because it positions the participant at the center of the team, collaborating with all of the providers regarding the person's care. The individual's life goals, aspirations, and ambitions drive treatment planning. Furthermore, the individual has a voice and a choice in deciding which treatment is best and what are considered good treatment outcomes (Bennett et al. 2017). It is important that providers allow a space for discussions to occur regarding what participants are experiencing and how they are making sense of their FEP, what it means in the context of their identity and life goals, and how to be part of the solution, instead of attempting to convince them of a diagnosis.

Normalizing the existential questions that program participants may be asking themselves while demonstrating humility about the providers' ability to predict course and outcomes is important. It is not uncommon for young people to attribute the experience of FEP to many different factors, question whether it is a one-time event or lifelong change, and remain skeptical that the services provided by the CSC team are actually what they need (Bennett et al. 2017). As such, when providers are able to walk alongside participants in this journey, using an inquisitive and open stance regarding the individual's and family's understanding about what is happening, participants and families tend to feel respected and valued and are able to build an alliance with the team that allows for better treatment.

Developing culturally competent practices enhances the team's ability to facilitate this process of finding common ground and sustaining an alliance throughout the time that the young person is receiving CSC treatment. Culture can be defined as an evolving process of meaning making that all individuals undergo on the basis of their background and experiences. Multiple aspects of people's social backgrounds can provide a basis for their cultural orientation, including their age, class, race or ethnicity, gender, sexual orientation, geographic culture (urban, suburban, or rural), occupation, language, and, for some, immigration and acculturation (Lewis-Fernandez et al. 2018).

With regard to FEP, culture is important because it guides how an individual and family understand the illness and what steps should be taken. Therefore, it is important that teams spend time developing an understanding of the cultural framework for each participant as well as how the culture of the team shapes the care that is provided. In doing so, the team becomes responsible for developing practices that incorporate relevant knowledge, skills, and attitudes that convey an appreciation for the role of the person and the family as experts on their own experiences and interpretation. The team should elicit the individual's preferences and terms that should be used to describe aspects of the young person's identity (Lewis-Fernandez et al. 2018). An important tool that can help with obtaining some of this information is the Cultural Formulation Interview in the *Diagnostic and Statistical Manual of Mental Disorders*, 5th Edition (DSM-5; American Psychiatric Association 2013). The key is genuinely understanding participants' self-identification and interpretation. The team should not presume that just because participants are of a specific race or religion they ascribe to the beliefs and norms associated with that culture.

Shared decision making then becomes the vehicle for putting together all of these concepts and practices because it provides a systematic framework for making treatment decisions that prioritize what matters most to participants and families by deliberately shifting the power dynamics between providers and participants. In essence, it consists of a process of deliberation whereby providers share their knowledge and the range and strength of the evidence on which their recommendations are based, while at the same time emphasizing how this knowledge aligns with the individual's preferences and values (Elwyn et al. 2017). At the center of shared decision making reside the principles of collaboration: an ability to share information in an accessible format that details all available options relevant to the decisions that program participants find important to make, inclusivity, and active listening to promote participation in treatment decisions.

Enacting shared decision making transcends being aware of or sensitive to what matters most to participants. It requires the use of specific steps to ensure that participants feel heard and are receiving all of the information needed to make informed choices. Shared decision making consists of a three-step process of shared decision making and details what should be happening at each step. The first step, team talk, consists of setting the framework for the collaborative approach, communicating support, and exploring an individual's goals. The second step, option talk, consists of describing the available options with all of the related evidence in an accessible format that allows for deliberation regarding the pros and cons of each option. The third step, decision talk, allows the individual to develop and share informed preferences and make a treatment decision (Elwyn et al. 2017). It is important to note that this process is not linear or final but rather cyclical as individuals progress through treatment and the need for various decisions to be made arises.

Case Example *(continued)*

When working with Jasmin, the team was able to keep her goal of returning to school at the forefront of her treatment. The team worked closely with Jasmin and her family while providing a hopeful message to help her find the best way to pursue her goal of becoming an engineer. Therefore, discussion around medications, therapy, and supported employment and education always connected back to how these treatments were instrumental in allowing Jasmin to pursue the life she wanted for herself.

Another important part of the treatment consisted of offering Jasmin and her family support and developing an understanding of their worldview. Jasmin's family is devout Christian, and it was important to them that Jasmin attend church and have the fellow parishioners pray for her recovery through prayer circles. This was something that Jasmin did not feel comfortable participating in, which led to frequent arguments. The team worked to develop a trusting relationship with Jasmin's supports. With Jasmin's permission, Martha attended a service and had an opportunity to have a discussion with the church's pastor, who has a close relationship with the family. Using the framework of shared decision making, Jasmin, her family, and the rest of the team were able to find some common ground around ways to incorporate other supports into her treatment that are important in the rest of the family's life and whose advice they value. Everyone discussed the options of attending church, meeting with the pastor, or going to a prayer circle and deliberated on the pros and cons of each. Jasmin decided that although she did not feel comfortable going to prayer circles or attending weekly services, she was willing to meet with her mom and the pastor on a more regular basis. Jasmin thought this would demonstrate respect toward her mother's cultural beliefs while also providing the pastor with information that could better help the family deal with Jasmin's difficulties and symptoms.

Thus far in this chapter, we have demonstrated the key components and the various ways in which a high-fidelity CSC program can work to provide services to young people and their families. At the same time, it is important to acknowledge that as the dissemination of CSC programs becomes more far reaching, adaptations will be necessary in order to meet the demands of specific communities and to work within the context of sometimes limited resources. This has become evident when services are implemented in rural settings.

Implementing Coordinated Specialty Care Services in Rural Settings

It is important to consider that distance and variability in available resources and infrastructure might inform the implementation of CSC services across geographic settings. This will impact several factors: 1) team training and functioning, 2) outreach activities, and 3) service delivery. The following subsections include recommendations for useful adaptations that can be implemented in each of these categories to help support the success of CSC teams delivering services in more rural areas.

Team Training and Functioning

As described earlier, CSC teams contain a very specific configuration of team members who require specialized training and support to help bolster their competencies in delivering specialized care. This can prove to be challenging in rural and underresourced areas where there is less access to financial resources, infrastructure, and workforce. Training a CSC team requires protected time and commitment, which can be difficult for agencies with staff who have multiple responsibilities with associated productivity requirements and that lack financial resources for engaging in training.

Creativity and flexibility go a long way toward overcoming some of these barriers. For example, one approach is to schedule trainings during times that are convenient for team members while taking into consideration whether this will lead to decreased productivity or affect their ability to perform other duties. Some organizations develop special productivity codes to account for the necessary training, consultation, and supervision time; others incentivize participation in these activities. In addition, the organization needs to plan resources for reimbursing travel and other costs associated with attending training, consultation, and supervision activities—especially when these activities are at a time or location when the team is not usually together. Conducting these activities face to face, with the entire team, helps to build collaborative relationships while providers acquire knowledge and skills.

Considerations about infrastructure are also necessary for facilitating learning during the training activities, particularly if done remotely.

Measured application of distance learning can be extremely useful. Organizations need to ensure that staff members have the proper equipment (e.g., computer, Web camera, microphone, speakers) to access the training materials. In addition, when using video technology, organizations need to ensure that Internet connections are robust enough to allow a smooth signal for uninterrupted interactions. Having a video freeze during a training or consultation session can break up the flow and interfere with learning.

A similar creative approach should be employed when considering team functioning. Rural and underresourced areas sometimes lack psychiatric providers; therefore, CSC teams should make an effort to attract and retain clinicians who are motivated to work with FEP and practice in a recovery-oriented framework. In addition, there are often logistical issues that might impede effective team functioning, such as when team members are not colocated. Teams may need to be flexible in the format of team meetings—either scheduling early enough in the day so that team members can spend the rest of the time in the community or using video or teleconferencing technologies. It takes extra effort to work as a team when members are not physically in the same place; however, it is not impossible.

Outreach Activities

Some of the most important activities performed by CSC teams are those associated with outreach because this helps to ensure appropriate and rapid referrals to the program. In rural and underresourced areas, it is vital that outreach activities are tailored to meet the individual needs of the community and its culture. When outreach activities are performed by staff members who are from the community and are keyed into the local network, their understanding of the culture, stakeholder priorities, and important relationships can help obtain buy-in from referral sources as well as more effectively engage potential participants. If, on the other hand, the team member performing outreach is not local, it is recommended that he or she take the time to develop effective working relationships with stakeholders within and outside typical health care settings (e.g., hospitals, schools, jails, chamber of commerce, Rotary Club, Knights of Columbus, faith-based organizations).

Service Delivery

The delivery of the CSC model can also require several adaptations and an added layer of flexibility and creativity in order for the team to effectively work with participants and their supports in rural and underresourced communities. One important consideration is that the number of participants being served by each team member and productivity expectations (if they exist) need to account for the additional time required to travel, sometimes long distances, to home or community sites where participants choose to meet with team members. Organizations need to recognize the additional time and effort needed by team members in order to adequately reach, engage, and work with participants and their families. This is especially relevant in rural areas where public transportation may not be readily available and the ability of team members to demonstrate flexibility in communication and scheduling is critical to developing a solid working alliance. Some recommendations include lowered productivity expectations to account for nonbillable travel time and adequate reimbursement for mileage or access to organization-provided vehicles.

When some team members are not able to meet in the community and participants are unable to get to the office, telehealth can be a useful tool. In fact, some younger people are more used to electronic communication and thus are more open to telehealth and other technology-associated communications. In addition to allowing for prescribers who are not co-located to serve participants, telehealth can also facilitate consultation and liaison between providers at the CSC program and others with experience and expertise in treating FEP.

However, as with other aspects of CSC, technology is useful only when it is consistent and reliable. Participants may not have reliable cellular service or Internet access where they live. Similarly, Internet service may be slow and may not support full video. Here again, flexibility and creativity are in order. Some organizations partner with resources closer to where participants live as a workaround. Having appointments at places such as recreation centers, libraries, businesses, or other health care providers or systems combines convenience, comfort, and the availability of more reliable Internet or cellular service. This serves the double task of providing reliable, convenient locations for participants and family members to receive services and building awareness and collaborative relationships with key community resources.

Conclusion

CSC is a treatment model for delivering team-based care for young people experiencing their first episode of psychosis, which has been demonstrated to improve outcomes. Although there are several variations for configuring this multi-element, multidisciplinary team approach, CSC includes several evidence-based practices that should be offered to individuals and families, including individual and group psychotherapy, family education and support, evidence-based psychopharmacology and wellness strategies, supported employment and education, and care management. It is important to remember that it is not solely the distinct interventions delivered but rather the process through which team members collaborate with each other and the underlying messages of hope, recovery, and empowerment that the team conveys to participants that seems to make a difference in young people's lives. Furthermore, it is important to note that even when adaptations to the model are needed, employing creativity and flexibility and appropriately adapting the implementation to meet the needs of the community being served ultimately lead to the success of the program and its participants.

KEY CONCEPTS

- Coordinated specialty care is an evidence-based multi-element early intervention treatment approach for young people experiencing a first episode of nonaffective psychosis. It is a time-limited intervention delivered by a team that has received specialized training.

- CSC provides participants with a suite of evidence-based practices that include individual and group psychotherapy, assertive care management, supported employment and education services, family education and support, and wellness and primary care coordination. Some teams provide additional services such as peer support.

- Recovery is viewed as a nonlinear "process of change over time through which individuals improve their health and wellness, live a self-directed life, and strive to reach their full potential" (Substance Abuse and Mental Health Services Administration 2011). Recovery for many individuals means learning to manage symptoms effectively and to use wellness strategies in order to achieve the things that matter in life: love, work, and community contribution.

- CSC relies on shared decision making, an approach to setting goals and making treatment decisions that relies on techniques such as decision aids, discussion of options, decisional balance exercises, comparing parallel ratings, and negotiating compromises. Shared decision making aims to increase knowledge, increase the individual's participation in and commitment to treatment, enhance the professional's understanding of the individual's values and preferences, and strengthen the therapeutic alliance.

- Professional practice providers are responsible for developing cultural competency, which is grounded in culturally relevant knowledge, skills, and attitudes.

Discussion Questions

1. What are some of the advantages associated with starting a CSC program in your community for both providers and young individuals experiencing FEP?

2. Given the range of services provided by CSC teams, what might be some ways in which an agency can support putting together this multidisciplinary treatment team?

3. Team collaboration is an important component of delivering effective CSC treatment. What are some concrete strategies that promote team collaboration and communication?

4. How might teams encourage and promote participant engagement with the treatment team across time? Are there any creative strategies that are unique to your community?

5. What steps can team members take to ensure that they remain recovery oriented and hopeful and that they are actively using formal shared decision-making steps?

Suggested Readings

Bennett M, Lee R, Watkins L, et al: OnTrackNY Team Manual. New York, Center for Practice Innovations, 2017. Available at: www.ontrackny.org/Resources. Accessed October 5, 2018.

Crisanti AS, Altschul D, Smart L, et al: Implementation of Coordinated Specialty Services for First Episode Psychosis in Rural and Frontier Communities. Albuquerque, NM, University of New Mexico, 2015. Available at: www.nasmhpd.org/sites/default/files/Rural-Fact Sheet-_1.pdf. Accessed October 5, 2018.

Dixon LB, Goldman H, Srihari V, et al: Transforming the treatment of schizophrenia in the United States: the RAISE initiative. Annu Rev Clin Psychol 14:237–258, 2018 29328779

Heinssen RK, Goldstein AB, Azrin ST: Evidence-Based Treatments for First Episode Psychosis: Components of Coordinated Specialty Care. Rockville, MD, National Institute of Mental Health, 2014. Available at:

www.nimh.nih.gov/health/topics/schizophrenia/raise/nimh-white-paper-csc-for-fep_147096.pdf. Accessed October 5, 2018.

Mueser KT, Gingerich S: NAVIGATE Team Members' Guide. Bethesda, MD, National Institute of Mental Health, 2014. Available at: http://navigateconsultants.org/manuals. Accessed October 5, 2018.

References

American Psychiatric Association: Diagnostic and Statistical Manual of Mental Disorders, 5th Edition. Arlington, VA, American Psychiatric Association, 2013

Azrin ST, Goldstein AB, Heinssen RK: Early intervention for psychosis: the recovery after an initial schizophrenia episode project. Psychiatr Ann 45(11):548–553, 2016

Bennett M, Lee R, Watkins L, et al: OnTrackNY Team Manual. New York, Center for Practice Innovations, 2017. Available at: www.ontrackny.org/Resources. Accessed October 5, 2018.

Correll CU, Galling B, Pawar A, et al. Comparison of early intervention services vs treatment as usual for early-phase psychosis: a systematic review, meta-analysis and meta-regression. JAMA Psychiatry 75(6):555–565, 2018 29800949

Dixon LB, Goldman HH, Bennett ME, et al: Implementing coordinated specialty care for early psychosis: the RAISE connection program. Psychiatr Serv. 66(7):691–698, 2015 25772764

Elwyn G, Durand MA, Song J, et al: A three-talk model for shared decision making: multistage consultation process. BMJ 359:j4891, 2017 29109079

Gafoor R, Nitsch D, McCrone P, et al: Effect of early intervention on 5-year outcome in non-affective psychosis. Br J Psychiatry 196(5):372–376, 2010 20435962

Grawe RW, Falloon IR, Widen JH, et al: Two years of continued early treatment for recent-onset schizophrenia: a randomised controlled study. Acta Psychiatr Scand 114(5):328–336, 2006 17022792

Heinssen RK, Goldstein AB, Azrin ST: Evidence-Based Treatments for First Episode Psychosis: Components of Coordinated Specialty Care. Rockville, MD, National Institute of Mental Health, 2014. Available at: www.nimh.nih.gov/health/topics/schizophrenia/raise/nimh-white-paper-csc-for-fep_147096.pdf. Accessed October 5, 2018.

Kane JM, Schooler NR, Marcy P, et al: The RAISE early treatment program for first-episode psychosis: background, rationale, and study design. J Clin Psychiatry 76(3):240–246, 2015 25830446

Lewis-Fernandez R, Jimenez-Solomon O, Bello I, et al: OnTrackNY Delivering Culturally Competent Care in FEP Manual. New York, Center for Practice Innovations, 2018

Srihari VH, Tek C, Kucukgoncu S, et al: First-episode services for psychotic disorders in the U.S. public sector: a pragmatic randomized controlled trial. Psychiatr Serv 66(7):705–712, 2015 25639994

Substance Abuse and Mental Health Services Administration: SAMHSA announces a working definition of "recovery" from mental disorders and substance use disorders. December 2011. Available at: www.samhsa.gov/newsroom/press-announcements/201112220300. Accessed October 5, 2018.

Psychopharmacology for People in Early Psychosis

Jian-Ping Zhang, M.D., Ph.D.
Douglas L. Noordsy, M.D.

Pharmacotherapy in First-Episode Psychosis

Antipsychotic medications are the mainstay of pharmacotherapy for people with schizophrenia and are also a key component of first-episode treatment. Because research has shown that duration of untreated psychosis (DUP) is correlated with worse outcome, successful treatment of the first psychotic episode is crucial for minimizing the cascading effects of social and vocational deterioration. In general, both typical, or first-generation, antipsychotics (FGAs) and atypical, or second-generation, antipsychotics (SGAs) are effective in improving positive symptoms. However, not all antipsychotics are created equal. Large clinical trials among people with first-episode psychosis (FEP) and meta-analyses have demonstrated that some antipsychotics are more efficacious than others. There are also significant differences in each medication's side-effect profile. Therefore, careful evaluation of a patient's symptomatology, family history, and prior medication exposure is the key to tailoring treatment to each individual in order to maximize efficacy and minimize potential side effects.

Although we can find guidance in the general schizophrenia treatment literature, it should be noted that randomized controlled trials (RCTs) of people with chronic schizophrenia have several limitations. These include confounding effects of prior medication use, potential overrepresentation of partially responsive or treatment-nonadherent patients, and a tendency to recruit patients with low pre-study functioning levels in whom ongoing illness and treatment effects might reduce overall treatment response. Conversely, some trials might enroll more responsive patients who are eligible for and willing to consent to participation in RCTs, thereby, again, potentially washing out differences between medications that would be apparent in more heterogeneous, real-life samples. Therefore, the results of large FEP clinical trials such as the European Union First Episode Schizophrenia Trial (EUFEST; Kahn et al. 2008), Comparison of Atypicals in First Episode of Psychosis (CAFE; McEvoy et al. 2007), and the Center for Intervention Development and Advanced Research (CIDAR) clinical trial (Robinson et al. 2015) provide useful information as to how we can best treat people in their first episode. These studies point to several issues that are unique to pharmacotherapy in FEP and should be considered in initial treatment planning and follow-up care.

Compared with treatment of individuals with chronic schizophrenia, treatment of first-episode patients is generally characterized by higher response rates, lower effective antipsychotic doses, and a higher sensitivity to drug-induced adverse effects. Hence, studies in first-episode populations offer the unique opportunity to examine the effectiveness and side effects of antipsychotics in patients who are more representative of the entire schizophrenia population and in whom important initial treatment effects can be observed. Furthermore, prior therapeutic and adverse response patterns to antipsychotics are largely unknown in individuals with FEP, so treatment recommendations must be based on information other than past treatment history.

Selection of an Antipsychotic Drug to Treat First-Episode Psychosis

The goal of antipsychotic treatment for people in FEP is to achieve significant treatment response, which will facilitate symptom remission and recovery from the illness and minimize drug-induced side effects, which will help treatment adherence and long-term treatment success. Unlike medication selection for patients with chronic illness, for whom selection of antipsychotic drugs can be guided by past treatment history, the choice of the first agent for patients in FEP needs to be based on evidence provided by clinical trials.

More than 20 published randomized clinical trials have been published comparing antipsychotic medications in people with FEP. One comprehensive meta-analysis examined the relative efficacy and tolerability of individual SGAs versus individual FGAs in 13 head-to-head trials with more than 2,500 patients (Zhang et al. 2013). Although there was no significant difference in overall efficacy between the two antipsychotic classes, SGAs had slight advantages in treating negative symptoms and improving cognitive function. Olanzapine seemed to outperform the FGA comparators in several outcome measures, but the effect sizes were relatively small (i.e., Hedges' $g=0.1$–0.3). SGAs were significantly better than FGAs in maintaining patients in treatment with lower all-cause discontinuation rate. As a class, FGAs caused more extrapyramidal effects (EPS) and tardive dyskinesia than SGAs, whereas SGAs were generally associated with more weight gain and cardiometabolic changes. In summary, SGAs, including olanzapine, risperidone, and quetiapine, may have a slight advantage over FGAs in treatment efficacy and persistence, although they are more likely to cause weight gain and metabolic side effects.

Recently, our group conducted another comprehensive meta-analytic review to compare the efficacy and side effects of various SGAs in treating FEP (Zhang et al. 2016). Twenty-two randomized acute treatment trials with more than 3,600 individuals in FEP using seven SGAs (olanzapine, risperidone, quetiapine, ziprasidone, aripiprazole, clozapine, and amisulpride) were included. Clozapine and amisulpride were used in only one study each, so the meta-analytic findings were based mostly on the other five drugs. Although there were no differences in treatment response rate and all-cause discontinuation, olanzapine and risperidone significantly outperformed quetiapine and ziprasidone in reducing overall symptoms as well as positive symptoms, with effect sizes ranging from 0.20 to 0.85 (all P values<0.05). Aripiprazole also had a slight advantage over quetiapine in total symptom reduction, but the difference was only approaching statistical significance. All drugs were similar in treating negative symptoms, except that in one study, aripiprazole was better than risperidone in treating negative symptoms such as avolition, apathy, asociality, and anhedonia (Robinson et al. 2015). Consistent with clinical experience, olanzapine caused significantly more weight gain than other drugs. Risperidone caused more EPS than olanzapine, whereas aripiprazole was more likely than quetiapine to induce akathisia.

On the basis of the meta-analytic findings and results from large FEP clinical trials, and after efficacy and side effects are carefully weighed, it seems that SGAs, especially risperidone and aripiprazole, should be considered as a first-line drug choice in treating people in FEP. Although olanzapine is as efficacious as risperidone, its weight gain liability and potential metabolic side effects make it less suitable as a first-line drug.

Quetiapine and ziprasidone may be considered as second-line drugs. Haloperidol and other FGAs may also be considered if a patient has failed or cannot tolerate first-line or second-line drugs. The evidence on using clozapine in FEP is limited. However, clozapine is certainly the drug of choice for patients whose illness proves to be treatment refractory, and there may be advantages to starting clozapine within the first year of illness when needed (Ballon et al. 2018). In addition, several newer antipsychotic medications, such as lurasidone, asenapine, and cariprazine, have shown relatively good tolerability in people with schizophrenia, a desirable characteristic in first-line medication. However, no clinical trials have been conducted to test the efficacy and tolerability of these medications in individuals with FEP.

Treatment Response Rate and Drug Dosing

The definitions of treatment response vary among medication treatment studies. Most studies use a percentage of total symptom score reduction, measured by either the Positive and Negative Symptoms Scale (PANSS; Kay et al. 1987) or the Brief Psychiatric Rating Scale (Woerner et al. 1988), or other equivalent instruments. RCTs among patients with chronic schizophrenia tend to use a 20% reduction of symptoms, whereas FEP trials usually use more stringent criteria, such as 40% or 50% reduction. It is generally agreed that patients in FEP need to have clinically significant symptom improvement to promote functional recovery; therefore, 50% or more reduction in total symptoms is more appropriate and a reasonable target for a substantial proportion of patients to achieve. A few studies have used even more stringent criteria, such as mild or lower rating on PANSS items and Clinical Global Impressions scale scores (Guy et al. 1976) of much improved or very much improved, which is close to the definition of symptom remission. Table 12–1 shows the average medication dose, response rate, definition of treatment response, and all-cause discontinuation rate (a measure of treatment effectiveness) in modern medication trials for FEP.

Overall, short-term treatment response rate in FEP clinical trials ranged widely from 9.1% to 76.2%, largely due to variations in medication used, treatment duration, and definition of treatment response. Averaging across multiple trials, risperidone, olanzapine, and aripiprazole had slightly higher response rates (44.8%, 45.1%, and 46.8%, respectively) than haloperidol and quetiapine (38.7% and 39.5%), with ziprasidone in between (41.2%). These numbers are slightly higher than the average response rate in people with chronic schizophrenia. Leucht and colleagues (2009) found in a meta-analysis of drug registration trials

TABLE 12–1. Medication used in large first-episode psychosis (FEP) clinical trials, dose, response rate, and all-cause discontinuation rate

Trials	N	Trial duration	Medication/mean dose	Short-term response rate	Response criteria	Time to response	Discontinuation rate (all-cause)	Time to discontinuation	Long-term response rate
Emsley and Risperidone Working Group 1999	183	6 weeks	Haloperidol 5.6 mg	56%	≥50% reduction on PANSS	NR	31.0%	NR	NR
			Risperidone 6.1 mg	63%			20.2%		
Lieberman et al. 2003a	160	52 weeks	Clozapine 400 mg	NR	≥50% reduction on BPRS + CGI-S ≤3 + ≤3 on BPRS positive symptoms (defined as "remission")	8 weeks	10%	NR	81%
			Chlorpromazine 600 mg (12 weeks)			12 weeks	11% (12 weeks) (15% and 22.5% at 52 weeks)		79%

TABLE 12–1. Medication used in large first-episode psychosis (FEP) clinical trials, dose, response rate, and all-cause discontinuation rate (*continued*)

Trials	N	Trial duration	Medication/ mean dose	Short-term response rate	Response criteria	Time to response	Discontin- uation rate (all-cause)	Time to discontin- uation	Long-term response rate
Lieberman et al. 2003b	263	104 weeks	Haloperidol 4.4 mg	46%	≥30% reduction on PANSS+ CGI-S ≥4+ mild or lower ratings of positive symptoms	8.4 weeks	46%	230 days	67.2%
			Olanzapine 9.1 mg (12 weeks)	55% (12 weeks)		7.9 weeks (within 12 weeks)	32% (12 weeks)	322 days (2 years)	59.9%
Early Psychosis Global Working Group; Schooler et al. 2005	555	104 weeks	Haloperidol 2.9 mg	76.2% (12 weeks) (9.1% for >50% reduction on PANSS)	>20% reduction on PANSS	22 days	22.4%	218 days	77.8%

TABLE 12–1. Medication used in large first-episode psychosis (FEP) clinical trials, dose, response rate, and all-cause discontinuation rate (*continued*)

Trials	N	Trial duration	Medication/mean dose	Short-term response rate	Response criteria	Time to response	Discontinuation rate (all-cause)	Time to discontinuation	Long-term response rate
			Risperidone 3.3 mg	73.6% (12 weeks) (10.6% for >50% reduction on PANSS)		26 days (12 weeks)	22.3% (12 weeks) (for 2 years: 36.5%, 42.1%)	192 days (2 years)	75.5%
PAFIP; Crespo-Facorro et al. 2006	172	6 weeks	Haloperidol 5.4 mg	57.1%	>40% reduction on BPRS	4.32 weeks	57.1%	7.9 months	96.4%
			Risperidone 4.0 mg	52.5%		4.85 weeks	43.9%	9.6 months	92.1%
			Olanzapine 15.3 mg	63.6%		4.36 weeks	32.7% (1 year)	10.0 months (1 year)	98.2% (6 months)

TABLE 12–1. Medication used in large first-episode psychosis (FEP) clinical trials, dose, response rate, and all-cause discontinuation rate (*continued*)

Trials	N	Trial duration	Medication/ mean dose	Short-term response rate	Response criteria	Time to response	Discontinuation rate (all-cause)	Time to discontinuation	Long-term response rate
Robinson et al. 2006	112	16 weeks	Risperidone 3.9 mg	54.3%	Mild or lower of SADS-C+PD positive symptoms+ CGI ≤2	10.4 weeks	26.7%	12.1 weeks	NR
			Olanzapine 11.8 mg	43.7%		10.9 weeks	28.3%	11.5 weeks	
CAFE; McEvoy et al. 2007	400	52 weeks	Risperidone 2.4 mg	NR	≤3 on all PANSS items+CGI-S ≤3	NR	71.4%	25 weeks	65%
			Olanzapine 11.7 mg				68.4%	28 weeks	64%
			Quetiapine 506 mg				70.9%	25 weeks	58%
EUFEST; Khan et al. 2008	498	52 weeks	Haloperidol 3.0 mg	34.0%	≥50% reduction on PANSS	NR	72%	0.5 months	37%

TABLE 12–1. Medication used in large first-episode psychosis (FEP) clinical trials, dose, response rate, and all-cause discontinuation rate (*continued*)

Trials	N	Trial duration	Medication/ mean dose	Short-term response rate	Response criteria	Time to response	Discontin-uation rate (all-cause)	Time to discontin-uation	Long-term response rate
			Amisulpride 451 mg	52.9%			40%	5.3 months	67%
			Olanzapine 12.6 mg	46.7%			33%	6.3 months	67%
			Quetiapine 499 mg	44.2%			53%	1.2 months	46%
			Ziprasidone 107 mg	37.8%			45%	1.1 months	56%
TEOSS; Sikich et al. 2008	119	8 weeks	Molindone 59.9 mg	50%	≥20% reduction on PANSS+ CGI-I ≤2	NR	39%	5.9 weeks	NR
			Olanzapine 11.4 mg	34%			53%	5.9 weeks	
			Risperidone 2.8 mg	46%			33%	6.4 weeks	

TABLE 12–1. Medication used in large first-episode psychosis (FEP) clinical trials, dose, response rate, and all-cause discontinuation rate (*continued*)

Trials	N	Trial duration	Medication/ mean dose	Short-term response rate	Response criteria	Time to response	Discontinuation rate (all-cause)	Time to discontinuation	Long-term response rate
German Research Network; Möller et al. 2008	289	8 weeks	Risperidone 3.8 mg	49.3%	>30% reduction on PANSS+ CGI-S ≤4+mild or better ratings of positive symptoms	41.0 days	38.5%	50.8 days	NR
			Haloperidol 3.7 mg	49.6%		38.6 days	54.1%	44.0 days	
Cuesta et al. 2009	100	26 weeks	Olanzapine 10.2 mg	NR	>50% reduction on SAPS	NR	45.5%	12.7 weeks	70.5%
			Risperidone 6.0 mg				50.0%	11.7 weeks	76.8%
San et al. 2012	114	52 weeks	Haloperidol 5.8 mg	19%	>50% reduction on PANSS	NR	85.7%	125 days	NR
			Olanzapine 16.2 mg	40%			40.0%	260 days	

TABLE 12–1. Medication used in large first-episode psychosis (FEP) clinical trials, dose, response rate, and all-cause discontinuation rate (*continued*)

Trials	N	Trial duration	Medication/ mean dose	Short-term response rate	Response criteria	Time to response	Discontin- uation rate (all-cause)	Time to discontin- uation	Long-term response rate
			Risperidone 5.1 mg	36%			56.5%	187 days	
			Quetiapine 672 mg	26%			64.0%	206 days	
			Ziprasidone 117 mg	30%			80.0%	143 days	
Zhang and Dai 2012	254	52 weeks	Paliperidone 6.4 mg	NR	NR	NR	22.2%	NR	NR
			Aripiprazole 14.5 mg				21.1%		
			Ziprasidone 65.3 mg				16.9%		

TABLE 12–1. Medication used in large first-episode psychosis (FEP) clinical trials, dose, response rate, and all-cause discontinuation rate (*continued*)

Trials	N	Trial duration	Medication/ mean dose	Short-term response rate	Response criteria	Time to response	Discontin- uation rate (all-cause)	Time to discontin- uation	Long-term response rate
PAFIP; Crespo-Facorro et al. 2013	202	12 weeks	Aripiprazole 16.8 mg	61.1%	≥50% reduction in BPRS	NR	23.1%	5.3 weeks	NR
			Ziprasidone 87.7 mg	36.5%			37.1%	5.1 weeks	
			Quetiapine 358.3 mg	50.0%			61.8%	5.1 weeks	
Ou et al. 2013	260	6 weeks	Ziprasidone 138.2 mg	NR	NR	NR	8.5%	NR	NR
			Olanzapine 19.0 mg				14.6%		

TABLE 12–1. Medication used in large first-episode psychosis (FEP) clinical trials, dose, response rate, and all-cause discontinuation rate (*continued*)

Trials	N	Trial duration	Medication/mean dose	Short-term response rate	Response criteria	Time to response	Discontinuation rate (all-cause)	Time to discontinuation	Long-term response rate
CIDAR trial; Robinson et al. 2015	198	12 weeks	Aripiprazole 14.8 mg	62.8%	Mild or lower of 4 BPRS positive symptoms + CGI-I ≤2	8.0 weeks	37.9%	8.3 weeks	NR
			Risperidone 3.2 mg	56.8%		8.2 weeks	43.9%	8.2 weeks	
Pagsberg et al. 2017	113	12 weeks	Aripiprazole 14.6 mg	23%	≥30% reduction in PANSS and CGI-I ≤2	NR	35%	9.3 weeks	NR
			Quetiapine ER 451.8 mg	23%			22%	10.4 weeks	

Abbreviations. BPRS=Brief Psychiatric Rating Scale; CAFE=Comparison of Atypicals in First Episode of Psychosis; CGI-I=Clinical Global Impressions—Improvement; CGI-S=Clinical Global Impressions—Severity; CIDAR=Center for Intervention Development and Advanced Research; CNFEST=Chinese First-Episode Schizophrenia Trial; EUFEST=European Union First Episode Schizophrenia Trial; NR=not reported; PAFIP=Programa Atención Fases Iniciales de Psicosis; PANSS=Positive and Negative Symptoms Scale; SADS-C=Schedule for Affective Disorders and Schizophrenia—Change; SAPS=Scale for the Assessment of Positive Symptoms; TEOSS=Treatment of Early-Onset Schizophrenia Spectrum Disorders.
Source. Adapted from Zhang et al. 2013.

(mostly in patients with chronic schizophrenia) that the average response rate was 41% for SGAs and 29% for haloperidol. In one large clinical trial comparing olanzapine and haloperidol (Lieberman et al. 2003b), 45% of patients with chronic schizophrenia ($n=1,913$) responded to olanzapine, compared with 67% of patients in their first episode ($n=83$) using the same criteria for response. Given the fact that many FEP trials used more stringent criteria to define treatment response, the response rate would have been much higher in patients with FEP than in patients who had had multiple episodes if the same criteria had been applied to both type of studies.

In contrast, effective doses of antipsychotic drugs used in individuals with FEP are relatively lower than in chronic patients. Across the large FEP clinical trials summarized in Table 12–1, the average daily dose is 4.0 mg for risperidone, 13.0 mg for olanzapine, 497 mg for quetiapine, 15.2 mg for aripiprazole, and 103 mg for ziprasidone. The average daily dose for haloperidol is 4.4 mg. Almost all of the FEP studies used a flexible dosing strategy. Therefore, these relatively lower doses were achieved while balancing efficacy and side effects. Many young people in FEP are sensitive to antipsychotic drugs because of lack of prior exposure, so they are more susceptible to developing side effects such as EPS, akathisia, and sedation. Rapid weight gain in young patients who are treated with antipsychotic drugs is very problematic, not only for metabolic health consequences but also for patients' self-image and social acceptance. Severe side effects from antipsychotic drugs may give patients a bad experience during their first treatment episode, which may lead to treatment nonadherence and worse long-term outcomes. Therefore, slow dose titration and close monitoring of drug-induced side effects are critical when treating a patient with FEP to ensure that patients will stay in treatment and obtain maximum benefits from treatment (Ballon et al. 2018).

Duration of Treatment

Clinicians treating patients with FEP will want to address the question of when improvement will be seen with both patients and their family. There is a large variation in how quickly a patient's psychosis responds to antipsychotic treatment. Unless psychosis is induced by substance use, which may quickly remit once the triggering substance is discontinued, it usually takes weeks for a patient's psychotic symptoms to improve. In studies listed in Table 12–1, the average time to response ranged from 4 to 11 weeks, with more studies in the range of 7–9 weeks. Patients will start to improve within the first 1–2 weeks of initiating treatment, often within days, but it is reasonable to estimate that many patients will need about 2 months of treatment to achieve significant improvement. In people with chronic schizophrenia, several studies have found that the amount of symptom improvement after 2 weeks of taking antipsychotic drugs is predictive of treatment response after 3 months. However, this phenomenon has not panned out in individuals with FEP. One study found that patients continued to improve week after week, up to 16 weeks of treatment, regardless how much they improve after 2 weeks (Gallego et al. 2011).

Note that these data resulted from monotherapy with a single antipsychotic medication. In clinical practice, clinicians often face pressure from health insurers and family members to get patients better quickly. Frequently, patients are treated with their first antipsychotic medication for 2–4 weeks, then switched to another if they do not improve fast enough. This practice may increase the chance of drug-induced side effects without actually helping patients improve faster. We recommend that patients continue to take their first antipsychotic medication for at least 8 weeks as long as they are able to tolerate it and show some response to treatment.

After significant improvement in psychosis with treatment (many individuals may have complete remission of all positive symptoms after their first episode), patients and their families often ask when they can stop taking medications. It is common for patients who have been hospitalized during their first psychotic episode to be taking high doses of multiple medications at discharge and experiencing significant, unfamiliar side effects. Patients may become nonadherent to the medication regimen, sometimes with the support of their family. In clinical trials conducted in North America and Europe, all-cause discontinuation rate within the short-term acute treatment phase (6–16 weeks) ranged from 20% to 57% (Table 12–1). The rate increased to 33%–81% within 1–2 years of treatment.

The question often arises whether a patient can be taken off medication without any further psychotic relapse, and if not, how soon a patient will have a relapse after stopping antipsychotic medication. Data on relapse after the first episode of psychosis are relatively scarce compared with data on treatment efficacy. However, both clinical experience and limited research data demonstrate that patients will be more likely to relapse into another psychotic episode when they are not taking antipsychotic medication than when they are. One study showed that after achieving responder status during the first year of treatment for psychosis, patients who adhered to their medication regimen had an 11.2% relapse rate, compared with a 26.9% relapse rate among patients who did not adhere to their medication regimen or stopped medication treatment (Crespo-Facorro et al. 2011).

Naturalistic follow-up studies of people with FEP up to 5 years after treatment commencement have suggested a progressive increment in the cumulative rate for relapse, from 16.2% at 1-year follow-up to 81.9%

at 5-year follow-up for a first episode of schizophrenia, and the top predictor of relapse is medication nonadherence (Robinson et al. 1999). Tiihonen and colleagues (2018) recently confirmed higher rates of treatment failure in patients who stop compared with those who continue antipsychotic medication following a first episode of schizophrenia in a large population sample across Finland with up to a 16-year follow-up; the study authors also found that time on medication prior to discontinuation is not protective against relapse. Therefore, it seems that the chance of relapse is substantial when a patient stops taking antipsychotic medication.

Preventing the second psychotic episode and helping individuals and families understand the risks of relapse and disease progression should be a large part of maintenance treatment. With each subsequent psychotic relapse, the risk of developing persistent psychotic symptoms increases. Recurrent psychotic episodes are associated with progressive loss of gray matter that may mediate cognitive impairment and treatment resistance. Moreover, relapse is likely to interfere with the social development and networks of young people suffering from psychosis, which may have a significant impact on long-term psychosocial and vocational functioning. The second edition of the American Psychiatric Association treatment guideline for schizophrenia, published in 2004 (no longer considered to be current), recommends indefinite antipsychotic drug treatment or, after at least 1 year of complete symptom remission, discontinuation of drug therapy with close follow-up and a plan of antipsychotic reinstitution with symptom recurrence (Lehman et al. 2004; see also Dixon et al. 2009 for update).

There are certainly controversies about the potential consequences of long-term antipsychotic use, but the general consensus is that for most people with first-episode psychosis, continued antipsychotic treatment will lower risks of relapse. However, regardless of practice guidelines and empirical evidence, many patients will attempt at least one trial of medication discontinuation after psychosis remission. For these individuals, it is critical that the treating clinician work closely with other members of the treatment team, the patient, and the patient's family on supervised medication discontinuation, perhaps first carefully tapering the medication to the lowest effective dose for maintenance to minimize side effects. When a patient chooses to stop medication, ensuring a slow tapering schedule with continuing engagement in other components of treatment and carefully monitoring for signs of relapse is advisable. Personalized early warning signs of relapse should be identified with the patient and family. Finally, it is also important to maintain an as-needed prescription after medication discontinuation so the patient can restart antipsychotic medication immediately on the first indication of relapse.

Shared Decision Making in Antipsychotic Drug Treatment

Successful treatment of FEP and complete recovery from the illness are not only critical to patients' long-term prognosis but also have significant impact on future treatment and relapse prevention (Kane et al. 2016). As discussed previously, many young people with FEP recover quickly, and thus, they frequently question whether they need to keep taking medications. Antipsychotic medications are not benign and carry multiple tolerability challenges. In addition, many people with FEP have used substances such as marijuana and may attribute their psychosis to substance use. They may hope that as long as they stop or control their substance use, they will not have another episode of psychosis. Developmentally, transition-age youth operate in a short time horizon and commonly underestimate risks. As such, lack of a disease framework for understanding their experience of psychosis can undermine logical recognition of need for treatment. Research has shown that lack of understanding regarding the nature of their illness is a predictor of treatment nonadherence and poor prognosis. Unless this is addressed effectively, treatment persistence is a significant problem for people after FEP.

Interestingly, medication refusal may at times serve patients' need for autonomy. Clinicians traditionally provide specific medical advice by consulting the biomedical literature and considering what is in the best interest of the patient. However, this approach to medical decision making may be experienced as paternalistic and does not take into account the perspective or preferences of the patient. Nonadherence may result from lack of patient input in medical decision making and dissatisfaction with the treatment relationship. A shared decision-making approach, in which clinicians and patients (as well as families and other support network members) work together to arrive at medical decisions after careful education about decision parameters and options and inclusion of patients' perspectives, values, goals, and preferences for treatment, is optimal. Research has shown that use of shared decision making in treatment of people with schizophrenia leads to higher patient satisfaction, resulting in better medication adherence and improved symptom regulation. Other studies have shown that shared decision making results in better quality of life, fewer unmet needs, and greater satisfaction with treatment.

Shared decision making is particularly relevant in treatment of people during and after their first episode of psychosis because of their unfamiliarity with their disorder, their developmental stage, and their sensitivity to medication-induced side effects. Antipsychotic medications are not easy to take. Bothersome side effects can quickly lead to a

negative experience of medication, thereby affecting long-term perceptions of medication treatment. Cultural attitudes toward Western medicine and medication taking must be considered and addressed as well.
There is little research specifically evaluating the effectiveness of shared
decision making in first-episode treatment. However, clinical experience in our early psychosis programs suggests that shared decision
making does help build therapeutic relationships with patients, increase treatment engagement of patients and their families, and decrease treatment dropout rate. Using a shared decision-making model
to work with patients in FEP usually involves the following steps:

1. Provide psychoeducation to patients and family regarding the nature of the illness, role of medication treatment, and possible long-
   term outcomes.
2. Discuss treatment options with various antipsychotic medications
   and explain benefits and efficacy and potential risks and side effects
   associated with each recommended option. Conduct a risk-benefit
   analysis with an emphasis on achieving and maintaining remission.
3. Listen to what the patient and family say regarding their needs and
   wishes for treatment and their cultural preferences and answer any
   questions that they may have about medications, other treatment,
   diagnosis, and prognosis.
4. Enter principled negotiation with the patient regarding medication
   choice, dosing, follow-up interval, laboratory tests, and other related
   issues, taking into account the patient's needs and requests.
5. When a patient chooses to stop taking medication, encourage him or
   her to stay in treatment and closely monitor for signs of relapse collaboratively to reduce risk for periods of untreated psychosis.

The goal of the shared decision-making approach is to keep patients
engaged with a strong sense of ownership over their treatment choices
and the relative merits of each option. Compromise is necessary at
times to meet the patient where he or she is and to increase patient satisfaction with treatment. This give-and-take occurs at every follow-up
visit, and the collaborative relationship between the clinician and the
patient continues when the clinician is evaluating treatment outcomes
and dealing with emerging issues in treatment. When a patient arrives
at a treatment decision after considering risks, benefits, and alternatives
with the help of the treating clinician, he or she is more likely to adhere
to the treatment choice, thus improving long-term outcomes.

Case Example

Dave was a 24-year-old graduate student when he experienced onset of
paranoia, ideas of reference, confusion, and disorganized thinking and be-

haviors. He was treated with olanzapine during an acute hospitalization. On referral to our early psychosis clinic, he was experiencing residual ideas of reference and fear of things getting out of control, as well as sedation and weight gain. Olanzapine had already been tapered from 20 mg to 5 mg nightly by his prior provider. After reviewing the rationale for maintenance antipsychotic treatment to prevent relapse and available medication options, we agreed to try switching to risperidone 1 mg nightly to address Dave's concern about the side effects he was experiencing. He returned reporting improvement in energy and normalization of appetite, but he was having difficulty falling asleep some nights as well as experiencing increased anxiety. We agreed to add risperidone 0.5 mg prn that Dave could take when he was having difficulty with anxiety or getting to sleep.

Dave responded well to psychotherapy and a physical exercise routine and rarely required the as-needed medication. His remaining symptoms faded, and his confidence improved over several months. When Dave obtained a full-time job, he found that subtle daytime sedation seemed to limit his cognitive performance at work. Because he was asymptomatic, we agreed to taper his scheduled risperidone dose to 0.5 mg and eventually 0.25 mg daily with resolution of cognitive impairment.

After about a year, Dave began to ask about whether continuing medication was necessary. His job was going well, and he had married his longtime partner. He reported no medication side effects, but he did not like the idea of taking medication. After reviewing risks of relapse and potential impact on life course, Dave chose a carefully monitored trial of medication discontinuation. We agreed that he could restart medication at any point and that he would call if there were any questions. At next visit he noted that suspiciousness, ideas of reference, and feelings of unease had developed within a week of stopping medication, so he had restarted risperidone and preferred to continue taking it to ensure his stability. He has remained in remission since.

Conclusion

Antipsychotic medication therapy is an essential component of first-episode psychosis treatment. Choosing an appropriate medication, carefully dosed on the basis of research evidence and individual characteristics to maximize efficacy and minimize side effects, is critical in helping patients to improve symptoms and maintain long-term stability. Risperidone and aripiprazole seem to have a balanced profile of efficacy and side effects and thus should be considered first-line medications for treatment of FEP. Other antipsychotics with a high margin of safety are reasonable alternatives and deserve specific evaluation in people with FEP. Treatment nonadherence and early discontinuation of medications are common, and using a shared decision-making approach in an integrated treatment team setting may help patients engage with and stay in treatment and achieve long-term recovery.

KEY CONCEPTS

- Antipsychotic medication treatment is central to early intervention for people with schizophrenia spectrum disorders.

- First-line treatments should ideally provide high tolerability with reasonable efficacy.

- Antipsychotic medications are typically difficult to tolerate and may constrict functioning but provide well-established protection against relapse, requiring careful shared decision making around acute and ongoing use.

- When people choose to stop taking antipsychotic medication after onset of psychosis, continued engagement in treatment and careful monitoring can minimize risks for relapse and ensure rapid response.

Discussion Questions

1. How do you educate people experiencing a first episode of psychosis (and their family) about duration of untreated psychosis, prevention of progression, and remission?

2. How do you discuss the role of antipsychotic medication treatment in preventing progression of psychosis?

3. How can you use shared decision making to address common side effects of antipsychotic medication?

4. How do you work with patients who have experienced a first episode of psychosis on optimizing their health, well-being, and long-term recovery?

5. How do you discuss ambivalence about treatment and desire to stop taking antipsychotic medications with patients (and families) in early psychosis?

Suggested Readings

International Early Psychosis Association Writing Group: International clinical practice guidelines for early psychosis. Br J Psychiatry Suppl 187(48):s120–s124, 2005

McGorry PD, Killackey E, Yung AR: Early intervention in psychotic disorders: detection and treatment of the first episode and the critical early stages. Med J Aust 187(7 suppl):S8–S10, 2007

Tiihonen JA, Tanskanen A, Taipale H: 20-year nationwide follow-up study on discontinuation of antipsychotic treatment in first-episode schizophrenia. Am J Psychiatry 175(8):765–773, 2018

Yung AR, Killackey E, Hetrick SE, et al: The prevention of schizophrenia. Int Rev Psychiatry 19(6): 633–646, 2007

Weller A, Gleeson J, Alvarez-Jiminez M, et al. Can antipsychotic dose reduction lead to better functional recovery in first-episode psychosis? A randomized controlled-trial of antipsychotic dose reduction. The reduce trial: study protocol. Early Interv Psychiatry Nov 29, 2018 [Epub ahead of print]

References

Ballon JS, Ashfaq H, Noordsy DL: Clozapine titration for people in early psychosis: a chart review and treatment guideline. J Clin Psychopharmacol 38(3):234–238, 2018 29659460

Crespo-Facorro B, Pérez-Iglesias R, Ramirez-Bonilla M, et al: A practical clinical trial comparing haloperidol, risperidone, and olanzapine for the acute treatment of first-episode nonaffective psychosis. J Clin Psychiatry 67(10):1511–1521, 2006 17107241

Crespo-Facorro B, Pérez-Iglesias R, Mata I, et al: Relapse prevention and remission attainment in first-episode non-affective psychosis. A randomized, controlled 1-year follow-up comparison of haloperidol, risperidone and olanzapine. J Psychiatr Res 45(6):763–769, 2011 21106207

Crespo-Facorro B, Ortiz-García de la Foz V, Mata I, et al: Aripiprazole, Ziprasidone and Quetiapine in the treatment of first-episode nonaffective psychosis: a 12-week randomized, flexible-dose, open-label trial. Schizophr Res 147(2-3):375–382, 2013 23643328

Cuesta MJ, Jalón EG, Campos MS, Peralta V: Cognitive effectiveness of olanzapine and risperidone in first-episode psychosis. Br J Psychiatry 194(5):439–445, 2009 19407274

Dixon L, Perkins D, Calmes C: Guideline Watch (September 2009): Practice Guideline for the Treatment of Patients With Schizophrenia. Arlington, VA, American Psychiatric Association, 2009. Available at: https://psychiatry-online.org/pb/assets/raw/sitewide/practice_guidelines/guidelines/schizophrenia-watch.pdf.

Emsley RA; Risperidone Working Group: Risperidone in the treatment of first-episode psychotic patients: a double-blind multicenter study. Schizophr Bull 25(4):721–729, 1999 10667742

Gallego JA, Robinson DG, Sevy SM, et al: Time to treatment response in first-episode schizophrenia: should acute treatment trials last several months? J Clin Psychiatry 72(12):1691–1696, 2011 21939612

Guy W, Bonato RR: CGI: Clinical Global Impressions, in ECDEU Assess Manual Psychopharmacol-Revised. Rockville, MD, MIMH Psychopharmacology Research Branch, Alcohol, Drug Abuse, and Mental Health Administration, U.S. Department of Health, Education and Welfare, 1976, pp 217–222

Han X, Yuan YB, Yu X, et al: The Chinese First-Episode Schizophrenia Trial: background and study design. East Asian Arch Psychiatry 24(4):169–173, 2014 25482837

Kahn RS, Fleischhacker WW, Boter H, et al; EUFEST study group: Effectiveness of antipsychotic drugs in first-episode schizophrenia and schizophreniform disorder: an open randomised clinical trial. Lancet 371(9618):1085–1097, 2008 18374841

Kane JM, Robinson DG, Schooler NR, et al: Comprehensive versus usual community care for first-episode psychosis: 2-year outcomes from the NIMH RAISE early treatment program. Am J Psychiatry 173(4):362–372, 2016 26481174

Kay SR, Fiszbein A, Opler LA: The positive and negative syndrome scale (PANSS) for schizophrenia. Schizophr Bull, 13(2), 261–276, 1987 3616518

Lehman AF, Lieberman JA, Dixon LB, et al: Practice guideline for the treatment of patients with schizophrenia, second edition. Am J Psychiatry 161(2 Suppl):1–56, 2004 15000267

Leucht S, Arbter D, Engel RR, et al: How effective are second-generation antipsychotic drugs? A meta-analysis of placebo-controlled trials. Mol Psychiatry 14(4):429–447, 2009 18180760

Lieberman JA, Phillips M, Gu H, et al: Atypical and conventional antipsychotic drugs in treatment-naive first-episode schizophrenia: a 52-week randomized trial of clozapine vs chlorpromazine. Neuropsychopharmacology 28(5):995–1003, 2003a 12700715

Lieberman JA, Tollefson G, Tohen M, et al; HGDH Study Group: Comparative efficacy and safety of atypical and conventional antipsychotic drugs in first-episode psychosis: a randomized, double-blind trial of olanzapine versus haloperidol. Am J Psychiatry 160(8):1396–1404, 2003b 12900300

McEvoy JP, Lieberman JA, Perkins DO, et al: Efficacy and tolerability of olanzapine, quetiapine, and risperidone in the treatment of early psychosis: a randomized, double-blind 52-week comparison. Am J Psychiatry 164(7):1050–1060, 2007 17606657

Möller HJ, Riedel M, Jäger M, et al: Short-term treatment with risperidone or haloperidol in first-episode schizophrenia: 8-week results of a randomized controlled trial within the German Research Network on Schizophrenia. Int J Neuropsychopharmacol 11(7):985–997, 2008 18466670

Ou JJ, Xu Y, Chen HH, et al: Comparison of metabolic effects of ziprasidone versus olanzapine treatment in patients with first-episode schizophrenia. Psychopharmacology (Berl) 225(3):627–635, 2013 22926006

Pagsberg AK, Jeppesen P, Klauber DG, et al: Quetiapine extended release versus aripiprazole in children and adolescents with first-episode psychosis: the multicentre, double-blind, randomised tolerability and efficacy of antipsychotics (TEA) trial. Lancet Psychiatry 4(8):605–618, 2017 28599949

Robinson D, Woerner MG, Alvir JM, et al: Predictors of relapse following response from a first episode of schizophrenia or schizoaffective disorder. Arch Gen Psychiatry 56(3):241–247, 1999 10078501

Robinson DG, Woerner MG, Napolitano B, et al: Randomized comparison of olanzapine versus risperidone for the treatment of first-episode schizophrenia: 4-month outcomes. Am J Psychiatry 163(12):2096–2102, 2006 17151160

Robinson DG, Gallego JA, John M, et al: A randomized comparison of aripiprazole and risperidone for the acute treatment of first-episode schizophrenia and related disorders: 3-month outcomes. Schizophr Bull 41(6):1227–1236, 2015 26338693

San L, Arranz B, Perez V, et al: One-year, randomized, open trial comparing olanzapine, quetiapine, risperidone and ziprasidone effectiveness in antipsychotic-naive patients with a first-episode psychosis. Psychiatry Res 200(2-3):693–701, 2012 22954905

Schooler N, Rabinowitz J, Davidson M, et al; Early Psychosis Global Working Group: Risperidone and haloperidol in first-episode psychosis: a long-term randomized trial. Am J Psychiatry 162(5):947–953, 2005 15863797

Sikich L, Frazier JA, McClellan J, et al: Double-blind comparison of first- and second-generation antipsychotics in early-onset schizophrenia and schizoaffective disorder: findings from the treatment of early-onset schizophrenia spectrum disorders (TEOSS) study. Am J Psychiatry 165(11):1420–1431, 2008 18794207 Erratum in Am J Psychiatry 165(11):1495, 2008

Tiihonen J, Tanskanen A, Taipale H: 20-year nationwide follow-up study on discontinuation of antipsychotic treatment in first-episode schizophrenia. Am J Psychiatry 175(8):765–773, 2018 29621900

Woerner MG, Mannuzza S, Kane JM: Anchoring the BPRS: an aid to improved reliability. Psychopharmacol Bull 24(1):112–117, 1988 3387514

Zhang Y, Dai G: Efficacy and metabolic influence of paliperidone ER, aripiprazole and ziprasidone to patients with first-episode schizophrenia through 52 weeks follow-up in China. Hum Psychopharmacol 27(6):605–614, 2012 24446539

Zhang JP, Gallego JA, Robinson DG, et al: Efficacy and safety of individual second-generation vs. first-generation antipsychotics in first-episode psychosis: a systematic review and meta-analysis. Int J Neuropsychopharmacol 16(6):1205–1218, 2013 23199972

Zhang JP, Gallego JA, Xia TX, et al: Relative efficacy and safety of individual second-generation antipsychotics in treating first episode psychosis: a systematic review and meta-analysis. Paper presented at the annual conference of the American Society of Clinical Psychopharmacology, Phoenix, AZ, June 2016

CHAPTER 13

Psychotherapeutic Interventions for Early Psychosis

Kate V. Hardy, Clin.Psy.D.
Yulia Landa, Psy.D., M.S.
Piper Meyer-Kalos, Ph.D.
Kim T. Mueser, Ph.D.

PROVIDING psychotherapy is a core component of early psychosis services. Only relatively recently has the contribution of psychotherapies in supporting recovery from psychosis been recognized. This change is due in part to a shift in our understanding of psychosis and the recognition of the stress-diathesis model (Zubin and Spring 1977) as an explanatory model for psychosis. The recognition of stressors in the model as a contributing factor to the development, and maintenance, of psychotic symptoms encouraged mental health professionals to develop interventions designed to help individuals with psychosis learn more adaptive coping strategies for managing potential stressors and distress. Additionally, the recognition that psychosis exists on a continuum (and is not a discrete entity as previously posited) allowed for increased normalization of psychotic symptoms and an understanding of psychosis within a recovery framework that facilitated more frank discussion of these symptoms.

Psychotherapy and Early Psychosis

Psychotherapy has been included as a core component of early psychosis service provision since the inception of these service packages. Two primary models of psychosocial interventions for psychosis have emerged that are frequently implemented in coordinated specialty care (CSC) services for first-episode psychosis (FEP) in the United States: cognitive-behavioral therapy for psychosis (CBTp) and individual resiliency training (IRT). These two models will be referred to collectively as *psychotherapies,* and both are described in detail in this chapter. Key elements of these interventions are consistent with the overarching principles of early intervention in psychosis (Table 13–1). Both approaches are evidence-based and, as all psychotherapeutic models do, rely on the development of a collaborative relationship to support the intervention. Both approaches recognize the potentially stigmatizing nature of a mental health diagnosis and address this through normalization and psychoeducation. In addition, the problems and goals that the young person identifies are prioritized in treatment with the aim of supporting functioning and resiliency, and both approaches can be adapted in response to cultural needs. However, there are also key differences between the CBTp and IRT models that will be highlighted in this chapter.

TABLE 13–1. Comparison of early intervention principles and key elements of psychotherapy interventions

Early intervention principles[a]	Psychosocial interventions
Provide interventions with demonstrated efficacy	Evidence-based approach
Provide services that actively partner with young people (shared decision making)	Collaborative approach (the "collaborative fence")
Challenge stigmatizing and discriminatory attitudes	Normalization and psychoeducation
Generate optimism and expectation of positive outcomes and recovery	Problem list and goals Focus on functional recovery and resiliency Development of skills and tools to support and maintain recovery Wellness planning
Culturally sensitive services	Individualized formulation

[a]Based on values and vision elaborated by Bertolote and McGorry (2005).

Frequently, talking therapies are provided in an outpatient setting by a single provider. However, within a CSC model, both CBTp and IRT are offered within the team setting, and providers of these models are integrated into the team approach. The core clinical competencies required for delivering these models are similar and are predicated on the principles of recovery orientation, respectful communication, collaboration, and shared decision making. Roth and Pilling (2013) describe competencies required for providers to effectively work with individuals with psychosis and highlight the need for knowledge of the presenting problems and diagnostic criteria of people presenting with psychosis; general therapy skills, including assessment, intervention, and collaboration; and comfort with *metacompetencies*, which they relate to "an ability to implement 'procedural rules'—using clinical judgment to decide when, how, and whether to carry out a particular action or set of actions…" (Roth and Pilling 2013, p. 25). In line with these core competencies is the need to ensure that providers are trained appropriately in the chosen intervention. However, it has been routinely observed that training alone is not sufficient to support the implementation of a practice, so it is important that trained clinicians have access to ongoing consultation with an expert in the model, where continued learning takes place, and that the consultation include review of taped examples of clinical interactions and provision of feedback on the competency of the individual clinician.

Psychotherapies in a Team Setting

Because CBTp and IRT for early psychosis are most often delivered in the context of a CSC team, the clinician collaborates extensively with the other members of the team to integrate psychotherapy as part of a comprehensive treatment. Weekly team meetings facilitate this collaborative process, although additional communication is often also necessary. Table 13–2 describes potential interactions between the clinician providing psychotherapy and the other team members related to common issues. However, this list is not exhaustive, and there are numerous creative ways in which a clinician may collaborate with other team members to provide holistic and integrated treatment for the young person.

Ideally, the clinician has the sole focus of providing psychotherapy, either CBTp or IRT, to the young person. However, in smaller teams with fewer resources, it may be necessary for the provider to hold the dual role of case manager and therapist. In this case, supervision should focus on this dual role and supporting the clinician to navigate the challenges associated with integrating these approaches.

TABLE 13–2.   Examples of team collaboration with psychotherapy clinician

Provider	Possible collaboration with psychotherapy provider
Medication management provider	• Address medication adherence and medication options through examination of beliefs about medications • Discuss timeline of development of symptoms and early warning signs of relapse to support medication planning
Supported education and employment provider	• Identify and address motivational and personal organizational barriers to following through on school or work leads.
Peer specialist	• Engage around normalization of symptoms. • Support young person to put in action skills discussed in therapy.
Family worker	• Develop wellness plan with family.

Cognitive-Behavioral Therapy for Psychosis

Cognitive-behavioral therapy for psychosis is an approach to improving symptoms and functioning in individuals with psychotic disorders. CBTp was adapted from cognitive-behavioral therapy (CBT) methods developed by Dr. Aaron T. Beck and used primarily for the treatment of depressive and anxiety disorders (Beck et al. 1979, 1985). Although the first documented application of CBT to psychotic symptoms was by Beck in the early 1950s and preceded most of the CBT applications to depression and anxiety (Beck et al. 2009), findings from standardized treatment programs (Chadwick et al. 1996; Kingdon and Turkington 1994; Morrison et al. 2004) and rigorous clinical trials of CBTp (Sensky et al. 2000) did not begin to be published until more than 40 years later by several different clinical research teams in the United Kingdom. Currently, more than 50 randomized controlled trials and multiple meta-analyses of the research literature on CBTp have been published documenting its beneficial effects on a range of symptoms and functional outcomes (Burns et al. 2014; Turner et al. 2014).

The goal of CBTp is to improve individuals' functioning and overall life satisfaction by reducing the distress and disability caused by delusions, hallucinations, negative symptoms, and thought disorder. An essential component of CBTp is its focus on the personal meaning of symptoms and anomalous experiences and on changing appraisals of these experiences in order to reduce distress. The key elements of CBTp include a shared understanding (or formulation) of psychosis between the client and therapist, identification of targeted symptoms that cause distress or interfere with the individual's functioning, and development of cognitive and behavioral strategies to cope with these symptoms. The therapeutic process of CBTp includes the following core components: 1) engagement, 2) identification of goals, 3) assessment and formulation, 4) interventions, and 5) relapse work.

Engagement

In CBTp, the development of a strong therapeutic alliance is essential to the success of the treatment. The therapist engages the client with empathy and normalizing and works to understand the problem as the client sees it. Rather than using an authoritative, directive, or expert style, the therapist uses what is called *Columbo style* (after the famous television detective) to gently help clients describe their experiences, how they arrived at their conclusions, and how they developed their specific beliefs. Engagement continues throughout the therapeutic relationship but can be thought of as the first step in the therapeutic process.

Identification of Goals

CBTp treatment starts with identification of the client's goals. The client generates a list of problems. The goals are based on the problem list and are usually written down so that each goal corresponds to a specific problem. Goals are specific, positive, realistic, achievable, measurable, and time limited.

After the problems and goals are identified, the therapist and client collaboratively decide which goal to address first. The factors considered in making certain goals a priority are the level of urgency, which is usually related to the level of distress caused by a problem, and the likelihood that the problem could be quickly and successfully resolved. The latter can provide the client with the experience of resolving problems successfully and therefore a sense of hope for treatment.

Assessment and Formulation

The individual's strengths and vulnerabilities and the possible effects of stress are discussed to develop a *formulation*—a model that explains the psychological mechanisms that underline the client's psychotic symptoms and related difficulties. This assessment is done in an empathic manner in which maintaining rapport with the client overrides the therapist's need to gain information. This formulation is developed collaboratively with the client and incorporates information about the cognitive, behavioral, affective, and physiological components of the individual's psychotic experiences. Cognitive components include information about cognitive intrusions (e.g., voices, visions, negative intrusive thoughts) and appraisal and interpretations of these intrusions, as well as cognitive biases (e.g., jumping to conclusions, attention to threat, externalizing). The client's life experiences that contributed to the formation of his or her current beliefs are also explored and integrated into the formulation. A narrative approach, constructing a story of what has been happening collaboratively with the client, is used when developing a formulation.

Interventions

Once the formulation is developed, therapist and client work collaboratively to identify appropriate interventions based on the client's goals. Interventions in CBTp can include exploring the evidence the client uses to support his or her delusional beliefs, verbal exploration of beliefs through discussion, and testing the validity of the beliefs. Verbal exploration of beliefs could involve looking for alternative explanations for the experiences that contributed to the formation of specific beliefs and comparing which explanations (beliefs) are better supported by evidence. Testing the validity of beliefs can involve encouraging the client to engage in specific behavior for the purpose of testing the belief, setting predictors for external events so that outcomes serve as tests of these predictors, and reviewing the outcomes. For example, an individual is more likely to be distressed by voices and to comply with command hallucinations if he or she believes that those voices have power or control over him or her. Clients are encouraged to explore alternative explanations of anomalous experiences (such as voices) that are less threatening, helped to engage in behavioral experiments to test out their belief about the power of auditory hallucinations, and helped to develop a more normalizing rationale for making sense of such experiences.

Similar to the IRT model, the stress-vulnerability model (Zubin and Spring 1977) is used to help individuals make sense of and normalize psychotic experiences. According to the stress-vulnerability model, various genetic predispositions and life events (e.g., early trauma, physical illnesses) make us vulnerable to developing certain symptoms (e.g., paranoia, hearing voices), and we tend to experience these symptoms when we are under stress. Thus, the stress-vulnerability model serves to highlight the relationship between stress and symptoms as well as to help normalize psychotic experiences by illustrating that at different levels of distress all people are capable of having such experiences. The therapist also helps the client become aware of whether or not his or her current coping behaviors are helping and develop better ways of coping. For example, a therapist could help identify strategies of coping with the voices that could diminish their frequency and intensity (e.g., talking to someone, reading aloud, listening to music, using earplugs). During the course of the treatment, the therapist and client collaboratively evaluate the effectiveness of these interventions. If the interventions are not successful, new interventions are tried until the treatment goal is achieved. CBTp is considered to be culturally responsive in that the influence of cultural background is integrated into the formulation, which aids the development of culturally responsive interventions (Rathod et al. 2015).

Relapse Prevention

Once both client and therapist decide that the goals of the treatment have been achieved, then relapse prevention is discussed. In the same manner in which the formulation of the client's difficulties is assessed and developed, the therapist assesses the relapse triggers and cognitions, and relapse prevention interventions are designed collaboratively with the client. CBTp treatment is intended to be provided weekly for at least 6 months. The treatment can also take longer depending on the client's symptomatology (e.g., it takes about 40 sessions to successfully work with systematized delusions). Once the treatment is complete, it is recommended that the client attend booster sessions (once a month, and then once in 3 and then 6 months) to reinforce the coping skills and cognitive strategies learned in therapy.

Case Example 1

Julio is a 20-year-old young man who was referred to CBTp after being hospitalized for FEP due to paranoia. Julio was afraid of being killed by the Mafia. He grew up in an Italian neighborhood in the Bronx in New York City, where he often felt unsafe. His father left when he was very young. He had witnessed several violent incidents at school and was hurt by older boys during one of these incidents, and as a result, he often felt vulnerable and unprotected. After Julio graduated from high school, he began working as a waiter in an Italian restaurant in his neighborhood. Around the same time, following the lead of his friends, he began using cannabis.

Initially, the CBTp therapist used empathy and a normalizing approach to understanding Julio's problems as Julio saw them in order to develop a therapeutic alliance and to begin to work collaboratively on formulating Julio's therapy goals. Julio wished that the Mafia "would leave me alone" and that he would be able to go out without the debilitating fear, make friends, and maybe even have a girlfriend. Rather than using an authoritative, directive, or expert style, the therapist used the

"Columbo style" of gently asking Julio to describe his experiences and how he arrived at his conclusion that the Mafia was out to kill him.

The therapist worked with Julio to better understand his experiences, thoughts, and feelings and to come up with a historical formulation—a model of symptom formation and maintenance (Figure 13–1). Julio's earlier life experiences contributed to his beliefs that he was worthless and weak, that people are dangerous, that he cannot trust anybody, and that paranoia is useful because it kept him on his toes. Growing up, Julio had also developed a tendency to personalize (to assume that what people are saying or doing relates to him), to jump to conclusions with little evidence, and to selectively pay attention to threatening information—thinking styles that contributed to the formation of delusional paranoid beliefs. The formulation also included information about a particular event that made Julio believe that the Mafia was after him: He had been working in the restaurant for several days and was getting little sleep in order to make more money. The restaurant owner made a negative comment about Julio's chatting with a customer, who turned out to be the restaurant owner's daughter. Julio then went to a party where he smoked cannabis and watched *The Godfather*, the classic tale of a Mafia family. On the way back home, Julio continued thinking about the restaurant owner's comment. He thought that the owner must belong to the Mafia and that he was mad at him for chatting with his daughter and might want to eliminate him. Suddenly, Julio heard loud sounds that he thought were gunshots. He began to think that these were warning messages for him sent by the Mafia. He became terrified and admitted himself to the hospital to escape. He continued hearing strange sounds, which he kept interpreting as gunshots by the Mafia to threaten him.

CBTp interventions were based on the formulation and Julio's goals. They included working with Julio to identify and reduce daily triggers of thoughts about the Mafia, including his use of cannabis. As part of the interventions, Julio's therapist provided education on cognitive distortions and thinking styles that contribute to the formation of delusions (including personalizing and jumping to conclusions) and taught him reasoning skills. She also worked with Julio on core beliefs contributing to paranoia (e.g., "I am helpless," "People are dangerous") and automatic thoughts of the same nature.

Throughout the treatment, the CBTp therapist continued to engage Julio, made efforts to protect and enhance his self-esteem, and explored the reasons Julio concluded that the Mafia was after him. She helped Julio question and reevaluate this belief by using a collaborative empiricism approach, in which she and Julio worked together to explore different possible explanations for his experiences and examined the evidence supporting or refuting each explanation (including those on which his beliefs were based). Julio's level of conviction that the Mafia was after him dropped from 99% to 5%. This enabled him to feel less scared and stressed, and he began to go out. As he went out and experienced being safe, he gradually stopped believing that the Mafia was after him.

After 20 sessions of CBTp, Julio decided that he had achieved his goals. Julio and his therapist discussed his thoughts about the possibility of relapse (the return of the debilitating fear of being killed by the Mafia), discussed relapse prevention, and formulated a plan. For 3 months, Julio continued to attend monthly booster sessions to reinforce skills learned in time-limited CBTp. After completing therapy, Julio met and moved in with a girlfriend, went to a culinary school, and opened his own restaurant.

Individual Resiliency Training

Individual resiliency training is a broad-based individual psychotherapeutic intervention that is part of the NAVIGATE program, a comprehensive treatment program for people recovering from a first episode of psychosis (FEP; Mueser et al. 2015). The NAVIGATE program was developed to be implemented by a five-person team of clinicians who provide four different interventions: 1) individualized medication management, 2) the family education program, 3) supported education and employment, and 4) individual resiliency training. The treatment philosophy of the program is based on a core set of clinical competencies that are cultivated among all the team members and are thought to be critical to the successful implementation of the program, including shared decision-making skills, a focus on strengths and resiliency, motivational enhancement, psychoeducational skills, and collaboration with natural supports. More information about NAVIGATE can be found in the article by Mueser et al. (2015).

The IRT program was designed as a psychotherapeutic approach aimed at achieving the following goals:

1. Establish personal goals of the client and make progress toward those goals over the course of the program
2. Support self-determination, build resiliency skills, and create positive emotional experiences in order to facilitate clients' ability to spring back from the adversity of FEP and regain control over their lives
3. Help individuals process the often-traumatic experience of FEP and reduce self-stigmatizing beliefs about mental illness that may accompany the episode
4. Teach basic information about FEP and the principles of its treatment in order to enable clients to participate in informed decision making about treatment for their disorder
5. Teach skills to clients for improving the management of their psychiatric disorder
6. Teach skills for improving clients' social relationships, leisure time, and health behaviors

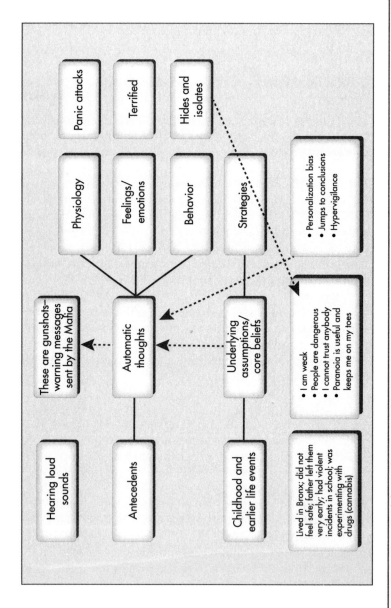

FIGURE 13–1.   Historical formulation: making sense of Julio's beliefs and experiences.

In IRT, people learn skills and strategies to manage their psychosis and take steps toward recovery. IRT is focused on helping people learn information and skills to address common concerns and problem areas such as substance use, social skills and interpersonal connections, negative feelings, and healthy lifestyles. IRT is tailored to meet individual needs by helping people identify personally meaningful goals at the beginning of treatment. Several unique considerations are embedded in IRT to address specific features of FEP, such as an awareness of developmental milestones in adolescence and early adulthood and a lack of experience with symptoms and treatment. IRT materials use plain language to increase engagement of persons with low insight and a brief history of psychosis.

In addition, responses to psychosis can be traumatic and stigmatizing and can lead to a syndrome of posttraumatic stress disorder (PTSD) symptoms (Mueser et al. 2010). IRT incorporates an approach designed to emotionally process upsetting and traumatizing experiences related to FEP and to address stigmatizing beliefs that clients may have about psychosis and their ability to achieve personal goals. IRT is inclusive of different cultural beliefs and traditions. An individualized assessment and treatment formulation allows for the integration of culture into personal definitions of recovery, individual goals, and illness management strategies and skills. Finally, to strengthen the focus of resilience in IRT, there are specific activities adapted from positive psychology interventions included throughout the intervention to increase positive emotions. These IRT elements are interwoven with client strengths and goals to help clinicians increase choice, respond flexibly to a person's concerns, and strengthen engagement.

Theoretical Underpinnings of IRT

The development of IRT was influenced by four general theories: theories of well-being, the stress-vulnerability model, the psychiatric rehabilitation model, and the theory of reasoned action. FEP is typically preceded by a gradual decline in psychosocial functioning, followed by a gradual worsening that occurs after the onset of psychosis but before the person is engaged in treatment, which traditionally focuses on addressing pathology and deficits rather than improving functioning and well-being. In order to reduce the demoralizing effects of this loss in functioning, and the impact of being diagnosed with a mental illness, IRT draws on *theories of well-being*, which posit that the cultivation of positive emotions and experiences leads to improvements in well-being, decreases in negative feelings, and a greater capacity to thrive despite the presence of adversity (Seligman 2012). For example, the broaden-and-build theory posits that experience of positive emotions leads to a broadening of one's personal and social resources and strengths, which can then be deployed in the service of achieving personal and functional goals (Fredrickson 2009). IRT adopted a specific focus on individual strengths (Rapp and Goscha 2006) while also incorporating specific strategies designed to enhance resiliency and positive emotional experiences.

The *stress-vulnerability model* of schizophrenia was used to guide the teaching of information and skills in IRT related to the management of psychosis and improving its long-term course (Zubin and Spring 1977). This model hypothesizes that psychosis, and its course, are influenced by the dynamic interplay between biological vulnerability, stress (including trauma), personal resources, and the social environment. On the basis of this model, a variety of factors can influence both biological vulnerability and stress, such as taking medication and minimizing substance use to reduce biological vulnerability and improving coping strategies and social support to reduce the effects of stress. More recently, this model has been modified to incorporate recovery skills as another personal factor that can influence the course of the illness, such as knowledge of psychosis and its treatment, involvement in treatment planning, and developing a relapse prevention plan (Mueser et al. 2013).

Psychiatric rehabilitation approaches were integrated into IRT to address the problem of impaired psychosocial functioning that is already prominent because of the FEP. Psychiatric rehabilitation directly targets improved psychosocial functioning through a combination of two broad approaches: teaching skills for achieving interpersonal and instrumental goals and providing environmental supports to facilitate optimal functioning and attainment of goals (Corrigan 2016). Skills training methods were incorporated into IRT to help participants achieve social goals (e.g., social skills training), and the provision of environmental supports is a primary focus of both the Family Education Program and Supported Employment and Education components of NAVIGATE.

Last, the *theory of reasoned action* was used as a general guide in IRT to understanding motivation to change one's behavior (Hale et al. 2002). This theory posits that the intention to engage in a behavior is the strongest determinant of behavior, and that intention is based on the expected outcomes of the behavior. Thus, people are more inclined to change their behavior when they view such change as in their own best interest. In IRT, the process of identifying and collaborating with clients on achieving personal goals creates natural opportunities to explore how improved illness self-management skills could help the individual achieve his or her goals, thereby harnessing motivation to actively participate in treatment.

Clinical and Technical Influences on the Development of IRT

The IRT program also drew on several previous interventions for the FEP or similar populations. The structure and organization of IRT information and skills training content into discrete modules, as well as the role of goal setting and tracking throughout the program and the teaching of illness self-management information and skills, was based on the Illness Management and Recovery program (McGuire et al. 2014). IRT also was modeled after the Graduated Recovery From Initial Psychosis (GRIP) program for people recovering from an FEP. GRIP is a flexible modular-based cognitive-behavioral therapy intervention that also includes goal setting and teaching of illness self-management skills (Penn et al. 2011).

The two resiliency modules in IRT were based on positive psychotherapy (Seligman et al. 2006) and the Positive Living intervention for people with schizophrenia (Meyer et al. 2012). Behaviorally based exercises from Positive Living were included in IRT to help people generate more positive emotions and incorporate these strategies into their daily lives.

Finally, the IRT program adopted the same basic session structure used in cognitive and behavioral therapies, including setting agendas, reviewing homework, teaching specific information and skills, and collaboratively developing home assignments to practice skills and foster generalization. Furthermore, many of the specific strategies used in cognitive and behavioral approaches were incorporated into the different IRT modules. For example, with respect to CBTp, the strategy of normalizing psychotic symptoms was incorporated into the Education About Psychosis module, the teaching coping strategies were incorporated into the Coping With Symptoms module, and cognitive restructuring was incorporated into the Processing the Psychotic Episode and Dealing With Negative Feelings modules. Similarly, social skills training strategies were incorporated into the Having Fun and Developing Good Relationships modules of IRT.

Structure and Organization of IRT

In IRT, clinicians (preferably with at least a master's degree) meet weekly to help people make progress toward a personally meaningful goal, learn illness management skills and information, and learn skills to build resiliency. IRT clinicians work closely with the other NAVIGATE team members to collaboratively develop treatment plans, enhance engagement in treatment, and practice IRT strategies.

The IRT manual is divided into 14 modules, each of which focuses on a specific topic area. The first 7 modules comprise the standard modules that target typical needs of persons with FEP and are designed to be delivered to everyone. Three IRT modules (Orientation, Education About Psychosis, and Relapse Prevention Planning) are coordinated with the Family Education program in NAVIGATE to encourage collaboration with family members and other supportive persons to ensure that family members are learning the same information and to offer flexibility on where people can learn illness management strategies and education. The individualized modules include an additional 7 modules that address special topics specific to persons with FEP. After the standard modules are completed, a decision is made by the client and clinician to focus on individualized modules that could help reduce distress or help the person achieve his or her goals. Usually, people complete the standardized modules before moving to the individualized modules, but the clinician has the option of teaching individualized modules at any point during IRT when the need arises (e.g., when significant suicidal ideation, co-occurring substance use, or distressing hallucinations are present and require immediate attention).

The IRT materials for each module include clinical guidelines that outline the goals of the module, teaching strategies, and strategies to solve common problems. The clinical guidelines are designed to help clinicians with varying levels of experience deliver IRT. Each set of clinical guidelines is accompanied by a set of worksheets that the IRT clinician uses in session to interactively discuss and practice skills and strategies. The IRT worksheets include discussion questions to elicit individual examples, opportunities to demonstrate and practice skills, and suggestions for home practice.

The IRT program relies on a core set of teaching strategies, including motivational, educational, and cognitive-behavioral methods. These strategies are used throughout the program to stimulate clients' interest and desire to learn information and skills related to the management of their psychosis and the attainment of personal goals, to teach critical information, and to help individuals acquire new skills and to transfer those skills to their daily lives.

Case Example 2

Ana, a 23-year-old woman, was referred to the NAVIGATE team after being hospitalized for wandering around her aunt's neighborhood screaming about the FBI monitoring the street with hidden cameras. Ana had moved in with her aunt in a small town about 3 months before being hospitalized because she had not been getting along with her grandmother, with whom she lived in a major metropolitan city. At the time that Ana was enrolled in NAVIGATE, she was often confused by what people were saying and had trouble putting together a full sentence. After being hospitalized, Ana described hearing voices talking to her, and her aunt said that she would stay in her room for several hours at a time.

Ana was introduced to Celia, the IRT clinician, when the NAVIGATE director, Terry, was enrolling her in the program. A week later, Ana started the Orientation module with Celia. In the beginning of IRT, Ana was hesitant to talk to her therapist. Celia focused on teaching and practicing relaxed breathing in session with Ana. Eventually, Celia worked with Ana to set small positive goals. In the beginning, Celia met with Ana twice a week for shorter sessions until she was more comfortable meeting weekly for 1 hour. Over the first 3 months of IRT, Ana shared her recent experiences at the hospital, including how uncomfortable she was with her voices and how she struggled with organizing her thoughts.

After completing module 2 (Assessment and Goal Setting), Ana identified her strengths as love of learning, kindness, gratitude, zest, and honesty. She started working on small goals such as earning some spending money to buy video games and to help her aunt with buying groceries. At the end of the Assessment and Goal Setting module, Celia reintroduced Ana to the supported employment and education specialist, Lin, in an IRT session to discuss how Lin could help Ana find short-term work to earn extra money.

When Celia started module 3 (Education About Psychosis) with Ana, she slowed down and broke each handout into two sessions because Ana needed to review the symptoms of psychosis and the stress vulnerability model in small chunks. After completing a relapse prevention plan in IRT, Ana shared the plan with her aunt in the family education meeting. Ana and Celia discussed completing module 5 (Processing the Episode) because Ana had repeatedly brought up how the hospitalization had upset her. After discussing the rationale with Ana, Celia decided to see if module 5, "Processing the Episode." could help Ana put together what had happened before she was hospitalized. During the completion of module 5, Ana identified "I will never recover" and "People will always believe I am dangerous" as self-stigmatizing beliefs that were very distressing to her. After telling her story of her experience with symptoms and being hospitalized for the first time, Ana updated her belief about her recovery, stating, "I had a difficult time, but I have family members who support me, and I am working hard to help my family and do things I enjoy." By the end of module 6, "Resiliency—Part 1," Ana had tried new ways to use her top five strengths in her daily life and had written down the good things that had happened to her at the end of every day.

Celia and Ana met collaboratively at the end of the standard modules to discuss Ana's progress to date and next steps for the individualized modules. In that session, Ana revealed to Celia that she had a new goal: she wanted to move back to the city to live with her grandmother so she could find a job and reconnect with her friends. On the basis of their discussion, Celia and Ana decided to move to module 8 (Dealing With Negative Feelings) to help Ana reduce her social anxiety, then review module 11 (Having Fun and Developing Relationships) to allow Ana to practice new skills to meet new people and reconnect with her friends when she returned to live with her grandmother.

CBTp and IRT: Comparing the Models

Table 13–3 summarizes the core components of psychotherapy for FEP and indicates how CBTp and IRT address each of them. Although there is significant overlap between the two approaches in terms of session structure, orientation toward goal attainments, and wellness and recovery, there are key differences as well. IRT is a highly manualized approach with extensive educational and worksheet materials in the form of handouts for clients and clinicians, whereas CBTp is less standardized and structured and consequently requires stronger clinical skills and experience to implement, offering greater flexibility for the experienced clinician. IRT is prescriptive in the sessions that are offered (with flexibility depending on the needs of the client), allowing for a consistent and systematic approach to treatment, whereas CBTp draws heavily on the collaboratively developed formulation to inform the direction of intervention, resulting in each client receiving different interventions.

Clients (and clinicians) may variably respond positively to one approach over the other in terms of preference for a structured, manualized treatment or a more flexible idiosyncratic process. IRT provides a strong psychoeducational basis to support treatment, thus ensuring the client has an understanding of psychotic symptoms. When clients are reluctant to engage in discussion regarding the experience of their psychotic symptoms, IRT encourages clinicians to use normalizing language consistent with the terminology being used by the client and to explore the client's understanding of his or her experiences. In addition to this approach, CBTp also encourages the clinician to sit on the collaborative fence, drop assumptions, and explore explanations other than an illness model or diagnosis to explain the distressing experiences. This does not preclude psychoeducation, but it does offer an additional way of engaging the individual who may not be initially open to considering his or her experiences within a mental health framework.

Common Challenges in Conducting Psychotherapeutic Interventions in Early Psychosis

Although psychotherapeutic interventions are routinely integrated into coordinated specialty care, there are a number of potential challenges in offering this approach to individuals with early psychosis. The importance of team coordination should not be underestimated, but it should also be recognized that this approach can be challenging in terms of resources and communication. Ensuring that there is protected time each week in the form of a case conference or team meeting may aid this process, and the use of remote teleconferencing capacity may be necessary to ensure that clinicians in remote geographical locations are able to be connected to the team virtually.

The clinician may also face challenges if a young person does not want to engage in services. Typically, both CBTp and IRT offer an alternative means of engaging a young person who may not be ready to discuss medications, and in some cases, the therapist may be the first point

TABLE 13–3. Goals, structure, organization, and methods of cognitive-behavioral therapy for psychosis (CBTp) and individual resiliency training (IRT)

Dimension	CBTp	IRT
General focus, structure, and format		
Target population	All persons with FEP	All persons with FEP
Aims of intervention	• Improve quality of life • Reduce distress and prevent future distress • Elicit hope in recovery • Assist the maintenance of a client's capacity to make informed decisions about his or her life • Help the client, over the course of therapy, work toward becoming his or her own therapist	• Increase strengths, resiliency, and self-determination • Teach information and skills to facilitate informed decision making about treatment and illness self-management • Teach information and skills and provide support for achieving personally meaningful goals
Session frequency and intervention duration	Frequency: adapted to the client's needs and speed of learning Duration: termination should include planning for long-term maintenance of gains after treatment	Frequency: weekly or biweekly Duration: 9–24+ months, depending on need

TABLE 13–3. Goals, structure, organization, and methods of cognitive-behavioral therapy for psychosis (CBTp) and individual resiliency training (IRT) *(continued)*

Dimension	CBTp	IRT
Organization	• *Engagement* • *Development of problem list and shared goals* • *Assessment (exploration of symptoms)* • *Development of collaborative formulation* • *Identification and implementation of cognitive and behavioral skills* • *Consolidation of skills* • *Relapse prevention* • *Booster sessions*	Curriculum-based program with information and skills organized into 14 different modules (or topic areas): • 7 standard modules provided to all clients • 7 individualized modules provided on the basis of client need and interest (taught whenever needed; do not require completion of standard modules)
Structure of sessions	• Session structure and content should be decided jointly between client and therapist • Client should be encouraged to prioritize items on the agenda • Major brief summaries should occur at the beginning and end of each session	Usual flow of sessions: • Set agenda • Review previous session • Review home practice • Follow up on goals • Teach new material • Summarize • Set new home practice
Materials for clinicians	*Numerous manualized CBTp interventions*	Manual and guidelines for teaching each module

TABLE 13–3. Goals, structure, organization, and methods of cognitive-behavioral therapy for psychosis (CBTp) and individual resiliency training (IRT) *(continued)*

Dimension	CBTp	IRT
Materials for clients	*Worksheets from manuals (may be included or may be developed idiosyncratically to meet needs of client)*	Educational handouts for each module, including the following: • Information about topic area • Prompt questions to facilitate discussion • Suggestions for in-session practice of skills • Tables completed in session • Suggestions for home assignments

Specific methods used and topic areas covered

Dimension	CBTp	IRT
Befriending and engagement	• Engage the client in the therapeutic relationship and take into account the client's perspective and world view • Explain the rationale of CBT to the client and demonstrate its use • Use client feedback to inform interventions • Encourage clients to express positive and negative reactions regarding therapy • Ensure consistent collaboration throughout sessions • Use collaborative feedback to engage the client	Emphasize engagement from the beginning of IRT in module 2 (Assessment and Goal Setting) when developing a definition of recovery and discussing different areas of life

TABLE 13–3. Goals, structure, organization, and methods of cognitive-behavioral therapy for psychosis (CBTp) and individual resiliency training (IRT) (*continued*)

Dimension	CBTp	IRT
Assessment	• Careful and collaborative exploration of current experiences through nonjudgmental, open questioning • Exploration facilitated by ability of clinician to sit on the "collaborative fence" • Symptom-specific measures used to track outcomes • Assessment of presenting symptomatology, past experiences of services, and cultural or family issues in engagement	• Brief Strengths Test • Satisfaction With Areas of My Life • Psychosocial history • Additional questions about medications and substance use
Team formulation	Formulation is used as part of team meetings and case consultation to support coordination around complex cases	IRT clinician participates in the weekly team meeting and regular treatment planning meetings to provide feedback on goals, strengths, and challenges
Goal setting and tracking	• Initial problem list • Development of SMART goals relating to problem list • Prioritization of goals based on need • Tracking of goals over time to assess progress	• Comprehensive review of life domains to set personally meaningful goals • Breakdown of long-term goals into shorter-term goals and steps • Use of a goal-tracking sheet to operationalize goals and track progress over time

TABLE 13–3. Goals, structure, organization, and methods of cognitive-behavioral therapy for psychosis (CBTp) and individual resiliency training (IRT) *(continued)*

Dimension	CBTp	IRT
Resiliency skills training	*Exploration of strengths and existing coping skills to support change*	• Covered in two modules (1 standard module and 1 individualized module) • Includes skills to identify character strengths and practice gratitude, mindfulness, and other positive emotions
Psychoeducation about FEP and its treatment (providing standard information about disorder in an interactive, flexible way to facilitate comprehension)	• *Psychoeducation is incorporated as needed but is not made a priority* • *Clinician remains open to pursuing alternative ways of understanding psychosis in a manner that allows reduced distress and increased functioning* • Clinician normalizes psychotic symptoms to reduce stigma and improve engagement	• Covered in Education About Psychosis module (standard) • Clinician maintains focus on understanding client's experience of psychosis • Clinician incorporates client's language to describe symptoms

TABLE 13–3. Goals, structure, organization, and methods of cognitive-behavioral therapy for psychosis (CBTp) and individual resiliency training (IRT) *(continued)*

Dimension	CBTp	IRT
Shared formulation and processing the psychotic episode	*Idiosyncratic formulation is developed for all clients:* • *Incorporates historical understanding of formation of psychotic symptoms and how client has reacted to them* • *Informs interventions* Formulation includes maintenance based in the here and now and a longitudinal formulation, to understand formation of psychosis symptoms: • A balanced conceptualization should highlight the client's strengths • Conceptualization should draw together current concerns, vulnerabilities, and precipitating and perpetuating factors • A cognitive-behavioral maintenance cycle should be devised and used to set targets for intervention • For effective CBT to occur, the conceptualization must be appropriate and shared	Formulation is covered in Processing the Episode module (standard): • Develop a narrative account of the episode • Identify and challenge self-stigmatizing beliefs about mental illness

TABLE 13–3. Goals, structure, organization, and methods of cognitive-behavioral therapy for psychosis (CBTp) and individual resiliency training (IRT) *(continued)*

Dimension	CBTp	IRT
Relapse prevention training (developing a plan to prevent future relapses)	*Wellness plan should be developed before terminating therapy*	Covered in Relapse Prevention Planning module (standard)
Enhancement of coping strategies (systematic enhancement of strategies for coping with problematic symptoms and teaching new coping strategies)	*Idiosyncratic coping strategies should be identified through the formulation and implemented as a behavioral intervention*	Covered in Coping With Symptoms module (individualized): • Address broad range of symptoms (psychotic symptoms, negative symptoms, depression, anxiety) • Incorporate behaviorally based coping strategies
Cognitive restructuring (teaching thought-feeling-behavior triad, recognizing thoughts underlying negative feelings, evaluating evidence for thoughts and changing when inaccurate)	• *Identify unhelpful thoughts and beliefs through the formulation, including examination of their impact on actions and emotions* • *Implement cognitive strategies to address unhelpful thoughts* • *Address core schema*	Briefly covered in Processing the Psychotic Episode module (standard) and Dealing With Negative Feelings module (individualized): • Address any negative feelings, including those related to psychotic symptoms, depression, suicidal thinking, anxiety, and PTSD symptoms (due to traumatic life events, psychotic symptoms, or coercive treatments) • Teach cognitive coping strategies

TABLE 13–3. Goals, structure, organization, and methods of cognitive-behavioral therapy for psychosis (CBTp) and individual resiliency training (IRT) *(continued)*

Dimension	CBTp	IRT
Interpersonal skills training (teaching social skills via breaking down skills, modeling, role play practice, feedback, home practice)	*Training incorporated as a behavioral intervention as needed on the basis of individualized formulation*	Covered in Having Fun and Developing Good Relationships module (individualized)
Substance use problems (education about substances and effects, motivational interviewing, decisional balance about using, plan for cutting down or preventing relapses)	*Interventions related to substance abuse incorporated as needed on the basis of client's goals and formulation*	Covered in Substance Use module (individualized)
Health issues (education about healthy lifestyles, guidance on changing habits)	*Interventions related to healthy living incorporated as needed on the basis of client's goals and formulation*	Covered in Making Decisions About Smoking, Nutrition, and Exercise module (individualized)

Note. CBTp column is based on Morrison and Barratt 2010. Italics indicate content added by chapter authors.
Abbreviations. FEP=first-episode psychosis; PTSD=posttraumatic stress disorder.

of contact with the team. These approaches allow a focus on personal goals and recognition of strengths and resiliencies that may be far removed from the presenting symptoms of psychosis. For a young person who is beginning to disengage with services, both approaches allow for a return to initial befriending and a focus on the therapeutic relationship to support ongoing continuation of care. Where a young person experiences an exacerbation of symptoms, it may also be necessary to return to rapport building, communicate concerns to the team, and liaise with other team members regarding appropriate support for the young person. Alternatively, when a young person is doing well and identifies that he or she needs less support, the provider, as well as the team, might want to engage the young person in shared decision making about the frequency of sessions potentially dropping to less frequent booster session contacts.

CBTp or IRT: Which Is the Best Fit?

CBTp and IRT are the two most common psychotherapy approaches for early psychosis used in the United States, although neither is broadly available. The structure of IRT sessions is grounded in cognitive-behavioral theory, offering a manualized approach to delivering psychoeducation and key skills, whereas CBTp may be seen as an extension of the traditional CBT model, emphasizing idiosyncratic formulation to inform intervention. At present, no formal guidance exists to support agencies in determining which of the two approaches is the most appropriate for their service. However, there are several principles that provide direction to agencies looking to train staff in psychotherapy approaches for this population. IRT was initially created in recognition of the need to support rapid workforce development in the provision of specialized psychotherapy for psychosis. Unlike other countries where early intervention in psychosis has been implemented, the United States lacks a training infrastructure that ensures clinicians are qualified in basic CBT for depression or anxiety on completion of postgraduate training. IRT offers a structure to support novice clinicians in providing key therapeutic interventions in a manualized manner, ensuring that clients are exposed to a range of interventions specific to early psychosis while also training the clinicians in the basic principles of CBT. IRT training assumes that clinicians may have a range of past experiences of CBT (including no previous exposure to CBTp) and supports the clinician in demonstrating fidelity to the approach through tape review and consultation. IRT materials may be used by novice and expert clinicians alike, with expert clinicians demonstrating greater flexibility in their use of the modules and increased familiarity with the materials.

In contrast, CBTp training typically assumes clinicians have at least an intermediate understanding of CBT and are comfortable with the core components of a CBT session, including agenda setting, collaboration, and homework development. This grounding in CBT is taken as a foundation on which CBTp is then built, supporting clinicians to learn the key skills specific to CBTp, including psychosis-specific formulation, normalization, and working from the collaborative fence. Training in CBTp may be aimed at the intermediate-level CBT practitioner, with consultation and tape review ensuring that clinicians develop competence in this approach.

Given the different orientations of these approaches in terms of the intended target audience of trainees, we recommend that services consider the skill level of their clinicians prior to engaging in training. For services in which clinicians lack significant experience either providing CBT or working with persons with psychosis, IRT offers a structured introduction to evidence-based practice. For agencies where clinicians are experienced in providing CBT and have at least several years' experience working with people with psychosis, CBTp may offer additional skills and insights to support the collaborative understanding of the client's presenting symptoms. In some cases, clinicians with extensive expertise in working with individuals with psychosis (but with less exposure to CBT) may be trained to competence in CBTp.

It is important that agencies considering training in these approaches conduct a thorough assessment of the strengths, skills, and needs of their staff team and consult with training experts regarding the best fit. In keeping with the current recommendations for tiered psychotherapy interventions for psychosis (Ince et al. 2016), an integrated approach in which both IRT and CBTp are available from clinicians trained to competence in both approaches may be warranted. For teams considering integrating both approaches at services where clinicians are unfamiliar with CBT or working with psychosis, we recommend initial training in IRT followed by CBTp training once IRT competence is achieved. The benefits of an integrated approach include the opportunity for clinicians to offer a range of services that match the needs of the client and for increased choice of services available to the client, thus further supporting shared decision making. Further investigation of the benefits and challenges of this integrated approach is justified.

Conclusion

Individual psychotherapy is a core component of early psychosis care and should be made routinely available to young people experiencing first episode of psychosis. Cognitive-behavioral therapy for psychosis and individual resiliency training are two evidence-based interventions that can be implemented within a team setting. Although there is overlap between these two approaches, each model also brings unique strengths, and the best fit for the service will be determined on the basis of resources, previous staff training, and overall service ethos.

KEY CONCEPTS

- Psychotherapy is a core intervention in early psychosis intervention.

- Individual resiliency training and cognitive-behavioral therapy for psychosis are two models of psychotherapy that have been integrated into coordinated specialty care services.

- Both models support recovery from psychosis through the development of key skills.

- Services considering implementing individual psychotherapy need to assess clinician skill and client preference.

Discussion Questions

1. How oriented is the staff team to providing evidence-based psychotherapeutic interventions for psychosis?

2. What is the skill level and training background of the clinicians in the service in relation to providing psychotherapy for psychosis?

3. What resources are in place to support training and consultation in evidence-based psychotherapeutic interventions for psychosis?

Suggested Readings

French P, Morrison A: Early Detection and Cognitive Therapy for People at High Risk for Psychosis: A Treatment Approach. New York, Wiley, 2004

Hardy KV: Fact sheet: Cognitive behavioral therapy for psychosis (CBTp). SAMHSA/CMHS, 2018. Available at: www.nasmhpd.org/sites/default/files/DH-CBTp_Fact_Sheet.pdf. Accessed October 9, 2018.

Kingdon D, Turkington D: Cognitive Therapy of Schizophrenia. New York, Guilford, 2005

Penn DL, Meyer PS, Gottlieb J, et al: Individual resiliency training (IRT). April 1, 2014. Available at: http://raiseetp.org/StudyManuals/IRT%20Complete%20Manual.pdf. Accessed October 9, 2018.

References

Beck AT, Rush AJ, Shaw BF, et al: Cognitive Therapy of Depression. New York, Guilford, 1979

Beck AT, Emery G, Greenberg RL: Anxiety Disorders and Phobias: A Cognitive Perspective. New York, Basic Books, 1985

Beck AT, Rector NA, Stolar N, et al: Schizophrenia: Cognitive Theory, Research, and Therapy. New York, Guilford, 2009

Bertolote J, McGorry P: Early intervention and recovery for young people with early psychosis: consensus statement. Br J Psychiatry Suppl 48:s116–119, 2005 16055800

Burns AMN, Erickson DH, Brenner CA: Cognitive-behavioral therapy for medication-resistant psychosis: a meta-analytic review. Psychiatr Serv 65(7):874–880, 2014 24686725

Chadwick P, Birchwood M, Trower P: Cognitive Therapy for Delusions, Voices, and Paranoia. Chichester, England, Wiley, 1996

Corrigan PW: The Principles and Practice of Psychiatric Rehabilitation: An Empirical Approach, 2nd Edition. New York, Guilford, 2016

Fredrickson BL: Positivity: Groundbreaking Research Reveals How to Embrace the Hidden Strength of Positive Emotions, Overcome Negativity, and Thrive. New York, Crown Publishers, 2009

Hale JL, Householder BJ, Greene KL: The theory of reasoned action, in The Persuasion Handbook: Developments in Theory and Practice. Edited by Dillard JP, Pfau M. Thousand Oaks, CA, Sage, 2002, pp 259–286

Ince P, Haddock G, Tai S: A systematic review of the implementation of recommended psychological interventions for schizophrenia: rates, barriers, and improvement strategies. Psychol Psychother 89(3):324–350, 2016 26537838

Kingdon DG, Turkington D: Cognitive-Behavioral Therapy of Schizophrenia. New York, Guilford, 1994

McGuire AB, Kukla M, Green A, et al: Illness management and recovery: a review of the literature. Psychiatr Serv 65(2):171–179, 2014 24178191

Meyer PS, Johnson DP, Parks A, et al: Positive living: A pilot study of group positive psychotherapy for people with schizophrenia. J Posit Psychol 7:239–248, 2012

Morrison AP, Barratt S: What are the components of CBT for psychosis? A Delphi study. Schizophr Bull 36(1):136-142, 2010 19880824

Morrison AP, Renton JC, Dunn H, et al: Cognitive Therapy for Psychosis: A Formulation-Based Approach. New York, Brunner-Routledge, 2004

Mueser KT, Lu W, Rosenberg SD, et al: The trauma of psychosis: posttraumatic stress disorder and recent onset psychosis. Schizophr Res 116(2–3):217–227, 2010 19939633

Mueser KT, Deavers F, Penn DL, et al: Psychosocial treatments for schizophrenia. Annu Rev Clin Psychol 9:465–497, 2013 23330939

Mueser KT, Penn DL, Addington J, et al: The NAVIGATE program for first-episode psychosis: rationale, overview, and description of psychosocial components. Psychiatr Serv 66(7):680–690, 2015 25772766

Penn DL, Uzenoff SR, Perkins D, et al: A pilot investigation of the Graduated Recovery Intervention Program (GRIP) for first episode psychosis. Schizophr Res 125(2–3):247–256, 2011 20817484

Rapp CA, Goscha RJ: The Strengths Model: Case Management With People With Psychiatric Disabilities, 2nd Edition. New York, Oxford University Press, 2006

Rathod S, Kingdon DG, Pinninti N, et al: Cultural Adaptation of CBT for Serious Mental Illness: A Guide for Training and Practice. Chichester, UK, Wiley, 2015

Roth AD, Pilling S: A competence framework for psychological interventions with people with psychosis and bipolar disorder. 2013. Available at: www.ucl.ac.uk/clinical-psychology//CORE/Docs/Working%20with%20 Psychosis%20and%20Bipolar%20Disorder%20background%20document %20web%20version.pdf. Accessed October 9, 2018.

Seligman ME: Flourish: A Visionary New Understanding of Happiness and Well-Being. New York, Simon & Schuster, 2012

Seligman MEP, Rashid T, Parks AC: Positive psychotherapy. Am Psychol 61(8):774–788, 2006 17115810

Sensky T, Turkington D, Kingdon D, et al: A randomized controlled trial of cognitive-behavioral therapy for persistent symptoms in schizophrenia resistant to medication. Arch Gen Psychiatry 57(2):165–172, 2000 10665619

Turner DT, van der Gaag M, Karyotaki E, et al: Psychological interventions for psychosis: a meta-analysis of comparative outcome studies. Am J Psychiatry 171(5):523–538, 2014 24525715

Zubin J, Spring B: Vulnerability—a new view of schizophrenia. J Abnorm Psychol 86(2):103–126, 1977 858828

CHAPTER 14

Substance Use and Early Psychosis

Jeffrey D. Reed, D.O.
Mary F. Brunette, M.D.

Case Example

James, a 19-year-old young man, went to his local emergency department with severe anxiety and the conviction that his family was in grave
danger. His parents (with whom he lived) related that he became increasingly irritable about 3 months ago. He reported "weird thoughts"
that his family was going to be murdered, that he was responsible for
the misfortunes of others, and that strangers could "see" his thoughts of
guilt. During the past month he slept poorly, was exhausted, and was
distracted at his cashier job.

When asked about substances, James said he had been using marijuana for about 4 years, increasing his use in the past year to a "few bong
hits with friends" each day. He realized that he felt more paranoid after
he smoked pot and said his supervisor was criticizing his work. Although he last used 2 weeks ago, he was now even more distressed.

While in the hospital, James started taking risperidone 0.5 mg each
evening for psychosis and melatonin 3 mg at bedtime for sleep. He and
his family met with his treatment team to discuss information about
psychosis and substance abuse, as well as options for care. His sleep and
distress from paranoia improved by 50% within 2 days. James stated
that his goals were to "get back to normal and to be able to go to work."
His team recommended continued medication, avoidance of alcohol
and marijuana, and counseling to work on skills to "do reality checks"
and manage anxiety and stress.

Following discharge, James attended monthly appointments with a psychiatrist and twice-monthly appointments with a therapist. His paranoia, irritability, and thought broadcasting progressively improved.

James's use of substances is similar to many individuals who are experiencing their first episode of psychosis. About half of people with early psychosis have recently used substances, and up to one-half of people with schizophrenia will develop a substance use disorder over their lifetime, a rate that is three to five times higher than general population rates (Addington et al. 2014; Brunette et al. 2018a). Although many people with schizophrenia report subjective pleasant effects with substance use, they also experience exacerbated psychotic symptoms (D'Souza et al. 2005). Persistent substance use or substance use disorder is associated with poorer treatment outcomes and worse course of illness in people with early psychosis (Hadden et al. 2018).

Given the adverse impact of substance use on an individual's symptoms and progress in treatment, in what ways can clinicians best support people who are in the early stages of psychotic illness and also using substances? The goals of this chapter are to 1) review facts about co-occurring early psychosis and substance use, 2) discuss how to screen and assess for substance use disorders and distinguish between early psychosis with co-occurring substance use disorders and substance-induced psychosis, and 3) describe stage-wise psychosocial and pharmacological interventions to treat people with early psychosis with co-occurring substance use disorders

Consequences of Substance Use in People with Early Psychosis

Among people with early psychosis, cannabis, tobacco, and alcohol use are particularly prevalent, and use of substances tends to follow the pattern seen in the general population, although people with schizophrenia are less likely to engage in heroin and other opioid abuse compared with the general population (Chiappelli et al. 2018). Heavy cannabis use in early adolescence has been shown to increase the risk of later developing schizophrenia (Murray et al. 2017); thus, cannabis likely precipitates schizophrenia in people who are at risk for developing the disorder.

When using substances, most people with a psychotic illness experience pleasant, relaxed, and "high" feelings and may also experience a sense of heightened sociability. These same individuals also experience transient increases in psychotic symptoms, despite taking antipsychotic medications. For example, in one study, about 70% of people with schizophrenia developed transient increases in psychotic symptoms after a single dose of a stimulant (Berman et al. 2009). Other studies have demonstrated that acute and chronic cannabis use exacerbates psychotic symptoms (D'Souza et al. 2005). Some reports have indicated that developing a substance use disorder is associated with higher levels of impulsivity, mood lability, and hostility in people with first-episode psychosis, which may place them at higher risk for unsafe behavior and legal problems (Brunette et al. 2018a). In people with schizophrenia, substance use disorder is related to more severe symptoms, reduced adherence to antipsychotic and psychological treatments, more relapses and hospitalizations, and lower levels of functioning (Drake et al. 2008).

Many clinicians ignore tobacco use disorder in individuals with first-episode psychosis because it does not appear to impede functioning or worsen symptoms in the way that alcohol and drugs do. However, people with psychosis are more likely to initiate smoking and have a higher level of dependence than smokers without psychosis (McClave et al. 2010). The problem with smoking is that it directly contributes to heart disease, lung disease, diabetes, and cancers—smoking is the leading preventable cause of these diseases in the United States. People with schizophrenia die 20–30 years earlier than the general population, and smoking is responsible for 50% of those deaths (Callaghan et al. 2014). Clinicians can provide information and resources to help clients cut down and quit smoking. A majority of young people with psychosis report *a desire* to quit smoking and will take steps to quit if provided clinical support (Brunette et al. 2017).

Distinguishing Between Substance-Induced Psychosis and First-Episode Psychosis

In the acute treatment setting, when an individual presents with both new psychosis symptoms and recent drug or alcohol use, the clinician will need to determine over time whether the client is experiencing a first episode of a primary psychotic illness, such as schizophrenia, or whether he or she is experiencing a substance-induced psychosis. Psychosis spurred by substance use may indicate an increased risk for additional psychotic episodes in the context of substance use or a more chronic psychotic illness. Providers and families should know that uncertainty exists and that close, longitudinal monitoring is necessary to distinguish between substance-induced and first-episode psychosis. In order to distinguish between substance-induced and primary psychoses, clinicians should consider whether the psychosis symptoms are consistent with the type of substances being used, the time course of the substance use and psychotic symptoms, and the person's personal and family history of substance abuse and psychosis (see Table 14–1).

Some substances of abuse are known to produce psychotic states in nonpsychotic people, especially when used in large amounts for long periods of time. *Substance-induced psychosis* is the presence of psychotic symptoms in the context of intoxication by or withdrawal from a substance that are not otherwise accounted for by a non-substance-related psychotic disorder (e.g., schizophrenia spectrum illness, affective disorders with psychotic features, delirium). People with substance-induced psychosis may also experience mood symptoms, abnormal behavior, disorganized speech, and impaired cognition. Substance-induced psychosis is most likely to develop in polysubstance users.

A number of abused substances can precipitate psychotic symptoms through intoxication or withdrawal in people with and without a psychotic disorder (Table 14–2). Stimulants and cannabis are the most commonly abused agents known to cause psychotic symptoms. For example, abuse of stimulants increases the risk of developing psychotic symptoms up to 11 times the risk in the non-using population (McKetin et al. 2006). Psychosis can also occur in the context of abusing phencyclidine, other hallucinogens, and inhalants. Psychosis symptoms typically seen with substance use, as well as other signs and symptoms associated with intoxication and withdrawal, are shown in Table 14–2. If a substance-using individual presents with psychosis symptoms that are not consistent with the substance, the clinician may be more concerned about the presence of a first episode of schizophrenia, but the diagnosis becomes clearer over time (Drake et al. 2011).

In the United States, many states are legalizing cannabis as *medical marijuana* and/or for recreational use, leading to more favorable attitudes and increased use of cannabis. Tetrahydrocannabinol (THC), the main psychoactive agent in naturally occurring cannabis and in synthetic cannabinoids (e.g., Spice, K2), can cause psychotic symptoms and exacerbate psychosis in people with schizophrenia who are taking antipsychotics (D'Souza et al. 2005), whereas cannabidiol (CBD), also in naturally occurring cannabis, may have calming, antipsychotic, and analgesic effects (D'Souza et al. 2016; Hahn 2018; Murray et al. 2017). The concentration of THC in cannabis has increased over the last 40 years. Some strains of high-THC cannabis precipitate psychotic symptoms among many people who use them. Cannabis-induced psychosis may be transient and remitting, but studies have reported that approximately 41% of people with cannabis-induced psychosis converted to having chronic schizophrenia (Starzer et al. 2018). Additionally, regular cannabis use causes changes in cognition (e.g., deficits in memory, disorganized thinking) as well as amotivation and impaired expression of affect.

TABLE 14–1. Distinguishing between first-episode psychosis and substance-induced psychosis

	First-episode psychosis without substances	First-episode psychosis triggered by substances	Substance-induced psychosis
Urine or blood toxicology	Negative[a]	Likely positive (stimulants, cannabis, alcohol, sedatives, phencyclidine, other hallucinogens, opioids)[a]	Likely positive (stimulants, cannabis, alcohol, sedatives, phencyclidine, other hallucinogens, opioids)[a]
Psychosis onset	Gradual or sudden and not coinciding with substance use[a]	Sudden onset during periods of acute substance use	Usually sudden during periods of acute or chronic substance use or withdrawal[a]
Resolution	Psychosis is nonremitting (may reduce in severity or resolve with antipsychotic medication)[a]	Psychosis may or may not remit during periods of abstinence[a]	Psychosis resolves during periods of abstinence or following withdrawal from acute or ongoing substance use[a]
Symptoms	Positive symptoms: mood incongruent hallucinations, delusions, thought disorder, agitation[a] Negative symptoms: avolition, apathy, reduced affect, poverty of speech, impaired cognition[a]	Symptoms may be characteristic of substance of abuse. May overlap with symptoms consistent with schizophrenia[a]	Dependent on substance of abuse (see Table 14–2)

TABLE 14–1.   Distinguishing between first-episode psychosis and substance-induced psychosis

	First-episode psychosis without substances	First-episode psychosis triggered by substances	Substance-induced psychosis
History	May have personal or family history of primary psychotic illness[a]	May have personal or family history of substance use disorder, primary psychotic illness, or substance-induced psychosis	May have personal or family history of substance use disorder or substance-induced psychosis[b]
Acute treatment	Antipsychotic medications, education, family engagement, ensuring safe environment, close monitoring, sleep regulation, abstinence from substances	Antipsychotic medications, reducing stimulation, providing reassurance and supportive care, education, close monitoring, sleep regulation	Reducing stimulation, reassurance and supportive care with close monitoring, antipsychotic and/or sedative-hypnotic medications (if behavior is dangerous)[c]

[a]American Psychiatric Association 2013.
[b]Brady et al. 1995.
[c]McIver et al. 2006.

TABLE 14–2. Signs and symptoms of acute intoxication and withdrawal for commonly abused substances

Substance	Acute intoxication	Acute withdrawal	Psychotic symptoms with intoxication	Psychotic symptoms with withdrawal	Exacerbates psychosis in schizophrenia spectrum disorders?
Alcohol and sedatives[a,b,c]	• Depression • Problematic behavior • Slurred speech • Poor coordination • Impaired cognition • Stupor	• Increased heart rate • Tremor • Insomnia • Nausea or vomiting • Hallucinations or illusions • Restlessness • Anxiety • Seizures	• Visual and tactile hallucinations • Auditory, visual, and tactile illusions	• Visual and tactile hallucinations • Auditory, visual, and tactile illusions	Sometimes

TABLE 14–2. Signs and symptoms of acute intoxication and withdrawal for commonly abused substances *(continued)*

Substance	Acute intoxication	Acute withdrawal	Psychotic symptoms with intoxication	Psychotic symptoms with withdrawal	Exacerbates psychosis in schizophrenia spectrum disorders?
Cannabis[a,b,c,e]	• Problematic behavior • Euphoria • Impaired learning and memory • Red or injected eyes • Increased appetite • Dry mouth • Increased heart rate	• Irritability • Anxiety • Insomnia • Decreased appetite • Restlessness • Depression • Physical complaints	• Paranoid delusions • Auditory and visual hallucinations and illusions	No	Yes
Stimulants[a,b,f]	• Heart rate abnormalities • Blood pressure abnormalities • Pupillary dilation • Sweating • Nausea or vomiting • Weight loss • Restlessness • Seizures and coma	• Depression • Fatigue • Vivid dreams • Insomnia or hypersomnia • Increased appetite • Motor slowing or agitation	• Paranoid delusions • Auditory, visual, and tactile hallucinations	No	Yes

Substance	Acute intoxication	Acute withdrawal	Psychotic symptoms with intoxication	Psychotic symptoms with withdrawal	Exacerbates psychosis in schizophrenia spectrum disorders?
TABLE 14–2.	Signs and symptoms of acute intoxication and withdrawal for commonly abused substances *(continued)*				
Opioids[a]	• Euphoria • Apathy • Pupillary constriction • Drowsiness and coma • Impaired cognition	• Depression • Nausea or vomiting • Diarrhea • Muscle pain • Pupillary dilation • Sweating • Piloerection • Yawning • Insomnia	No	No	Unknown

TABLE 14–2. Signs and symptoms of acute intoxication and withdrawal for commonly abused substances (*continued*)

Substance	Acute intoxication	Acute withdrawal	Psychotic symptoms with intoxication	Psychotic symptoms with withdrawal	Exacerbates psychosis in schizophrenia spectrum disorders?
Phencyclidine (PCP)[a,g]	• Impulsivity • Aggression • Abnormal balance • Restlessness • High blood pressure or heart rate • Reduced response to pain • Seizures • Sensitivity to sound and volume	• Headaches • Increased appetite • Fatigue • Depression	• Paranoid and other delusions • Auditory, visual, and tactile hallucinations	No	Unknown

TABLE 14–2. Signs and symptoms of acute intoxication and withdrawal for commonly abused substances (*continued*)

Substance	Acute intoxication	Acute withdrawal	Psychotic symptoms with intoxication	Psychotic symptoms with withdrawal	Exacerbates psychosis in schizophrenia spectrum disorders?
Other Hallucinogen[a,g]	• Pupillary dilation • Palpitations • Sweating • Blurred vision • Tremor • Poor coordination	Unknown	• Ideas of reference • Depersonalization • Derealization • Auditory, visual, and tactile hallucinations • Illusions or synthesthesias	Persisting hallucinations consistent with those experienced during intoxication	Unknown

[a]American Psychiatric Association 2013.
[b]Ouellet-Plamondon et al. 2017.
[c]Noordsy et al. 1991.
[d]D'Souza et al. 2005.
[e]Sherif et al. 2016.
[f]Berman et al. 2009.
[g]National Institute on Drug Abuse 2018.

To determine whether psychosis symptoms occur independent of substance use, clinicians can help clients draw a timeline of psychosis symptoms alongside a timeline of substance use, including type, frequency, and severity. If psychotic symptoms continue during periods of abstinence, a primary psychotic illness is likely. Clinicians may need to monitor individuals prospectively for symptoms and substance use to observe whether psychosis persists during periods of abstinence, taking into account that when clients are taking antipsychotic medication, psychosis may be controlled or in remission, and it may take months for psychosis to recur once people are no longer taking medications. People with substance-induced psychosis can be advised that they may develop a chronic psychotic disorder and should be provided appropriate monitoring and treatment.

Management of Acute Substance-Induced Psychosis

People with an acute episode of substance-induced psychosis may require reassurance and a calm, quiet, low-stimulation, supportive environment. Those with substantial psychological or behavioral agitation may require oral or intramuscular sedative-hypnotic or sedating antipsychotic medications. Individuals with psychotic symptoms that are substantially distressing or disruptive should be treated with antipsychotic medications, with or without sedative-hypnotic medications (McIver et al. 2006). Once the crisis is stabilized, clients and their families can be provided education, monitoring, and additional intervention as described below. If psychotic symptoms occur solely with substance use and resolve completely with abstinence from substance use, tapering off of antipsychotic medication may be indicated.

Screening and Evaluation of Substance Use Disorder in People With Psychosis

All clinicians treating individuals with psychosis can screen for substance use initially, periodically evaluate them for substance use disorders, and provide basic education about the impacts of substance use. The National Institute on Drug Abuse (NIDA) offers a "quick screen" (https://www.drugabuse.gov/publications/resource-guide-screening-drug-use-in-general-medical-settings/nida-quick-screen), including the NIDA-Modified ASSIST (https://www.drugabuse.gov/sites/default/files/pdf/nmassist.pdf), that systematically assesses the type and frequency of substances used. The NIDA-Modified ASSIST, which is based on the World Health Organization's Alcohol, Smoking and Substance Involvement Screening Test (ASSIST), obtains a more detailed history of all substance use and severity of use. As in the case of James, obtaining an initial comprehensive history of substance use and presence of use disorder relative to the onset of psychotic symptoms is an important part of the initial and ongoing evaluation.

Clinicians can ask clients whether they have ever used alcohol, street drugs, or tobacco and also whether they have used prescribed medications or medical marijuana to relax, deal with stress, or get high. Among those who have used, clinicians can then ask about recent use (we recommend past year) of each substance, including amount, method of use, frequency of use, and context of use (e.g., people, places), in a curious and nonjudgmental fashion. The clinician should assess perceived benefits and consequences of use, such as inclusion in peer groups; anxiety reduction; impacts on school or work and family relationships; and legal problems. Such an evaluation should be completed at the time of initial contact and periodically thereafter. Because people generally underreport substance use, obtaining information about substance use from family, friends, clinicians, and other supports is also important. Many clinics obtain urine drug screens when behavior suggests that substance use may be contributing to a person's illness.

Peer Influences on Substance Use in Psychosis

In addition to direct genetic and environmental effects on substance use in young people, peer substance use is influential, both through selection (choosing to be with people whose behavior is similar to one's own) and via direct influence (creating or changing perceptions and expectancies, facilitating access, using social modeling, and other mechanisms) (Edwards et al. 2016). Given the importance of peer influence on behavior in young people, including peers in team care may increase engagement and acceptability of interventions for people with early psychosis (Deutsch et al. 2017).

Integrated Stagewise Treatment for Substance Use Disorders in Early Psychosis: Assessing Motivation for Recovery

Integrated treatment consolidates components of treatment for early psychosis and treatment for substance use disorders into a single setting and team (Addington et al. 2014; Drake et al. 2008). This approach ensures that all clients receive a consistent message about how substance use impacts their psychotic symptoms and also ensures access to both treatments and individualization of these treatments to best fit the needs of the client (Drake et al. 2008; Mueser et al. 2003). Ideally, treatments are tailored to an individual's level of motivation to change and recovery goals.

Stagewise substance use treatment for people with schizophrenia yields functional improvements over time (Xie et al. 2005). This approach employs Osher and Kofoed's (1989) Model of Recovery Supports applied strategically for individuals at each level of motivation (Mueser et al. 2003):

1. For clients who are in precontemplation, interventions focus on *engagement*. Engagement interventions include developing a therapeutic relationship, providing practical help, assessing substance use and related problems, and providing education on risks of substance use and effects on psychiatric symptoms.
2. For clients who are in contemplation, interventions are encompassed by the term *persuasion*. In this phase, clinicians continue with education, provide motivational interventions, help clients set meaningful personal goals, and then help them identify the pros and cons of substance use and how substance use may affect their ability to attain these goals.
3. For clients who are in the action stage of change, clinicians provide *active treatment interventions*. Active treatment includes helping people learn skills to reduce and stop substance use and to cope with symptoms and stress. Most people in this phase still need motivational support.
4. For clients in the *relapse prevention* phase, clinicians help them avoid relapse and maintain recovery. During this phase, clinicians provide assistance in learning skills to maintain sobriety and expand recovery to other areas of life, such as school, fitness, social networks, and work.

Interventions for Substance Use Disorders in Early Psychosis

Psychosocial Interventions

Individuals entering treatment for a first episode of early psychosis need intensive supports to stabilize their psychosis, as described in the second half of this book (see Chapters 10–20). Early on, clinicians provide engagement-stage interventions, assessing level of substance use and whether a substance use disorder is present. Clinicians educate all clients and families about psychiatric symptoms and prognosis and provide an overview of treatment as described in Chapter 6 ("Engaging Families and Individuals in Care") and Chapter 17 ("Implementing Peer Support in Early Psychosis Programs"), as well as about the negative impact of substance use on psychosis recovery. Individuals who persist in using substances and experience negative consequences from using after the first 3–6 months of coordinated specialty care for psychosis may need additional treatment for substance use disorders.

Motivational interviewing is a form of counseling in which clinicians help clients increase their interest in making change (Miller and Rollnick 1991). It can focus on substance use, antipsychotic medication, or any behavior. Among individuals who are misusing substances, brief motivational interviewing can help them use skills to reduce their substance use in the early stages of psychotic illness (Kavanagh et al. 2004). Among others, it may simply increase a client's willingness to engage in counseling to learn new skills to cut down and stop using substances. Incorporating families into motivational counseling may enhance the efficacy of this approach (Horsfall et al. 2009).

Cognitive-behavioral therapy (CBT) is a type of counseling that involves teaching people skills to cope with urges to use substances, avoid high-risk situations, manage social interactions effectively, and engage in replacement activities such as hobbies and sports. This action-stage intervention can be provided to individuals, families, and groups of individuals. Among clients who are motivated to change their substance use, CBT can be tailored to help clients manage both their psychosis and their substance use disorder (see Chapter 13, "Psychotherapeutic Interventions for Early Psychosis"). CBT provided in groups offers the advantage of developing and practicing social skills with peers, access to peer feedback about substance use, and exposure to peer role models who have been able to take positive steps forward (Mueser et al. 2003).

Contingency management combined with psychosocial interventions such as community reinforcement therapy is an effective approach to addressing addiction (Sigmon 2007). Contingency management involves providing agreed-on reinforcers for behaviors such as abstinence based on clear evidence of that behavior (e.g., drug-free urine) (Horsfall et al. 2009; Sigmon 2007). For example, effective contingent reinforcers could include small and increasing amounts of cash, gift cards for movies or meals, or drawings for prizes based on negative urine drug screens, treatment attendance, or both. Teams can work with clients and their families or representative payees to provide such incentives using money from the person's social security benefits in situations where other resources are not available for incentives (Ries et al. 2004). Recent evidence supporting use of this strategy shows success in treating alcohol use disorder and tobacco use disorder in people with schizophrenia and other severe mental illnesses (Brunette et al. 2018b; McDonell et al. 2013).

Medication Management

Medications are important preparation-, action-, and maintenance-stage interventions for people with early psychosis and substance use disorders. Antipsychotic medications reduce or eliminate psychosis symptoms, enabling people to participate in school and work; engage in naturally rewarding, healthy activities; and participate in substance use disorder treatment if needed. Addiction treatment medications aim to reduce craving and reduce substance use. In the following subsections, we review the impact of antipsychotic medications and other medications on substance use in schizophrenia.

ANTIPSYCHOTICS AND SUBSTANCE USE DISORDERS

Antipsychotic medications are targeted at psychosis but may have differential impacts on substance use behavior (Akerman et al. 2014). Maintaining good control of psychotic symptoms is important for people with co-occurring substance use disorder because this enables them to participate in substance use disorder treatment. However, drugs with strong dopaminergic blockade, such as high-potency typical antipsychotics (e.g., haloperidol), have been associated with worse outcomes, worsening substance use in patients with co-occurring disorders, perhaps due to reduced brain reward circuit function (Green 2007). Drugs with partial dopaminergic blockade, such as aripiprazole, or with a relatively low level of dopamine D_2 receptor blockade and stronger α_2-adrenergic receptor antagonism and noradrenergic reuptake inhibition, such as clozapine and quetiapine, may reduce substance use, perhaps by improving brain reward function. More research is needed to establish whether one medication provides clear advantage over another for people with co-occurring schizophrenia and substance use disorder.

Long-acting injectable (LAI) formulations of antipsychotics simplify medication for patients and enable clinicians to be aware of when patients discontinue antipsychotic medications. Several studies indicate that people with chronic schizophrenia assigned to receive LAI risperidone or paliperidone had better substance-related outcomes than those assigned to receive oral medications (Green et al. 2015; Lefebvre et al. 2017). Long-acting injectable antipsychotics are an important option for patients who have difficulty taking oral medications.

MEDICATIONS USED TO TREAT SUBSTANCE USE DISORDERS

In this subsection, we discuss medication options in the treatment of substance use disorders and, where data are available, in the treatment of people with co-occurring psychosis (Akerman et al. 2014).

Alcohol use disorder. The first-line pharmacological treatments for alcohol use disorder include naltrexone and acamprosate, which reduce craving for alcohol and are appropriate for people with heavy drinking (Lyon 2017). These medications may be used safely in combination with antipsychotic medication. Naltrexone has been shown to have a promising impact on reducing drinking in people with schizophrenia and alcohol use disorder (Petrakis et al. 2004).

Disulfiram is a medication that blocks metabolism of alcohol, resulting in aversive and potentially dangerous side effects if a person drinks. Anticipating these effects can be a deterrent to drinking. This medication is most effective when its use is monitored daily by family or clinicians of motivated patients (Mueser et al. 2003). Varenicline has been shown to reduce drinking in people with alcohol use disorder (Litten et al. 2013). One small trial was promising in people with schizophrenia and alcohol use disorder, but the effectiveness was limited by low tolerability (primarily abdominal pain) (Meszaros et al. 2013).

Cannabis use disorder. N-acetylcysteine may offer some positive effects in reducing cannabis use in adolescents with cannabis use disorder (Deepmala et al. 2015), but it has not been studied in people with schizophrenia and cannabis use disorder. Oral THC as a replacement therapy does not reduce cannabis use in people with cannabis use disorder (Haney et al. 2008); however, early research indicates that the combination of high doses of THC and CBD in nabiximols combined with motivation enhancement therapy and CBT may be helpful (Trigo et al. 2018). Early research has shown that CBD reduces symptoms of psychosis in people with schizophrenia (Hahn 2018), but it is not clear whether CBD alone has an impact on cannabis use in individuals with cannabis use disorder.

Tobacco use disorder. Three U.S. Food and Drug Administration–approved treatments for tobacco use disorder have all been shown to be safe and effective in people with schizophrenia: varenicline (Chantix), bupropion (Zyban), and nicotine replacement therapy (nicotine gum, patch, lozenge, or inhaler) (see Cather et al. 2017 for review). Current treatment guidelines recommend providing cessation counseling with the use of varenicline or bupropion alone or with nicotine replacement therapy in smokers with schizophrenia. Continued maintenance treatment with counseling and medications may also reduce relapse in this population.

Opioid use disorder. Medication-assisted treatments dramatically improve outcomes and reduce overdose deaths for people with opioid use disorder. The current recommended opioid agonist therapies include buprenorphine, which can be prescribed by office-based providers, and methadone, available only from licensed clinics. These medications occupy brain opioid receptors, preventing people from getting high when they use opioids, thus reducing drug-seeking behavior and enabling people to engage in treatment and recovery activities. Naltrexone occupies opioid receptors without agonism, also preventing intoxication. This medication has lower rates of success than buprenorphine and methadone in the general population. These medications have not been studied in people with schizophrenia and opioid use disorder, but their use is safe and should be encouraged (American Society of Addiction Medicine 2015). Close monitoring and avoiding medication interactions, such as with benzodiazepines, enhances safety and adherence.

Maintenance Treatment, Relapse Prevention, and Recovery

Once individuals with early psychosis and substance use disorder are managing symptoms of psychosis and are abstinent or without symptoms of substance use disorder, preventing relapse is the primary goal of treatment (Drake et al. 2008). Relapse prevention skills training helps clients identify *triggers*—situations, people, and places that may increase risk for relapse—and to develop a plan to address them.

People with psychosis and co-occurring substance use disorders are better able to maintain sobriety when they have stable housing in a supportive environment, are socially connected with abstinent peers, and have adopted self-monitoring attitudes around their substance use and mental health. Regular structured activities, such as school, exercise, and paid or volunteer work, are key to developing a meaningful life as young people maintain their recovery. Involvement in self-help groups such as Alcoholics Anonymous may provide support and an avenue for developing a social network that does not involve substance use.

Case Example *(continued)*

A few months after James's discharge, he returned to work. There, he reconnected with friends and started smoking marijuana with them. A week later, he stopped his medication. Over the next few weeks, he became increasingly anxious. With his therapist, he explored the pros and cons of smoking marijuana in relation to being with his friends and in relation to anxiety and paranoia. They also explored the pros and cons of using antipsychotic medication in relation to James's symptoms and his ability to function at work. Additionally, he talked with his doctor about weight gain—he had gained 20 pounds. His newly stated personal goals were to look good in order to get a girlfriend, to avoid feeling anxious, and to be able to keep his job so he could have money. After reviewing these goals, James realized he probably should use medication to keep the anxiety low. He agreed to restart an antipsychotic with lower risk for weight gain and developed a plan for regular exercise.

James noticed feeling calmer within a few days of starting the medication. He decided he would commit to taking the medication for a year. After a month of ongoing discussions with his therapist about whether smoking marijuana "was worth it," especially related to his work performance, James decided to avoid smoking pot and to focus on one friend at work who did not smoke marijuana. Over the next 12 months, James worked his way up to an assistant manager position at his place of employment.

Conclusion and Recommendations

Many people with early psychosis experiment with stopping medications and trying substance use again after a period of abstinence. James's presentation demonstrates the challenges that can be worked through to engage and treat clients with co-occurring disorders. His treatment team continued to regularly assess for substance use and engage in therapeutic work to rebuild motivation to manage psychosis symptoms and avoid using substances. They supported him in finding sober peers, listened to his concerns about his psychiatric treatment, and worked with him to find a tolerable medication that would enable him to make progress toward his personal goals.

A team-based approach that involves client-centered psychosocial and medical interventions enables assessment, prevention, and management of substance use disorders in individuals with early psychosis. Teams deliver the following treatment components to help clients effectively manage their substance use:

- Early and accurate identification of psychosis and psychosis-risk syndromes
- Psychoeducation for clients and families that promotes understanding of psychosis and substance use and their interactions
- Screening for substance use and diagnosis of use disorders
- Stagewise psychotherapeutic interventions to increase motivation and skills to reduce and stop substance use
- Peer support to improve social connectedness and model responsible substance use and abstinence
- Careful medication management that targets both psychosis and substance use

With these treatment components in coordinated specialty care, clients can develop the skills needed to manage both their substance use and psychosis to better meet their personal goals and achieve recovery.

KEY CONCEPTS

- Substance use is common in people presenting with early psychosis, with bidirectional interactions.

- Longitudinal observation is often required to distinguish substance-induced psychosis from early psychosis triggered by substance use.

- Ongoing substance use is associated with lower likelihood of remission from psychosis and worse outcomes.

- Integrated treatment for psychosis and substance use within a coordinated specialty care framework is recommended in order to improve outcomes.

Discussion Questions

1. Why might diagnostic uncertainty between substance-induced psychosis and primary psychosis be a good prognostic sign? How would you discuss this with families eager to know the diagnosis?

2. Why would degree of reduction in positive and negative symptoms in response to antipsychotic medication and abstinence be helpful in clarifying diagnosis?

3. How could discussion of long-term functional goals facilitate motivation for treatment of substance abuse? For treatment of psychosis?

4. Why might integration of substance abuse treatment into the coordinated specialty care team have advantages?

Suggested Readings

Brunette MF, Noordsy DL, Green AI: Co-occurring substance use and other psychiatric disorders, in Textbook of Schizophrenia. Edited by Lieberman JA, Stroup TS, Perkins DO. Washington, DC, American Psychiatric Press, 2006, pp 223–244

Drake RE, O'Neal EL, Wallach MA: A systematic review of psychosocial research on psychosocial interventions for people with co-occurring severe mental and substance use disorders. J Subst Abuse Treat 34(1):123–138, 2008 17574803

Mueser KT, Noordsy DL, Drake RE, et al: Integrated Treatment for Dual Disorders: A Guide to Effective Practice. New York, Guilford, 2003

Ziedonis DM, Smelson D, Rosenthal RN, et al: Improving the care of individuals with schizophrenia and substance use disorders: consensus recommendations. J Psychiatr Pract 11(5):315–339, 2005 16184072

References

Addington J, Case N, Saleem MM, et al: Substance use in clinical high risk for psychosis: a review of the literature. Early Interv Psychiatry 8(2):104–112, 2014 24224849

Akerman SC, Brunette MF, Noordsy DL, et al: Pharmacotherapy of co-occurring schizophrenia and substance use disorders. Curr Addict Rep 1(4):251–260, 2014 27226947

American Psychiatric Association: Diagnostic and Statistical Manual of Mental Disorders, 5th Edition. Arlington, VA, American Psychiatric Publishing, 2013

American Society of Addiction Medicine: National Practice Guideline for the Use of Medications in the Treatment of Addiction Involving Opioid Use. Chevy Chase, MD, American Society of Addiction Medicine, 2015

Berman SM, Kuczenski R, McCracken JT, et al: Potential adverse effects of amphetamine treatment on brain and behavior: a review. Mol Psychiatry 14(2):123–142, 2009 18698321

Brady KT, Sonne S, Randall CL, et al: Features of cocaine dependence with concurrent alcohol abuse. Drug Alcohol Depend 39(1):69–71, 1995 7587977

Brunette MF, Feiron JC, Aschbrenner K, et al: Characteristics and predictors of intention to use cessation treatment among smokers with schizophrenia: young adult compared to older adults. J Subst Abus Alcohol 5(1):1055, 2017 29881770

Brunette MF, Mueser KT, Babbin S, et al: Demographic and clinical correlates of substance use disorders in first episode psychosis. Schizophr Res 194:4–12, 2018a 28697856

Brunette MF, Pratt SI, Bartels SJ, et al: Randomized trial of interventions for smoking cessation among Medicaid beneficiaries with mental illness. Psychiatr Serv 69(3):274–280, 2018b 29137560

Callaghan RC, Veldhuizen S, Jeysingh T, et al: Patterns of tobacco-related mortality among individuals diagnosed with schizophrenia, bipolar disorder, or depression. J Psychiatr Res 48(1):102–110, 2014 24139811

Cather C, Pachas GN, Cieslak KM, et al: Achieving smoking cessation in individuals with schizophrenia: special considerations. CNS Drugs 31(6):471–481, 2017 28550660

Chiappelli J, Chen S, Hackman A, et al: Evidence for differential opioid use disorder in schizophrenia in an addiction treatment population. Schizophr Res 194:26–31, 2018 28487076

Deepmala SJ, Slattery J, Kumar N, et al: Clinical trials of N-acetylcysteine in psychiatry and neurology: a systematic review. Neurosci Biobehav Rev 55:294–321, 2015 25957927

Deutsch AR, Wood PK, Slutske WS: Developmental etiologies of alcohol use and their relations to parent and peer influences over adolescence and young adulthood: a genetically informed approach. Alcohol Clin Exp Res 41(12):2151–2162, 2017 29083505

Drake RE, O'Neal EL, Wallach MA: A systematic review of psychosocial research on psychosocial interventions for people with co-occurring severe mental and substance use disorders. J Subst Abuse Treat 34(1):123–138, 2008 17574803

Drake RE, Caton CLM, Xie H, et al: A prospective 2-year study of emergency department patients with early phase primary psychosis or substance-induced psychosis. Am J Psychiatry 168(7):742–748, 2011 21454918

D'Souza DC, Abi-Saab WM, Madonick S, et al: Delta-9-tetrahydrocannabinol effects in schizophrenia: implications for cognition, psychosis, and addiction. Biol Psychiatry 57(6):594–608, 2005 15780846

D'Souza DC, Radhakrishnan R, Sherif M, et al: Cannabinoids and psychosis. Curr Pharm Des 22(42):6380–6391, 2016 27568729

Edwards AC, Gardner CO, Hickman M, et al: A prospective longitudinal model predicting early adult alcohol problems: evidence for a robust externalizing pathway. Psychol Med 46(5):957–968, 2016 26670459

Green AI: Pharmacotherapy for schizophrenia and co-occurring substance use disorders. Neurotox Res 11(1):33–40, 2007 17449446

Green AI, Brunette MF, Dawson R, et al: Long-acting injectable vs oral risperidone for schizophrenia and co-occurring alcohol use disorder: a randomized trial. J Clin Psychiatry 76(10):1359–1365, 2015 26302441

Hadden KL, LeDrew K, Hogan K, et al: Impact of comorbid cannabis use on outcome in first episode psychosis. Early Interv Psychiatry 12(5):848–855, 2018 27592556

Hahn B: The potential of cannabidiol treatment for cannabis users with recent-onset psychosis. Schizophr Bull 44(1):46–53, 2018 29083450

Haney M, Hart CL, Vosburg SK, et al: Effects of THC and lofexidine in a human laboratory model of marijuana withdrawal and relapse. Psychopharmacology (Berl) 197(1):157–168, 2008 18161012

Horsfall J, Cleary M, Hunt GE, et al: Psychosocial treatments for people with co-occurring severe mental illnesses and substance use disorders (dual diagnosis): a review of empirical evidence. Harv Rev Psychiatry 17(1):24–34, 2009 19205964

Kavanagh DJ, Young R, White A, et al: A brief motivational intervention for substance misuse in recent-onset psychosis. Drug Alcohol Rev 23(2):151–155, 2004 15370020

Lefebvre P, Muser E, Joshi K, et al: Impact of paliperidone palmitate versus oral atypical antipsychotics on health resource use and costs in veterans with schizophrenia and comorbid substance abuse. Clin Ther 39(7):1380–1395, 2017 28641996

Litten RZ, Ryan ML, Fertig JB, et al: A double-blind, placebo-controlled trial assessing the efficacy of varenicline tartrate for alcohol dependence. J Addict Med 7(4):277–286, 2013 23728065

Lyon J: More treatments on deck for alcohol use disorder. JAMA 317(22):2267–2269, 2017 28538998

McClave AK, McKnight-Eily LR, Davis SP, et al: Smoking characteristics of adults with selected lifetime mental illnesses: results from the 2007 National Health Interview Survey. Am J Public Health 100(12):2464–2472, 2010 20966369

McDonell MG, Srebnik D, Angelo F, et al: Randomized controlled trial of contingency management for stimulant use in community mental health patients with serious mental illness. Am J Psychiatry 170(1):94–101, 2013 23138961

McIver C, McGregor C, Baigent M, et al: Guidelines for the Medical Management of Patients With Methamphetamine-Induced Psychosis. Adelaide, Australia, South Australia: Drug and Alcohol Services, 2006

McKetin R, McLaren J, Lubman DI, Hides L: The prevalence of psychotic symptoms among methamphetamine users. Addiction 101(10):1473–1478, 2006 16968349

Meszaros ZS, Abdul-Malak Y, Dimmock JA, et al: Varenicline treatment of concurrent alcohol and nicotine dependence in schizophrenia: a randomized, placebo-controlled pilot trial. J Clin Psychopharmacol 33(2):243–247, 2013 23422399

Miller WR, Rollnick S: Motivational Interviewing: Preparing People to Change Addictive Behavior. New York, Guilford, 1991

Mueser KT, Noordsy DL, Drake RE, et al: Integrated Treatment for Dual Disorders: A Guide to Effective Practice. New York, Guilford, 2003

Murray RM, Englund A, Abi-Dargham A, et al: Cannabis-associated psychosis: neural substrate and clinical impact. Neuropharmacology 124:89–104, 2017 28634109

National Institute on Drug Abuse: Commonly abused drugs. January 2018. Available at: https://d14rmgtrwzf5a.cloudfront.net/sites/default/files/commonly_abused_drugs.pdf. Accessed October 9, 2018.

Noordsy DL, Drake RE, Teague GB, et al: Subjective experiences related to alcohol use among schizophrenics. J Nerv Ment Dis 179(7):410–414, 1991 1869869

Osher FC, Kofoed LL: Treatment of patients with psychiatric and psychoactive substance abuse disorders. Hosp Community Psychiatry 40(10):1025–1030, 1989 2807202

Ouellet-Plamondon C, Abdel-Baki A, Salvat É, Potvin S: Specific impact of stimulant, alcohol and cannabis use disorders on first-episode psychosis: 2-year functional and symptomatic outcomes. Psychol Med 47(14):2461–2471, 2017 28424105

Petrakis IL, O'Malley S, Rounsaville B, et al; VA Naltrexone Study Collaboration Group: Naltrexone augmentation of neuroleptic treatment in alcohol abusing patients with schizophrenia. Psychopharmacology (Berl) 172(3):291–297, 2004 14634716

Ries RK, Dyck DG, Short R, et al: Outcomes of managing disability benefits among patients with substance dependence and severe mental illness. Psychiatr Serv 55(4):445–447, 2004 15067161

Sherif M, Radhakrishnan R, D'Souza DC, Ranganathan M: Human laboratory studies on cannabinoids and psychosis. Biol Psychiatry 79(7):526–538, 2016 26970363

Sigmon SC: Investigating the pharmacological and nonpharmacological factors that modulate drug reinforcement. Exp Clin Psychopharmacol 15(1):1–20, 2007 17295581

Starzer MSK, Nordentoft M, Hjorthøj C: Rates and predictors of conversion to schizophrenia or bipolar disorder following substance-induced psychosis. Am J Psychiatry 175(4):343–350, 2018 29179576

Trigo JM, Soliman A, Quilty LC, et al: Nabiximols combined with motivational enhancement/cognitive behavioral therapy for the treatment of cannabis dependence: a pilot randomized clinical trial. PLoS One 13(1):e0190768, 2018 29385147

Xie H, McHugo GJ, Helmstetter BS, et al: Three-year recovery outcomes for long-term patients with co-occurring schizophrenic and substance use disorders. Schizophr Res 75(2–3):337–348, 2005 15885525

Role of Aerobic Exercise in the Treatment of Early Psychosis

Luz H. Ospina, Ph.D.
Jacob S. Ballon, M.D., M.P.H.
David Kimhy, Ph.D.

MOST psychotic disorders, including schizophrenia spectrum disorders, begin with a prodromal period characterized by attenuated positive and negative symptoms as well as altered functioning before the onset of a full psychotic episode (Yung et al. 2004). These subthreshold symptoms differ from symptoms associated with full psychotic episodes in their intensity, frequency, and/or duration. Nevertheless, these symptoms, in combination with additional risk factors, may increase the likelihood of developing a psychotic disorder and may predict clinical severity and general functional outcome. For example, deficits in neurocognition (e.g., memory, attention, executive functioning, perceptual processes) appear during the prodromal stage and remain present throughout illness progression and may represent a core feature of psychosis-related disorders (Rund 1998). Furthermore, cognitive impairments remain after psychopharmacological intervention (Keefe et al. 2007) and symptomatic stabilization (Bilder et al. 2000) and have been shown to be a main predictor of functional outcome in individuals with early and chronic psychosis (Green et al. 2004). Additionally, negative clinical symptoms such as anhedonia, blunted affect, avolition, and apathy occur during the high-risk period and remain persistent through-out the course of illness, and these symptoms typically respond poorly to psychopharmacological intervention (Hasan et al. 2012). These clinical and affective impairments negatively influence individuals' disability levels and ability to function in all areas of daily life, including social and occupational areas, and do not appear to be treatable using traditional antipsychotic medications (Hasan et al. 2012).

Although pharmacological intervention is widely used in psychotic disorders and may treat specific symptoms (such as hallucinations or other positive symptoms), very few, if any, interventions exist that reliably improve neurocognition and functioning in this population. Therefore, it is imperative to develop intervention strategies that target neurocognitive deficits in people experiencing early psychosis, which may subsequently improve general functional outcome. One recent intervention that targets these factors for both chronic and early psychosis includes using the benefits of increased physical activity or exercise. *Exercise* refers to structured, planned, and repetitive physical movement to maintain or improve one or more mechanisms of physical fitness. In this chapter, we detail the potential benefits of physical activity, primarily aerobic exercise interventions, for cognitive and negative symptoms in people with psychotic disorders.

Impact of Physical Exercise on Cognition in Early Psychosis

Although a significant number of studies have assessed the influence of exercise on cognition in individuals with chronic psychosis, few studies have examined this relationship in individuals with early psychosis, including individuals with first-episode psychosis (FEP) and persons at clinical high risk (CHR) of psychosis. An early meta-analysis by Dauwan et al. (2016) of individuals with chronic psychosis (29 studies with 1,109 schizophrenia spectrum patients) found no reliable effect of general exercise on neurocognition. However, the large heterogeneity in the results suggested that type, frequency, and intensity of exercise may differentially influence cognitive performance. Addressing this issue, a subsequent review and meta-analysis by Firth et al. (2017) of 10 trials with 385 individuals diagnosed with schizophrenia indicated that aerobic exercise improved global cognition, demonstrating a moderate-level effect size and no statistical heterogeneity. Exercise was found to improve specific cognitive domains, including working memory, social cognition, and attention/vigilance—domains typically known to be deficient in people with psychotic disorders. No significant benefits were shown for processing speed, verbal and visual memory, and reasoning and problem solving. Also, a greater amount of exercise (in minutes per week) and exercise interventions supervised by physical activity professionals were associated with greater global cognitive improvements (Firth et al. 2017). Evidence from other studies indicated that intensity of aerobic exercise also predicted cognitive improvement (Kimhy et al. 2016). Overall, meta-analytic results suggest that exercise of moderate to vigorous intensity confers the greatest benefits on mental and physical health, as well as aspects of neurocognition.

Studies examining potential benefits of physical exercise on cognition in individuals with early psychosis have generated similar results (see Table 15–1). One early study including 14 individuals with FEP compared groups on the basis of low or high physical activity levels (without an exercise intervention) on brain volume, cortical thickness, and cognitive performance (McEwen et al. 2015). The results showed that individuals with FEP and low physical activity presented with reduced brain volume and cortical thickness, as well as a trend-level tendency toward poor social cognition (using the MATRICS Consensus Cognitive Battery), when compared with individuals with FEP and high physical activity.

In another study, Lin et al. (2015) implemented aerobic exercise and yoga therapy of 12 weeks duration to 124 women diagnosed with schizophrenia spectrum disorders (within 5 years of onset) to determine possible improvements in cognition. Both yoga and aerobic exercise conditions demonstrated enhancement in working memory, with moderate to large effect sizes, in comparison with the control group. Additionally, the yoga group also displayed significant improvements in attention and verbal acquisition.

Firth and colleagues also conducted a number of aerobic exercise intervention studies to assess the effects of exercise on cognition, particularly in people with FEP. In their feasibility study, Firth et al. (2018a) administered a 10-week exercise program to 31 individuals with FEP; their exercise regimen aimed to achieve at least 90 minutes of weekly moderate to vigorous activity using aerobic and resistance training (e.g., treadmills, rowing, cycle ergometers). Cognitive results indicated the greatest change for verbal memory scores, with moderate improvements in social cognition, processing speed, executive functioning, and inhibitory control. Firth et al. (2018b) conducted a subsequent longitudinal study assessing the effects of their previously described exercise program on cognition at 6-month follow-up. Although improved scores in processing speed were maintained at 6-month follow-up, verbal memory had reverted to baseline performance at 6-month assessment. This finding is supported by prior literature, which suggests that exercise-induced enhancements in verbal memory persist only when physical activity is maintained (Bowie et al. 2014); in Firth et al.'s (2018b) longitudinal study, only 55% of the sample continued to exercise independently after termination of the study.

TABLE 15–1. Studies assessing effects of exercise on cognition in early psychosis

	Sample characteristics				Exercise intervention			Cognitive domains
	Exercise (*n*)	Control (*n*)	Mean age (years)	Population	Activity	Duration and frequency		Cognitive domains
Lin et al. 2015	31 (aerobic) 38 (yoga)	33 waitlist	24.56	Onset within 5 years	60 minutes of either yoga therapy or aerobic exercise (i.e., walking or cycling)	12 weeks, 3 times per week		Verbal memory Working memory Attention Executive function
McEwen et al. 2015	7	7	23.35	FEP	Low and high physical activity according to the IPAQ	—		Processing speed Attention/ vigilance Working memory Verbal learning Visual learning Reasoning/ problem solving Social cognition

TABLE 15–1. Studies assessing effects of exercise on cognition in early psychosis (*continued*)

	Sample characteristics			Exercise intervention		Cognitive domains
	Exercise (*n*)	Control (*n*)	Mean age (years)	Population	Activity	Duration and frequency	
Firth et al. 2018a	31	7 TAU	25.35	FEP	45–60 minutes of moderate to vigorous activity using aerobic (e.g., treadmill, rowing, cycle ergometer) and resistance exercises	10 weeks, 2 times per week	Processing speed Verbal memory Executive function Inhibitory control Motor function Social cognition
Firth et al. 2018b	28	—	26.96	FEP	Longitudinal follow-up of previous study 6 months later	10 weeks, 2 times per week	Verbal memory Processing speed Executive function Inhibitory control Social cognition

TABLE 15–1. Studies assessing effects of exercise on cognition in early psychosis *(continued)*

	Sample characteristics			Exercise intervention		
	Exercise (*n*)	Control (*n*)	Mean age (years)	Population	Activity	Duration and frequency	Cognitive domains
Nuechterlein et al. 2016	7 (with CT)	9 CR	22.65	FEP	150 minutes/week of moderate to vigorous aerobic exercise (i.e., calisthenics) in conjunction with CR	10 weeks, 4 times per week	Processing speed Attention/ vigilance Working memory Verbal learning Visual learning Reasoning/ problem solving Social cognition

TABLE 15–1. Studies assessing effects of exercise on cognition in early psychosis (*continued*)

	Sample characteristics				Exercise intervention		
	Exercise (*n*)	Control (*n*)	Mean age (years)	Population	Activity	Duration and frequency	Cognitive domains
Dean et al. 2017	12	—	19.42	CHR	Two exercise conditions: 1) moderate (65% intensity 2 days/week) or 2) vigorous (85% intensity 3 days/week), including treadmill, bikes, and elliptical machines	12 weeks, 2–3 times per week	Processing speed Attention/vigilance Working memory Verbal learning Visual learning Reasoning/problem solving Social cognition

Abbreviations. CHR=clinical high risk; CR=cognitive remediation; CT=cognitive training; FEP=first-episode psychosis; IPAQ=International Physical Activity Questionnaire; TAU=treatment as usual.

Finally, Nuechterlein et al. (2016) conducted a combined 10-week intervention pilot study examining the effects of aerobic exercise in conjunction with cognitive training, compared with cognitive training alone, in individuals with FEP. For the first 5 weeks, neurocognitive training consisted of computerized exercises aimed at improving perceptual processing and verbal learning and memory; the remaining weeks focused on social cognitive training exercises to improve cognitive processes underlying social and emotional interactions. The combined intervention group also completed a concurrent aerobic exercise training program, which consisted of a series of calisthenics for a total of 150 minutes over 4 days per week. Results indicated that persons in the combined exercise and cognitive training condition improved notably more (with large effect sizes) than did individuals in the cognitive training alone group, with the largest increase in scores for social cognition, working memory, processing speed, and attention/vigilance domains. The combination of cognitive training and physical exercise may allow for the beneficial effects of aerobic exercise training by enhancing improvements yielded from cognitive training alone, which has been previously demonstrated (Wykes et al. 2007). Therefore, these results suggest possible improvements in cognition as a result of moderate-intensity (i.e., aerobic) exercise in individuals with early psychosis.

To date, only one study has used an exercise intervention in persons at CHR for psychosis. In Dean et al.'s (2017) pilot study, 12 CHR individuals were assigned to one of two aerobic exercise regimens: 1) a moderate-intensity program, exercising twice per week at 65% intensity of their maximal oxygen consumption for 12 weeks ($n=7$), or 2) a vigorous-intensity program, exercising 3 days a week at 85% intensity of their maximal oxygen consumption for 12 weeks ($n=2$). Both groups were given the choice to use treadmills, stationary bikes, or elliptical machines, and each session lasted approximately 30–45 minutes. Results indicated considerable improvement in cognitive performance for both groups, specifically, working memory, verbal learning, visual learning, processing speed, attention/vigilance, and reasoning and problem solving (with moderate to large effect sizes). There was also a significant increase in the cognitive composite score after completion of the intervention.

One possible explanation for the positive effects of exercise on neurocognition relates to increases in brain volume, particularly in the hippocampus. The hippocampus has been largely implicated as a major brain region impaired in psychosis and plays a significant role in controlling both the physiological stress response and higher-order cognition (Harrison 2004). A number of studies using physical exercise programs have demonstrated increases in hippocampal volume in individuals with schizophrenia (Pajonk et al. 2010). Similarly, studies in individuals with early psychosis have also shown concurrent increases in brain volume and improved neurocognitive scores, particularly volumetric increases in hippocampal and prefrontal cortex, in response to physical exercise. Also, reduced cortical brain thickness in the prefrontal cortex has been evidenced in individuals with FEP with low physical activity (McEwen et al. 2015). Finally, one study assessing functional connectivity in CHR individuals showed increased functional connectivity between the left hippocampus and occipital cortex after a 12-week aerobic exercise intervention (Dean et al. 2017).

Another possible explanation for the beneficial effects of physical exercise on neurocognition relates to brain-derived neurotrophic factor (BDNF), a neural growth factor that is highly expressed in the hippocampus and is associated with facilitating neurogenesis, synaptic plasticity, memory, and learning (Gomez-Pinilla et al. 2008). Although no studies to date have assessed changes in BDNF expression in response to an exercise intervention in individuals with early psychosis, one study did demonstrate a significant relationship between BDNF upregulation and improved neurocognition in people with chronic schizophrenia. Using a 12-week moderate-to-vigorous aerobic exercise intervention in 33 people with schizophrenia, Kimhy et al. (2015) found significant improvement in neurocognitive scores, particularly social cognition and visual learning. Additional regression analyses also determined that increases in BDNF and enhancement in aerobic fitness significantly predicted neurocognitive improvement. Taken together, these results suggest that aerobic exercise upregulates the production of BDNF, which is believed to be associated with brain neuroplasticity and neurogenesis, thereby promoting growth of specific brain regions, such as the hippocampus, that are critical for neurocognitive performance (Vakhrusheva et al. 2016).

Impact of Physical Exercise on Positive and Negative Symptoms in Early Psychosis

A number of meta-analyses and reviews have examined the influence of physical activity on positive and negative symptoms in individuals with chronic schizophrenia spectrum disorders. In Firth et al.'s (2015) early meta-analysis, 16 out of 17 studies monitored the effects of exercise on overall mental health, focusing on positive and negative symptoms. Although low-intensity exercise did not affect change scores for clinical symptom assessments, moderate to vigorous exercise exhibited a strong effect on total psychiatric symptoms, with significant reductions in both positive and negative scales. Dauwan et al.'s (2016) review also demonstrated reductions in total symptom severity, although their results had high heterogeneity. Their analysis of positive symptoms (15 studies, $N=641$), negative symptoms (18 studies, $N=765$), and general symptom severity (10 studies, $N=436$) indicated significant reductions in overall clinical symptoms as a result of exercise, specifically yoga and aerobic interventions, compared with control groups. Finally, a review by Tarpada and Morris (2017) included eight intervention studies ($N=301$) using the Positive and Negative Syndrome Scale (PANSS) as the outcome measure; physical activity regimens included yoga, dance, and aerobic exercises and resistance training. They discovered that physical activity significantly improved total and positive PANSS symptom scores when compared with control groups. Also, there was a trend for improvement in PANSS negative symptom scores, although this finding did not achieve significance.

Most studies assessing exercise and symptom severity in early psychosis also demonstrated improvements in positive, negative, and total symptom scores. In one early study, Mittal et al. (2013) examined 29 CHR individuals and 27 matched controls on physical activity (using actigraphy monitors), clinical symptoms, and brain structure. They found that CHR individuals engaged in less physical activity than did the nonclinical control group. Furthermore, physical activity was observed to correlate significantly with bilateral parahippocampal gyrus volumes and occupational functioning. However, Mittal and colleagues did not detect any relationship between physical activity level and clinical symptoms.

Regarding exercise intervention studies, Lin et al. (2015) showed improvement of overall symptom severity in response to 12-week yoga and aerobic exercise interventions. Interestingly, negative symptoms decreased for those in the yoga condition, whereas positive symptoms did not improve for either the yoga or aerobic exercise groups. Also, Firth et al. (2018a) demonstrated a significant reduction in PANSS scores, particularly for negative and general symptoms, for individuals with FEP assigned to a 10-week aerobic exercise program, compared with a control (treatment as usual) group. Similarly, positive symptoms in the exercise group did not decrease and were statistically similar to symptoms in the control group. Results for Firth et al.'s (2018b) follow-up longitudinal study suggested that individuals who continued to exercise on a weekly basis after completion of the intervention study continued to show symptomatic reductions in PANSS total scores, compared with individuals who ceased exercising after supervised intervention. In fact, non-exercisers' total PANSS scores *increased* (i.e., worsened) after the intervention period. Finally, Dean et al.'s (2017) aerobic exercise intervention in 12 CHR individuals exhibited significant medium-to-large decreases in positive symptoms and a small-to-medium decrease in negative symptoms at termination of the 12-week trial. Overall, these results implicate potential beneficial effects of physical exercise on symptoms, particularly negative and total symptom scores, in individuals with early psychosis.

Although the specific mechanisms by which physical activity may affect positive and negative symptoms in early and chronic psychosis remain unclear, a number of hypotheses attempt to explain this relationship. One frequently proposed explanation includes enhanced synaptic neuroplasticity due to upregulation of BDNF. As mentioned in the previous paragraph, BDNF is related to neurogenesis and neuroplasticity. One meta-analysis (Green et al. 2011), which included 16 studies, demonstrated moderately reduced blood BDNF levels (Hedges' $g=-0.458$) in drug-naïve and medicated patients with schizophrenia, both male and female. Neurodevelopmental models of schizophrenia (van Haren et al. 2008) suggest that reduced BDNF underlies the core behavioral signs and symptoms of the disorder; as such, upregulation of BDNF as a result of physical activity may lead to reductions in many of the clinical symptoms associated with psychosis.

Most studies in individualindividuals with early and chronic psychosis reflected reductions in negative and total symptoms, with one study (Dean et al. 2017) including CHR individuals showing reductions in both negative and positive symptoms. Although it remains unclear why physical activity specifically reduces negative symptoms more than positive symptoms, this observation is important given that prior studies have revealed significant associations between negative symptoms and functional outcome, whereas positive symptoms are less strongly correlated with overall functioning in schizophrenia spectrum disorders (Ventura et al. 2009). Therefore, reducing negative symptoms, which may partially mediate the association between neurocognition and general functioning, may improve both neurocognition and functional outcome in individuals with early and chronic psychosis.

Impact of Physical Exercise on Affective Symptoms in Early Psychosis

Studies assessing the impact of physical activity on affective symptoms in both chronic and early psychosis are limited. Regarding chronic patients, Firth et al.'s (2015) meta-analysis demonstrated that physical exercise decreased depressive and anxiety scores within broader mental health assessments in 3 of 17 trials, although only in relation to baseline scores and not comparison groups. Dauwan et al.'s (2016) review presented overall significant reductions in depressive symptomatology, with a large effect size (Hedges' $g=0.71$), in response to exercise interventions. Finally, one recent study examining factors that motivate and sustain exercise in schizophrenia spectrum patients who were already independently and regularly exercising ($n=14$) showed 7%–11% average decreases in anxiety and depressive symptoms in response to individual exercise sessions (Dahle and Noordsy 2018). Therefore, physical exercise interventions also appear to confer beneficial reductions in affective, particularly depressive, symptoms, in chronic psychosis.

Exercise studies in individuals with early psychosis also generally demonstrate potential improvements in clinical affective symptomatology. For example, Lin et al. (2015) showed a significant decrease in depressive symptoms for both yoga and aerobic exercise groups after a 12-week intervention; importantly, these effects on affective symptoms remained stable at 12-month follow-up. Also, in the study by Firth et al. (2018b), results exhibited trend-level reductions in depressive and anxiety symptoms after a 10-week moderate-to-vigorous aerobic exercise intervention.

Although evidence for the effects of physical exercise on affective symptoms in psychosis is scant, numerous studies have assessed these effects in depressive disorders. In individuals with depression, exercise has been observed to lead to physiological changes such as increased release of specific neurotransmitters that have been linked to enhanced mood (e.g., serotonin and endorphins) (Ströhle 2009). Other possible mechanisms for the beneficial effects of physical activity on affective symptomatology and mental health in individuals with psychosis include changes in psychological factors such as increased social support and improved perceptions of self-efficacy, competence, and autonomy (Gorczynski and Faulkner 2010).

Impact of Aerobic Exercise on Functional Outcome in Early Psychosis

Studies in chronic psychosis have overwhelmingly demonstrated the beneficial effects of physical activity, particularly moderate to vigorous aerobic exercise, on functional outcome. The meta-analysis by Firth et al. (2015) showed significant improvements in functional disability and quality of life in two trials that used moderate- to vigorous-intensity exercise, and two studies that used low-intensity exercise demonstrated mild improvements in social functioning. Similarly, Dauwan et al.'s (2016) review also suggested that exercise improves global functioning scores, with a moderate effect size (Hedges' $g=0.32$). In individuals with early psychosis, various types of exercise have been associated with enhanced global functioning and quality of life. Results from Lin et al. (2015) demonstrated greater physical and psychological health as a result of both yoga and aerobic exercise programs.

Other studies have demonstrated beneficial effects of moderate- to vigorous-intensity physical exercise on specific aspects of functioning, such as socio-occupational functioning, in individuals with FEP as well as CHR individuals. Furthermore, one longitudinal study (Firth et al.

2018b) assessing follow-up 6 months after an exercise intervention continued to show improvements in socio-occupational functioning after the intervention had ended, regardless of exercise adherence after supervised intervention. A combined aerobic exercise and cognitive training pilot study (Nuechterlein et al. 2016) revealed enhanced functional outcome, specifically in such domains as independent living, family network relationships, and working productivity, above and beyond improvements elicited in individuals who received cognitive training alone. Finally, physical exercise of moderate to vigorous intensity has also been observed to improve both social and role functioning in CHR individuals (Dean et al. 2017). Similar to explanations of exercise's enhancing effects on affective symptoms, theories attempting to explain the beneficial effects of physical activity on functional outcome relate to psychological improvements in self-esteem and confidence, which may lead to further engagement in the world and better well-being (Vancampfort et al. 2011).

Conclusion

Overall, numerous studies have found beneficial effects of physical activity, particularly moderate to vigorous aerobic exercise, on cognition and negative symptoms, as well as functional outcome in early and chronic psychosis. Importantly, studies have found that physical exercise interventions improved cognition, attenuated psychotic symptoms, ameliorated negative symptoms, decreased depressive symptoms, and improved social and role functioning. A number of biological markers may partially explain these enhancement effects, including increased release and upregulation of BDNF, which may subsequently promote neurogenesis and neuroplasticity, leading to volumetric increases in key brain regions (such as the hippocampus) associated with cognition. Although most studies implicate the importance of moderate- to vigorous-intensity level of exercise in order to maximize benefits, a few studies do suggest that lower-intensity training, such as yoga, may also ameliorate symptoms and improve neurocognition and functioning. Additional studies are necessary to ascertain the specific mechanisms by which various forms of physical exercise improve cognition, symptoms, and functioning in early and chronic psychosis.

KEY CONCEPTS

- Aerobic exercise training has been observed to improve cognitive functioning and clinical symptoms in individuals with psychosis disorders.

- Preliminary results suggest that aerobic exercise training may also improve cognition, clinical and affective symptoms, and overall functioning in individuals at high risk for psychosis.

- Neurobiological studies associate aerobic exercise with the increased release and upregulation of brain-derived neurotrophic factor, a neural growth factor, in specific brain regions related to neurocognition and functioning.

Discussion Questions

1. Most studies have assessed the effects of aerobic exercise on cognition and clinical symptoms in individuals with psychosis disorders. Would other types of exercise (strength training, high-intensity interval training, yoga, or stretching) confer similar effects on aspects of cognition or clinical symptom severity? If so, what are the possible neurobiological mechanisms for such enhancement effects?

2. Psychosis disorders that are treated early during illness progression (i.e., during the first psychotic episode) have better illness prognosis. Would this phenomenon also occur when using an aerobic exercise intervention? What would the course of illness look like for individuals with a psychosis disorder who engaged in aerobic exercise treatment during their first episode?

Suggested Readings

Firth J, Rosenbaum S, Stubbs B, et al: Motivating factors and barriers towards exercise in severe mental illness: a systematic review and meta-analysis. Psychol Med 46(14):2869-2881, 2016

Rosenbaum S, Lederman O, Stubbs B, et al: How can we increase physical activity and exercise among youth experiencing first-episode psychosis? A systematic review of intervention variables. Early Interv Psychiatry 10(5):435-40, 2016

Stubbs B, Rosenbaum S (eds): Exercise-Based Interventions for Mental Illness. London, Academic Press, 2018

References

Bilder RM, Goldman RS, Robinson D, et al: Neuropsychology of first-episode schizophrenia: initial characterization and clinical correlates. Am J Psychiatry 157(4):549–559, 2000 10739413

Bowie CR, Grossman M, Gupta M, et al: Cognitive remediation in schizophrenia: efficacy and effectiveness in patients with early versus long-term course of illness. Early Interv Psychiatry 8(1):32–38, 2014 23343011

Dahle D, Noordsy D: Factors motivating spontaneous exercise in individuals with schizophrenia-spectrum disorders. Schizophr Res 199:436–437, 2018 29656908

Dauwan M, Begemann MJ, Heringa SM, et al: Exercise improves clinical symptoms, quality of life, global functioning, and depression in schizophrenia: a systematic review and meta-analysis. Schizophr Bull 42(3):588–599, 2016 26547223

Dean DJ, Bryan AD, Newberry R, et al: A supervised exercise intervention for youth at risk for psychosis: an open-label pilot study. J Clin Psychiatry 78(9):e1167–e1173, 2017 29178684

Firth J, Cotter J, Elliott R, et al: A systematic review and meta-analysis of exercise interventions in schizophrenia patients. Psychol Med 45(7):1343–1361, 2015 25650668

Firth J, Stubbs B, Rosenbaum S, et al: Aerobic exercise improves cognitive functioning in people with schizophrenia: a systematic review and meta-analysis. Schizophr Bull 43(3):546–556, 2017 27521348

Firth J, Carney R, Elliott R, et al: Exercise as an intervention for first-episode psychosis: a feasibility study. Early Interv Psychiatry 12(3):307–315, 2018a 26987871

Firth J, Carney R, French P, et al: Long-term maintenance and effects of exercise in early psychosis. Early Interv Psychiatry 12(4):578–585, 2018b 27587302

Gomez-Pinilla F, Vaynman S, Ying Z: Brain-derived neurotrophic factor functions as a metabotrophin to mediate the effects of exercise on cognition. Eur J Neurosci 28(11):2278–2287, 2008 19046371

Gorczynski P, Faulkner G: Exercise therapy for schizophrenia. Schizophr Bull 36(4):665–666, 2010 20484521

Green MF, Kern RS, Heaton RK: Longitudinal studies of cognition and functional outcome in schizophrenia: implications for MATRICS. Schizophr Res 72(1):41–51, 2004 15531406

Green MJ, Matheson SL, Shepherd A, et al: Brain-derived neurotrophic factor levels in schizophrenia: a systematic review with meta-analysis. Mol Psychiatry 16(9):960–972, 2011 20733577

Harrison PJ: The hippocampus in schizophrenia: a review of the neuropathological evidence and its pathophysiological implications. Psychopharmacology (Berl) 174(1):151–162, 2004 15205886

Hasan A, Falkai P, Wobrock T, et al; World Federation of Societies of Biological Psychiatry (WFSBP) Task Force on Treatment Guidelines for Schizophrenia: World Federation of Societies of Biological Psychiatry (WFSBP) Guidelines for Biological Treatment of Schizophrenia, part 1: update 2012 on the acute treatment of schizophrenia and the management of treatment resistance. World J Biol Psychiatry 13(5):318–378, 2012 22834451

Keefe RS, Sweeney JA, Gu H, et al: Effects of olanzapine, quetiapine, and risperidone on neurocognitive function in early psychosis: a randomized, double-blind 52-week comparison. Am J Psychiatry 164(7):1061–1071, 2007 17606658

Kimhy D, Vakhrusheva J, Bartels MN, et al: The impact of aerobic exercise on brain-derived neurotrophic factor and neurocognition in individuals with schizophrenia: a single-blind, randomized clinical trial. Schizophr Bull 41(4):859–868, 2015 25805886

Kimhy D, Lauriola V, Bartels MN, et al: Aerobic exercise for cognitive deficits in schizophrenia—the impact of frequency, duration, and fidelity with target training intensity. Schizophr Res 172(1–3):213–215, 2016 26852401

Lin J, Chan SK, Lee EH, et al: Aerobic exercise and yoga improve neurocognitive function in women with early psychosis. NPJ Schizophrenia 1(0):15047, 2015 27336050

McEwen SC, Hardy A, Ellingson BM, et al: Prefrontal and hippocampal brain volume deficits: role of low physical activity on brain plasticity in first-episode schizophrenia patients. J Int Neuropsychol Soc 21(10):868–879, 2015 26581798

Mittal VA, Gupta T, Orr JM, et al: Physical activity level and medial temporal health in youth at ultra high-risk for psychosis. J Abnorm Psychol 122(4):1101–1110, 2013 24364613

Nuechterlein KH, Ventura J, McEwen SC, et al: Enhancing cognitive training through aerobic exercise after a first schizophrenia episode: theoretical conception and pilot study. Schizophr Bull 42(suppl 1):S44–S52, 2016 27460618

Pajonk FG, Wobrock T, Gruber O, et al: Hippocampal plasticity in response to exercise in schizophrenia. Arch Gen Psychiatry 67(2):133–143, 2010 20124113

Rund BR: A review of longitudinal studies of cognitive functions in schizophrenia patients. Schizophr Bull 24(3):425–435, 1998 9718634

Ströhle A: Physical activity, exercise, depression and anxiety disorders. J Neural Transm (Vienna) 116(6):777–784, 2009 18726137

Tarpada SP, Morris MT: Physical activity diminishes symptomatic decline in chronic schizophrenia: a systematic review. Psychopharmacol Bull 47(4):29–40, 2017 28936008

Vakhrusheva J, Marino B, Stroup TS, et al: Aerobic exercise in people with schizophrenia: neural and neurocognitive benefits. Curr Behav Neurosci Rep 3(2):165–175, 2016 27766192

Vancampfort D, Probst M, Sweers K, et al: Relationships between obesity, functional exercise capacity, physical activity participation and physical self-perception in people with schizophrenia. Acta Psychiatr Scand 123(6):423–430, 2011 21219266

van Haren NE, Cahn W, Pol HH, Kahn RS: Schizophrenia as a progressive brain disease. Eur Psychiatry 23(4):245–254, 2008 18513927

Ventura J, Hellemann GS, Thames AD, et al: Symptoms as mediators of the relationship between neurocognition and functional outcome in schizophrenia: a meta-analysis. Schizophr Res 113(2–3):189–199, 2009 19628375

Wykes T, Reeder C, Landau S, et al: Cognitive remediation therapy in schizophrenia: randomised controlled trial. Br J Psychiatry 190:421–427, 2007 17470957

Yung AR, Phillips LJ, Yuen HP, et al: Risk factors for psychosis in an ultra high-risk group: psychopathology and clinical features. Schizophr Res 67(2–3):131–142, 2004 14984872

CHAPTER
16

Supported Employment and Education for People in Early Psychosis

Deborah R. Becker, M.Ed., CRC
Robert E. Drake, M.D., Ph.D.

EMPLOYMENT and education are normal and expected life activities for adolescents and young adults. Young people with a first episode of psychosis desire to fit into society like their peers in the general population. Furthermore, holding a job and/or going to school—once thought to be goals for people *after* a lengthy stabilization period following early psychosis—are paths to recovery from behavioral health disorders. Work and school provide opportunities for young people to use their skills, meet people, earn income, have a positive identity and social status, and be like other young people. Team members of coordinated specialty care teams that serve young adults with early psychosis provide the hope and support for these individuals to secure functional roles as workers and/or students.

The most effective vocational intervention for people with behavioral health conditions, including people with first-episode psychosis, is evidence-based supported employment, also known as individual placement and support (IPS; Drake et al. 2016; Marshall et al. 2014). Service delivery systems sometimes use the term *supported employment* differently, and therefore the term IPS is used to clearly differentiate the evidence-based practice, which includes the strongest research base, implementation manuals, a fidelity scale and manual, and an international network of providers. More than 25 randomized controlled trials of IPS conducted worldwide by different investigators have demonstrated that IPS is more effective than any other vocational intervention (for more information, see www.ipsworks.org).

We use the term *IPS specialist* (rather than employment/education specialist) to identify clearly the person who directly provides these services. Although the initial focus of IPS in the late 1990s was on people with serious mental illness and therefore mostly on competitive employment, IPS is now provided to people with early psychosis as well as to transitional-age youth with mental health conditions. When serving a young population, IPS includes support for education and further schooling as part of building a career path (Swanson et al. 2017). By helping young adults return to functional roles (i.e., worker, student), IPS services help divert people from a life of disability.

IPS uses a strengths-based approach by drawing on the person's skills, talents, interests, and previous experiences. Although the IPS specialist takes the lead on providing employment and education support, other members of the coordinated specialty care team support the participant's efforts toward building a career path. They ask questions that help young people consider employment or furthering their education: "What job would you like the most? What skills do you have that would transfer to that type of work? What about that job interests you?" Team members focus on what the person can do rather than on limitations. Through a strengths-based approach, practitioners demonstrate their belief in the person's capabilities and resilience.

Engaging People With Early Psychosis in Work and School

The IPS specialist on the coordinated specialty care team engages people when they say they are ready to think about going to work or school. They build rapport on the basis of each person's level of interest. The rapid job search principle helps in this regard; participants do not want to be delayed by lengthy assessments. IPS specialists ask program participants how often they want to meet, where they want to meet, and for how long: "What are we working on that you find helpful? What else could we be doing that would be helpful to you? What would you like to be doing in 3 or 4 years? What would be a good first step in reaching that goal?" People are more likely to stay in services when the focus is on their strengths and their interests (Maraj et al. 2019).

When engaging young people, IPS specialists limit the amount of time completing paperwork and forms. They have discussions that focus on jobs, schooling, and careers and minimize talking about mental health problems. IPS specialists build credibility with the people they serve when they demonstrate knowledge of the local labor market and educational institutions. In order to maintain engagement and a working relationship, IPS specialists are flexible to changes in direction that the person may present. They may spend small amounts of time talking about other topics and interests as part of relationship building but always return to the topics of employment, education, and careers.

Technology provides various ways to communicate and maintain engagement with young people. Many young people respond more quickly to texts, instant messaging, and e-mails rather than by phone. By using modern technology, IPS specialists can connect with young people frequently and reach out when they miss appointments.

Including Family Support for Employment and Education

With permission from the young person, the IPS specialist invites family members to their meetings. Family is defined broadly and may include immediate family, friends, and other supporters. The IPS specialist should ask whether the young person would like a friend to be part of one of the meetings to talk about work and career plans. To expand the pool of people who are important to the individual, the IPS specialist may ask who would the person want to tell if he or she just became employed or aced a test in school.

Family members are an important resource for information about the person's skills, interests, and experiences that may relate to work and career goals. Family members want to be involved and to know about the services and plans. The IPS specialist educates the family that young people often try several jobs that last brief periods of time before settling into a job. Young people change their minds frequently about their plans, and team members and family members may sometimes be frustrated by this uncertainty. IPS specialists help young people explore options of employment and schooling, continue to engage them during periods of uncertainty, and support family in adjusting expectations in terms of career plans (Table 16–1).

Snapshot of IPS Services

Team-Based Approach

The IPS specialist is the primary team member of the coordinated specialty care team who provides direct employment and education support. The IPS specialist attends all team meetings to encourage consideration of work and/or school for all participants, to report on each participant's progress

TABLE 16–1. Core principles of IPS supported employment and education

Principle	Description
Zero exclusion for eligibility	All young adults with early psychosis who are interested in work and school are eligible, regardless of symptoms, substance use, or other characteristics.
Mainstream competitive employment and education	The focus is on regular jobs and mainstream educational programs that are available to people on the basis of their qualifications rather than disability status or participation in social services.
Individual preferences and strengths	Services are based on participants' preferences and choices rather than providers' judgments.
Integrated services	Team members provide employment and educational support through a team approach. IPS specialists participate in team meetings to review and coordinate client progress.
Rapid job/school search	Rapid job search and career/educational exploration begin soon after entry into IPS.
Job development	IPS specialists meet employers to learn about their business needs and hiring practices. They may give the information to job seekers or directly introduce qualified job seekers to employers, depending on the job seeker's preference.
Individual and time-unlimited supports	Team members provide individualized job and educational supports as long as needed and desired by program participants.
Personalized financial counseling	Young adults are referred for personalized counseling to learn how earned income affects entitlements and how to finance their education.

in his or her return to work or school, and to ask about those who are not pursuing work or school: "How are they spending their time? What do they want to be doing in 2 years? What are their interests?"

During the intake assessment, the team asks participants about their work history, interest in working, education background, and interest in furthering their education. The team supports and nurtures participant goals in part because they are related to functional outcomes. Young adults often value work or school above addressing problems related to low energy, social relations, confusion and poor concentration, and symptoms and side effects. In addition, having school and work interests leads to greater work or school participation 12 months later (de Waal et al. 2018).

Young people who express an interest in support around employment and/or education are referred directly to the IPS specialist. The IPS specialist meets with participants individually to learn about their interests, build relationships, review their history, and develop a plan. All team members should attend to the person's interests and goals and view structured activity as vital to illness management by providing anchors to keep attention away from symptoms. Team members gently encourage vocational planning and provide support to individuals who are actively seeking employment and to those who have gained employment. Some young people may want to postpone pursuing employment and/or education. Team members have brief discussions with them over time to keep the topic of conversation current and demonstrate that they can pursue these goals in the future.

During team meetings, team members provide input about each person's skills, experiences, and preferences that may relate to an individualized job search or support plan. For example, a social worker might say to the IPS specialist, "I learned from Sharon's mother that Sharon loves to bake. Have you thought about exploring a job related to baking?" Team members may offer information about the type of environments where the young person feels comfortable and other aspects of the person's preferences that could transfer to a work setting. For example, a psychiatrist might say, "Matthew is less preoccupied with symptoms when he has structured time. A job may help him distance from symptoms." Team members may have leads for potential employers and can recommend specific job types and locations that are a fit for specific individuals.

Team members provide suggestions for problem solving and remind participants of individualized coping strategies to use in stressful situations at work or school. Medication prescribers tailor medications to best fit the needs of a young person's functioning at work and/or school. The peer specialist on the team may provide motivation by telling how he or she moved forward in his or her recovery through work or school and may accompany the participant to increase comfort and confidence (e.g., on a visit to the campus where the young person will attend classes). Team members help with socialization and communication skills in the context of work and/or school and provide general encouragement.

Many participants are likely to have current alcohol or drug use (see Chapter 14, "Substance Use and Early Psychosis"). The team helps these young people reflect on how their use may impact employment and learning at school. They help to identify a job type and work environment that will support recovery. Money is often a trigger for alcohol and drug use; therefore, the IPS specialist helps to develop a plan for managing paychecks. Many young people with early psychosis experience cognitive difficulties that may interfere with learning, and substance use can further complicate education experiences. Over time, interest in school and/or a job that they find rewarding can provide motivation to reduce alcohol and drug use for many young people with early psychosis.

Career Profile and Employment and Education Plan

Case Example 1

Jack is a 19-year-old who developed a psychotic illness just as he was finishing high school. As he recovered, he thought about college but was certain that he was not ready. Talking with his IPS specialist, Zeke, Jack decided he would like to find a job instead, but he had no idea what kind of job. They discussed lots of options, but Jack kept coming back to the theme that he liked playing music with his friends in a local band and spending time with his dog. Jack decided to continue meeting his friends in the evening for "jam sessions" and to find a job during the day working with dogs. Zeke and the team checked with veterinary clinics and pet stores before one team member talked with a friend of his who had a business as a dog walker. This friend needed an assistant to expand his business and was delighted to hire Jack soon after he met him. The two of them walk dozens of dogs each day, and Jack makes a good salary for 4 hours of work each day. He naps in the afternoon and plays with his band in the evening.

The IPS specialist begins meeting right away with the young person who has expressed interest in employment and/or school to gather information about the person's interests, goals, hobbies, experiences, and transferable skills. The information is documented in the career profile or other similar assessment tool. During these meetings, the IPS specialist builds a collaborative relationship with the participant. The IPS specialist assesses the participant's tolerance for these discussions and makes adjustments accordingly. Sometimes the meetings are brief and geared to other interests of the participant. Occasionally, IPS specialists use interest inventories to help identify career choices. The IPS specialist and job seeker use the information along with suggestions from the family and team members to develop ideas for jobs, types of preferred work environments, number of work hours, and interest in further education and training.

Information from the career profile is the foundation for building an employment and/or education plan. The young person's short- and long-term goals are documented on the plan in his or her own words. Steps and timeframes to reach the goals are outlined, as well as the people who will provide supports to help achieve the steps. The IPS specialist and participant share the plan with the team and family members in order to build support and collaboration.

Conducting an Individualized Job Search

The IPS specialist and the participant begin to explore job possibilities from the employment plan within 30 days. They explore jobs quickly, which demonstrates to participants that the IPS specialist and coordinated specialty care team are honoring their goals and taking action. The IPS specialist makes at least six in-person direct employer contacts with hiring managers per week to learn about their business and hiring practices. They develop relationships with employers who have positions that are consistent with the skills and interests of people they are serving.

Prior to the start of the job search, the IPS specialist explains to the participant how he or she contacts employers to learn about hiring practices and positions. If the IPS specialist speaks to an employer about a specific job seeker, the job seeker needs to agree to disclosure beforehand. Through discussions about disclosure and confidentiality, the young person weighs the advantages and disadvantages of an employer having information about his or her needs and the job support team. For example, many people feel that there is a stigma about having a mental health condition and fear they will be treated differently by employers. The participant decides what if any information may be disclosed to an employer. If the participant does not wish to disclose information about his or her mental health condition, the IPS specialist does not contact employers directly but instead gives information about positions and hiring practices to the job seeker. With this information, the job seeker can apply for positions independently without the IPS specialist.

In addition to discussions about disclosure, the IPS specialist offers participants access to a trained benefits counselor who explains information about possible entitlements such as Social Security disability benefits. Family members or clinicians may consider applying for benefits if they fear that work is too stressful and will exacerbate symptoms, but participants and family need to know that securing disability benefits may have unintended consequences. For some people, disability benefits may be helpful in the short term but harmful over the long term. In any given year, less than 0.5% of Social Security Disability Insurance and Supplemental Security Income (SSI) beneficiaries leave the disability rolls and return to work. Monthly SSI checks are below the poverty level, so the team should encourage participants to consider jobs and careers, avoiding the path of dependence on the mental health system and poverty. If the young person is interested in applying for benefits, team members help the individual consider the advantages and disadvantages. For example, the peer specialist may explain his or her choice of employment over disability benefits. If the participant then chooses to apply for benefits, the team should continue to encourage education and work to build a path to independence.

People with early psychosis may have little or no work experience. They may have never gone on a job interview and might be unfamiliar with expected work behaviors. Some people know what they want to do, but others will want to explore different options. The IPS specialist and job seeker may visit job sites to learn about different types of jobs and interview people in those positions to help make decisions about work. Young people explore the world of work in different ways that sometimes include volunteer work, internships, certificate programs, and additional schooling. When the individual expresses interest in an internship, the IPS specialist should suggest options that are related to the person's job goals. The IPS specialist listens carefully to all of the person's ideas and supports trying different opportunities.

IPS specialists also help young people with criminal justice backgrounds apply for jobs. IPS specialists coach job seekers on how to describe their skills and characteristics in relation to the position. Because most employers conduct a background check that reveals a person's legal history, job seekers are encouraged to prepare a brief statement explaining regret for past actions and commitment to corrected ways to encourage employers to consider hiring them. In these situations, some employers consider having a support team to be an advantage.

Providing Job Supports

The IPS specialist and the rest of the coordinated specialty care team provide individualized supports when participants start working. The IPS specialist coaches the employee about going to work on time, how to get to work, what to wear, and other matters for the first day on the job. Recently hired employees need to know when they will receive paychecks and for what time period. The new employee and the IPS specialist develop a support plan that will help the person be a successful worker. Team members help workers with communication skills with their fellow employees and supervisor. Family members and other members of the coordinated specialty care team provide support and encouragement as well.

The IPS specialist and coordinated specialty care team members provide ongoing support to enable successful work experiences. Sometimes, when young people start jobs, they no longer see the need for continued support. They are striving for independence and may want to disengage from services, believing that they have recovered from their problems. In these situations, the IPS specialist may reduce the number of contacts but should maintain some engagement to give support until the person has demonstrated the ability to stay employed.

Advancing Careers

The IPS specialist helps people end jobs and provides support to start new jobs. Most young people work multiple jobs over time as they are developing a career path. When someone wants to leave a job, the IPS specialist counsels the worker to give advanced notice to the employer and to include the work experience on his or her resume. The IPS specialist reviews the positive and negative aspects of the job experience: "What did you learn about yourself as a worker and your preferences for the future? What will you do differently on the next job?" New short-term or long-term job goals are incorporated into career plans, and the IPS specialist should ask the young person whether he or she wants further education or training to gain skills and knowledge to advance his or her career.

Supported Education

Case Example 2

Rebecca is a 20-year-old who became ill during her sophomore year of college. After a brief hospitalization, she returned to her hometown, where she joined an early psychosis program. Meeting with her IPS specialist, Lucia, Rebecca insisted that her only goal was to return to college as a full-time student. Together with Lucia, she explored the local community college and filled out an application for the next term. Following admission, Rebecca signed up for a full course load and declined any disclosure with the college's academic services office. One month into the term, however, she realized she was unable to concentrate in class, was falling behind, and was headed for disaster. She asked Lucia for help. Lucia and Rebecca rapidly negotiated with the college academic dean to reduce Rebecca's course load to one class and with the academic services office to allow her to tape lectures and have extra time for tests. Lucia also helped Rebecca find a quiet place to study in the college library. After these accommodations, Rebecca did well in her first class and decided to increase her college workload gradually.

Education is developmentally appropriate for adolescents and young adults and therefore is an important part of IPS. Some young people, particularly those with attenuated symptoms, are in high school when they first experience psychosis (see Chapter 8, "Assessment and

Targeted Intervention for Individuals at Clinical High Risk for Psychosis"). Others are in postsecondary education or are considering education or vocational skills training to develop careers.

Just as IPS specialists develop relationships with employers in the
community, they also learn about different educational institutions and
training programs in the local area. The IPS specialist should tour college campuses to see where students attend classes, study, and gather
socially. The IPS specialist makes appointments to meet with guidance
counselors and staff from offices for special services who can help to arrange accommodations if needed. In addition, the IPS specialist should
learn about vocational certificate training programs (e.g., pharmacy
technician, home health aide) that are offered in community colleges
and other educational resources such as short-term training programs
(e.g., graphic design programs, culinary programs).

IPS for Students in High School

Level of education relates to employment and financial security over
time; therefore, the team should always encourage young people to
complete high school or obtain the equivalent certificate. To earn the
certificate, students must pass four general educational development
(GED) tests in the areas of language arts, math, science, and social studies. Students may attend free classes to prepare for the test. The IPS specialist may talk with an instructor to find out about a student's progress
and help the student structure ways to study. For high school students,
the IPS specialist may contact a school counselor to obtain guidance on
how to support the student. IPS specialists never fill the role of a tutor,
but they may help students develop good study habits. If a tutor is indicated, the IPS specialist may help to make arrangements.

In the United States, high school students with a disability that affects
their ability to learn may be eligible for an Individualized Education Program (IEP). Special education teachers, parents, the student, and others
(e.g., a school psychologist or other specialist) develop a written plan that
includes academic and functional goals and objectives, the student's
strengths, and possible accommodations to help the student succeed. Ongoing meetings occur to discuss the student's progress, and the plan is
updated at least yearly. If the student is determined ineligible for an IEP,
he or she may request a 504 plan, which has less restrictive eligibility requirements and includes opportunities for accommodations and services
to enhance learning and school performance.

Postsecondary Education

The IPS specialist helps the young person identify a course of study
based on the young person's ideas about careers. How does the career

choice fit with the person's interests, strengths, and preferred work environment? The IPS specialist can help the young person meet people working in the field, observe them working, and interview them about their job. What do they like about the work? What skills are needed? Young people need to consider their options carefully. Making decisions about which classes to enroll in after high school is important because time and financial resources are invested in education. The IPS specialist helps the young person identify possible universities or community colleges, visit the schools, and learn about financial alternatives to pay for school and can accompany the young person to appointments with guidance counselors and academic advisors. IPS specialists are flexible when working with young people and understand that changing directions is normal for most young people.

The IPS specialist coaches the young person about college applications, which are typically online, and may accompany the young person to meetings with financial counselors and help with federal student aid applications if financial support is needed. The IPS specialist helps the young person with class registration and discusses the course load. Many young students are eager to take a full course load, but starting with a reduced course load allows the person who has been away from school for an extended period to adjust to the student role. Students who experience onset of psychosis in high school or college may use a reduced course load to support staying in school. Student support groups such as Students With Schizophrenia (www.sws.ngo) may also be helpful.

Providing Education Supports

The IPS specialist and the student develop an education plan, which outlines the student's goals and steps to achieve the goals. Because many young people complain of poor attention, the team should focus on ways to optimize cognitive function to support learning by addressing medications, substance use (see Chapter 14), exercise (see Chapter 15, "Role of Aerobic Exercise in the Treatment of Early Psychosis"), nutrition, cognitive skills training, and technology supports (see Chapter 20, "Using Technology to Advance Early Psychosis Intervention"). The team helps the student identify stressors, individualized coping techniques, and potential accommodations. Other members of the team as well as family members support the student and provide encouragement, and family members are reminded to refrain from having high expectations too soon.

IPS specialists ensure that students have a system for keeping track of homework assignments and test dates and may suggest using a calendar to keep track of due dates as well as time devoted to completing homework. They help students develop good study skills and an individualized plan for learning. For example, a student who has difficulty with concentration may plan to focus for 15 minutes, take notes, and take a break. The student and IPS specialist discuss places to study that will minimize distractions. Postsecondary schools have offices for students with disabilities where students who have disabilities may request accommodations to help them succeed in school. Documentation of the disability is required prior to receiving approval for an accommodation. Examples of accommodations include extra time on tests; extra breaks during classes; tutoring; permission to record lectures; preferential seating, such as sitting at the front of the room to minimize distractions; help with notetaking; extended deadlines for projects; and receiving an incomplete grade to finish coursework late because of a hospitalization. Additionally, an IEP from high school may carry over to postsecondary education to address specific learning issues.

Supported Employment and Supported Education

Case Example 3

Dwight is a 21-year-old who developed a psychotic illness during his first year of college. He returned home and tried several jobs, but they were short-lived because of arguments with his coworkers and supervisors. Dwight joined an early psychosis program knowing that he would have help with employment. He was introduced to the team's IPS specialist, Nick, who asked him about his interest in work, previous work experiences, schooling, how he spends his time, and other background information. They discussed opportunities to use Dwight's computer skills and the possibility of taking a computer course at the local community college. Members of the treatment team also talked with Dwight about his alcohol and marijuana use and the possible impact of this use on work and school. Dwight and Nick identified several entry-level computer positions and practiced job interviewing. At his second interview, Dwight received a job offer. The job was a good fit for him, and after 4 months he registered for a computer course with Nick's help. Dwight was excited about building his skills to prepare for a more advanced computer job in the future.

The IPS specialist, other team members, and family support students as they gain knowledge and skills to advance their careers. Young people may take time off from school and return when they feel ready to continue their studies. They may go back and forth between employment and education. For some young people, short-term certificate programs give them the opportunity to advance with technical skills. Each young person makes decisions about how best to build his or her career path as part of recovery from early psychosis.

Conclusion

People who work a job or take a class are moving forward in their recovery. The whole coordinated specialty care team supports their efforts and continues to provide hope and support during difficult periods. The team helps the young person learn from missteps at work and/or school to improve his or her next experiences. For people with early psychosis, work and school provide the opportunity to gain confidence and control of their life. A major responsibility of coordinated specialty care teams is to help people with early psychosis to experience opportunity, develop their aspirations, and build successful careers. Employment and education are central areas to address in supporting young people with early psychosis in achieving recovery.

KEY CONCEPTS

- Work and school are important to young adults in early psychosis.

- Early psychosis programs engage young adults in employment and school using a strengths-based approach.

- Family members are included in supported employment and education to expand support.

- Key elements of supported employment and education include a team-based approach, developing an employment and/or education plan, conducting an individualized search, providing supports, and advancing careers.

- All members of coordinated specialty care teams support people in work and school as part of their care.

Discussion Questions

1. Why are work and school important to young adults with early psychosis?

2. How might the vocational and education needs of a teenager with attenuated psychosis syndrome differ from those of a young adult with schizophrenia?

3. How might you help a young person who has unrealistic school goals? How might you help a young person who has no job experience?

4. How might you help a young person who uses marijuana and wants to seek employment?

Suggested Readings

Bond GR, Drake RE, Luciano A: Effectiveness of individual placement and support for young adults. Epidemiology and Psychiatric Services 24(5):446–457, 2015

Corrigan PW: The disabling effects of mental illness on my education. Psychiatr Serv 69(8):847–848, 201829716448

Di Capite S, Upthegrove R, Mallikarjun P: The relapse rate and predictors of relapse in patients with first-episode psychosis following discontinuation of antipsychotic medication. Early Interv Psychiatry 12(5):893–899, 201827734591

Dixon LB, Goldman HH, Bennett ME, et al: Implementing coordinated specialty care for early psychosis: The RAISE Connection Program. Psychiatr Serv 66(7):691–698, 201525772764

Kane JM, Robinson DG, Schooler NR, et al: Comprehensive versus usual community care for first-episode psychosis: 2-year outcomes from the NIMH RAISE early treatment program. Am J Psychiatry 173(4):362–372, 201626481174

References

de Waal A, Dixon LB, Humensky JL: Association of participant preferences on work and school participation after a first episode of psychosis. Early Interv Psychiatry 12(5):959–963, 2018 29052948

Drake RE, Bond GR, Goldman HH, et al: Individual placement and support services boost employment for people with serious mental illness, but funding is lacking. Health Aff (Millwood) 35(6):1098–1105, 2016 27269028

Maraj A, Mustafa S, Joober R, et al: Caught in the "NEET trap": the intersection between vocational inactivity and disengagement from an early intervention service for psychosis. Psychiatr Serv Feb 5, 2019 [Epub ahead of print] 30717644

Marshall T, Goldberg RW, Braude L, et al: Supported employment: assessing the evidence. Psychiatr Serv 65(1):16–23, 2014 24247197

Swanson SJ, Becker DR, Bond GR, et al: The IPS Supported Employment Approach to Help Young People with Work and School: A Practitioner's Guide. Lebanon, NH, IPS Employment Center at the Rockville Institute, 2017

CHAPTER 17

Implementing Peer Support in Early Psychosis Programs

Megan Sage, M.S.W., LCSW
Tamara Sale, M.A.
Nybelle Caruso, B.S., PSS
Michael Haines, QMHA, PSS
Ryan Melton, Ph.D.
Ally Linfoot, PSS

ALTHOUGH professional peer support has not traditionally been a part of all early psychosis programs, it is rapidly evolving as a core discipline within early psychosis teams. Fortunately, this addition is informed by a large history and thriving peer support movement. Peer support specialists play essential roles in all aspects of program service delivery and decision making, and effective inclusion of peer support helps organizations to become truly recovery oriented. The combination of lived experience as a source of relevant knowledge along with scientific inquiry enables early psychosis programs to create more effective, humane, and relevant responses to their participants.

Marcus's Story

Our story begins with Marcus, a peer support specialist in the local early psychosis program, as he makes a presentation for Mental Health

Awareness Week at the local library. As part of the presentation, Marcus shares his own story:

> For a long time, I was hallucinating and was caught up in my own beliefs, and no one really helped me. I was homeless for a while and wandering the streets. I was arrested and put in jail. But once I found a team of people who were kind and understood what I was going through, I was able to recover. The turning point for me was meeting a peer support specialist at the hospital. I thought I was all alone and that there was no hope for me or my future. I was grieving over being broken and everything I had lost. The peer support specialist shared that he had had similar experiences and feelings, that someone else had told him that sometimes others must hold on to your hope for you. He said that step by step, he had found his way from there to a very good place, a place where he felt stronger and wiser for his struggles. He expressed confidence that I would get there too. I had been told that I would never work and that I had a lifelong condition, but his words allowed me to begin to trust and to try, step by step, to get my life back. And I did. Three years ago, I got married. I graduated from college. I realized that I could help people as much from my own lived experience as from any theory, so I became a peer support specialist myself. The people I meet every day are remarkable—they are scientists, artists, musicians, researchers, teachers, writers. They're sensitive, honest, humorous, creative. They teach me so much. If you have ever been told that psychosis is a condition you can never get over, you have been told wrong. With the right support and people who believe in you, the experience of psychosis can create greater awareness, compassion, and understanding. But when you experience it, you feel like the only one. It's our job to make sure no one is left feeling alone.

History of Peer Support in Early Psychosis

Marcus's story is reflective of the broad history of peer support. Peer support is an emerging field with increasing evidence of its effectiveness (Chinman et al. 2014) and has a long history with a growing body of research, spanning cultures and health care conditions (Tang 2013). One study (Davidson et al. 2012) compared individuals in hospital settings who received care as usual with those who received care as usual and support from a peer recovery mentor. This study demonstrated "statistically significant main findings for the number of hospitalizations and the number of days spent in the hospital, with participants assigned recovery mentors doing significantly better than those without a recovery mentor" (Davidson et al. 2012, p. 125). Other findings from this study concluded that participants assigned a peer recovery mentor experienced a "significant decrease in substance use," as well as a "decrease in depression and increases in hope, self-care, and a sense of well-being" (Davidson et al. 2012, p. 125).

The peer support movement in the United States arose alongside other civil rights movements in the 1960s and 1970s, including the Independent Living movement, which brought civil rights to individuals with a range of disabilities (Deegan 1992). Many leaders in the mental health peer support movement have stories of profound indignities and injustices: being ignored until they were held against their will and forced into demeaning and harmful care or being told that they were unemployable, that their hopes and ambitions were not realistic, that their actual truths were delusional, or that they should expect to be disabled for life.

Historically, despite negative attitudes and beliefs in the larger society, individuals with psychosis found their way to recovery because of their own resilience, the caring of people who believed in them, and mental health clinicians who had positive attitudes despite the system barriers they faced. As individuals with lived experience found each other, they began to recognize the importance of working through their trauma regarding the injustices they experienced as consumers. They also recognized and advocated for the idea that recovery exists, is achievable, and does not necessarily require an absence of all symptoms. By creating local informal support networks and alternatives developed and delivered by peers, leaders in the consumer movement (also known as the psychiatric survivor movement) provided informal support systems and began to challenge pathology-driven practices. They focused on supporting the person in a holistic healing and growth process in the community (Mead 2003). Individuals with lived experience have played central roles in advocating for change and have won formal systemic recognition that recovery exists and is achievable, as well as highlighting the importance of peer support as a core element of care (Frese and Davis 1997).

Family peer support emerged in the United States in the 1970s as a result of many of the same injustices, although family members' perspectives were different as they struggled to find help for their loved ones. During that time, families were commonly told, "There's nothing we can do until he's an imminent threat to himself or others." Much of the early family peer support movement focused on basic concerns for survival, safety, and access to services for loved ones and was a reaction to predominant theoretical models that held that families caused schizophrenia. Family members of loved ones with mental health diagnoses largely embraced the medical model and the treatment system, whereas advocacy by the individual consumer movement focused on the system's coercive injustices and dehumanizing approach to care. Ultimately, both the individual and family peer support movements were fueled by recognition of and belief in each person's importance and capabilities. According to the College for Behavioral Health Leadership Peer Services Toolkit, the peer support movement has "continued to evolve to connect people to their communities, and offer information on rights, advocacy, services and supports, recovery, and whole health" (Hendry et al. 2014, p. 11).

Since the 1990s, peer support has become mainstream both for its informal community role and as a professional discipline that is widely viewed as a central element of effective community-based treatment. Peer support specialist services are currently considered best practice by the Substance Abuse and Mental Health Services Administration, are available in all 50 states, and are reimbursable by Medicaid in 35 states (www.mentalhealthamerica.net/peer-services). Peer support certification programs have been developed in most states and nationwide to allow for billing, with careful attention to ethical considerations, supervision, and training needs. Earlier models of early psychosis intervention did not include professional peer support as an identified element. However, with an emphasis on feedback and participatory decision making, along with advocacy, many early psychosis programs now include individual and, to a lesser degree, family peer support within their coordinated specialty care teams (Jones 2015; Thurley et al. 2014).

Core Roles and Attributes of Peer Support

Peer support is based on nonhierarchical sharing of common experience not defined by clinical language or concepts. Individual peer support specialists are receptive to the individual's viewpoint without predetermined clinical assumptions. They support the individual in making meaning from his or her own reality and supporting constructive assertion of power. They refrain from participation in diagnostic decision making and decision making related to involuntary care, except as an advocate for the individual and family (Mead 2003; Mead et al. 2001). Peer support can occur in any setting (e.g., outpatient, crisis, hospital, employment, housing) and may incorporate a broad range of foci, including mental health recovery, medical wellness, and community integration.

Peer support specialists have the unique role of being able to relate to individuals on a personal level and address fears, confusion, uncertainty, and/or anxiety about receiving mental health services. They are nonjudgmental, try not to overreact, and remain attuned to the perspective of the person with whom they are working. In the words of one peer support specialist, the role is to be "endlessly curious about their client's thoughts, activities, values and worldview. They remain 'unimpressed' when meeting a highly symptomatic client, thereby providing acceptance, understanding, encouragement and normalization. They are equally unimpressed when a previously symptomatic client 'clears.'" (T.Casebeer, personal communication, March 2018). In other words, the individual is fully accepted as an important and interesting person whose point of view matters regardless of his or her mental state.

Peer support specialists on early psychosis teams contribute to all aspects of care and treatment and emphasize that individuals are not defined by their diagnosis or symptoms. They offer a point of view that is holistic and focuses on the individual's beliefs, culture, and values. As a current early psychosis peer support specialist stated, "They know from life experience that no one can be reduced to a particular set of symptoms or a diagnosis" (T.Casebeer, personal communication, March 2018).

In contrast to individual peer support specialists, family peer support specialists partner with family members and their support systems throughout the assessment process to provide education and information specific to their needs. Both individual and family peer support specialists focus on helping individuals discover and build on their personal resources and strengths and feel empowered to make the changes they desire. As noted by a current peer support specialist, "Many people will respond well to an interaction with a peer that is driven by intention to create a human connection, give the person space to be heard in a nonjudgmental manner, and to lessen power imbalances as much as possible. A person told me they liked working with peers because we never told her what to do; we just listened" (N.Caruso, personal communication, March 2018).

Peer support specialists play a vital role in shared decision making. They encourage individuals to learn about the multiple treatment options available to them within the program, understand the pros and cons, and collaborate with their team and support system to decide what option is best for them individually. They rely on their own lived experience and practical knowledge to support the individual in making informed decisions about the most appropriate and helpful treatment for them. Peer support specialists and other members of the team work with individuals to understand their preferences and what is important to them on the basis of their goals. As noted by a current peer support specialist, they "act as a subtle stimulus for their clients' self-actualization" (T.Casebeer, personal communication, March 2018). Peer support specialists assist individuals in weighing benefits and risks with regard to decisions about changing jobs, starting medication or switching to a different medication, or moving out of their parents' home to live on their own.

Peer support specialists safeguard the importance of individuals being heard by others and of making their own decisions and choices on the basis of the information that they have regarding risks and benefits, while remaining actively concerned for the person's safety and well-being. Family peer support specialists help family members understand and express their own values and concerns, as well as navigate differences in perspective and decisions by their loved ones. Individual peer support specialists can also be helpful in encouraging parents to allow their young person a certain amount of space for risk taking, and family peer support specialists can provide a different point of view for young people as well as help them navigate developmental changes within family roles.

Individual and family peer support specialists also play a critical role in engaging individuals and families in psychoeducation and in delivering these interventions with a focus on empowerment. Peer support specialists engage with the individual, listen, and "allow their clients a place to unroll and explore their story/experience and share aspects of their own life history where relevant" (T. Casebeer, personal communication, March 2018). They use their own lived experience to share information on multiple topics, including but not limited to coping skills, relationships, communication, normalization of grief related to experiencing symptoms, medications, self-advocacy, treatment options, typical adolescent and young adult development, substance use, legal rights, benefits, relapse prevention, and early and late stages of recovery. Individual psychoeducation is tailored to the person's values, needs, and goals. Peer support specialists share their own lived experiences within these topic areas from a strengths-based perspective that focuses on recovery. Their perspective allows individuals to hear messages of hope and to understand that the recovery process can vary and is not linear.

Marcus Meets William

Denise, who attended the early psychosis community education event at the public library where Marcus was a presenter, calls the program because of her concerns about her boyfriend, William. William is a 23-year-old African American young man who has become fearful that others are trying to hurt him, is disorganized, and is unable to go to his job. As a result, William was fired. He has been sleeping throughout the day and staying up all night. He told Denise he thinks she can read his thoughts, and he has started talking to himself. Denise is fearful to leave him alone at home but must get to her full-time job to pay the bills. William and Denise have been living together for 2 years and have a small dog named Mac.

Denise arranges for Marcus and Sadie, the early psychosis intervention screener, to visit their home and meet William. An initial conversation with Denise and William identifies William's many strengths. William is a high school graduate who has been studying to enter medicine. He loves animals and has continued taking Mac out for walks on days when he feels safe in the neighborhood. William reports that listening to music sometimes helps him feel better. William's grandparents live in the area and have some intermittent contact with him. William is willing to talk but does not want to sign any paperwork to receive services through the early intervention program. He does not understand why no one else can see that he is being followed when he leaves the home and does not see a reason for mental health treatment. He expresses concern that he is being watched by the police and worries about his safety. He and Denise argue frequently, and William expresses frustration that no one believes that what he is experiencing is real. William's sleep has been worsening. He spends most of his time isolated in the basement, listening to music or playing video games.

During the home visit, Marcus listens nonjudgmentally and empathetically, and he and William connect over a similar taste in music. William sets up another appointment with Marcus to listen to music together the following day. In the meantime, Marcus, Sadie, and other early intervention team members provide education and information about symptoms of psychosis to Denise. Shameka, the early intervention family peer support specialist, sets up an appointment to meet with Denise later that week, in which she shares her own experiences as the mother of a young woman who developed symptoms of psychosis. Shameka speaks to the unique challenges in supporting a loved one who is struggling while at the same time addressing one's own self-care and personal needs. Shameka assists Denise in coming up with ideas about how to reduce her own stress levels and how she can get her own support.

William and Marcus meet a couple more times at William's home, and Marcus discusses his own past struggles with paranoia and difficulty sleeping and talks about what has been helpful to him. Marcus is open about his own path to finding understanding and recovery. Through multiple conversations, William begins to feel less anxious about leaving the house and agrees to sign paperwork to engage in ongoing services with the early intervention team. William and Denise work with Marcus, Shameka, and William's primary clinician, Miranda, to come up with strengths-based, recovery-oriented treatment goals. Denise notes that the support of the team has helped to reduce conflict between her and William and increase their positive communication.

William's most pressing goal is that he wants a job but is unsure if he will be able to keep the job because he was fired previously for not showing up to work. Marcus empathizes with William around this concern and says that he and his team members will support William in getting a job as well as keeping a job once he is hired. He and William meet with the supported employment specialist, Jorge, to talk about what type of job William may be interested in and to discuss the pros and cons of different work environments and schedules.

William is frightened of taking medications and fearful of being put in the hospital against his will. He is reluctant to talk to the psychiatrist, Louise, but is more comfortable being open with Marcus. Marcus empathizes, reminds William about the shared decision-making process, and helps William think through his goals and fears. Marcus and William meet with Louise together. William is surprised that Louise shares an interest in some of his favorite musical artists and is easier to talk to and a more receptive listener than he had expected. He decides to try a low dose of antipsychotic medicine.

As time goes on, William participates in treatment and periodically confides in Marcus about decisions he is making and things that are bothering him. He continues to express concern that the police are watching him and fears being harmed by police when he leaves home. Marcus helps William express this concern to the team. This leads to a broader discussion about times in the past when William felt he was targeted by police on the basis of his race, and the whole team engages with Denise, William, and William's grandparents about this topic. William feels it would be helpful to check out his feelings of being targeted with Denise, Marcus, his grandparents, or other team members when he feels this way. Marcus and the rest of the early intervention team view a person's symptoms through a social and cultural lens, paying attention to their individual experiences and how they make sense of these experiences. As a result, the team and William's loved ones agree that William's feelings of being targeted by police might not be related to his symptoms of psychosis and might be based in reality.

With Marcus's help, William feels more and more comfortable expressing his perspectives and needs to the team and advocating for himself. Marcus encourages William to participate in opportunities to share his perspective, such as a focus group about how to improve the program. Marcus invites William to attend a meet-up group in the community and offers to attend the group with him. He also offers to connect William to an advocacy group that meets monthly, which William says he will think about. He likes the idea of working with others to improve services for young people and has gained confidence in his ability to speak with others about his own experiences through his work with Marcus.

Defining "Peer" in Early Psychosis Programs

Just as with all roles in early psychosis intervention teams, peer support services must be modified to address the unique developmental and cultural needs of adolescents and young adults. One active debate is whether *peer* is defined by experience of psychosis or other mental health condition, age, or some other criterion such as prior participation in community mental health services. The experience of psychosis is different from other mental health conditions, and an individual whose lived experience does not include psychosis may not be as able to relate to individuals who are experiencing this condition as would an individual who has experienced psychosis. However, even when individuals have experienced psychosis, in their training and practice they must recognize that experiences are widely variable and that there is no single "right" answer.

The optimal combination for peer support specialists working in early psychosis intervention programs likely includes mentoring and engagement by individuals with some psychosis experience, as well as the ability to relate to individuals developmentally. Many of the challenges faced by individuals in early psychosis programs relate to normal developmental changes associated with changing roles and relationships, emergence of an adult identity, and increased pressure to learn new skills and take on adult responsibilities. Thus, peer support may also focus on the developmental challenges and tasks of being a young adult.

Peer support specialists also play a significant role in the transition process as individuals prepare for discharge from early psychosis intervention services. Through their participation in mental health services, individuals often become interested in continuing in advocacy work after they complete the program. Peer support specialists help individuals identify their strengths and build on them to tell their stories and practice receiving feedback in a safe and supportive environment. Peer support specialists are key in assisting individuals in creating and revising personal wellness or relapse prevention plans and building their support networks. They connect individuals and families with opportunities for continued engagement as graduates of the early psychosis program, as well as opportunities to explore other informal and formal prospects outside the program. In addition, they act as role models for those who want to become peer support specialists themselves.

Creating an Environment Conducive to Peer Support

The peer support core values and practices of nonjudgment, empathetic listening, reciprocal learning, consciousness of the dynamics of power, advocacy for voice and rights, and fundamental belief in each person challenge and infuse clinical cultures with a more humanistic, positive way of thinking and operating. It is important for clinicians, administrators, and policy makers to understand the unique history, values, and approach of peer support to facilitate rather than diminish its impact. In addition, authentic inclusion of peer support often involves profound and personal rethinking of explicit and implicit biases, negative assumptions, reactivity to symptomatology, and overly medicalized and pathologizing approaches to care. When peer support on early psychosis intervention teams is done well, it can transform a team's understanding and capacity to engage with and support the individuals and family members it serves.

Peer support certification curricula and job descriptions sometimes leave out the values and principles of peer-developed peer support (Kaufman et al. 2016; Penney 2018). Negative attitudes and clinical cultures within existing care systems that do not align with the principles of peer support jeopardize the discipline (Stastny and Brown 2013). Thus, it is important to focus on maintaining the integrity of peer support at all levels of conceptualization, implementation, decision making, and practice and to proactively educate policy makers, administrators, clinicians, and other staff about the core principles and practices of peer support. Supervision should support a careful thought process around intentional self-disclosure. Other team members should be conscious of, and challenge, statements and assumptions that might suggest that individuals and/or families experiencing psychosis are somehow "less than" others.

It is also very important for early psychosis intervention teams to understand and value the peer support role and not assign tasks that minimize or are inconsistent with their role. An example of this would be looking to the peer support specialist on a team as a transportation provider outside his or her typical peer support role. As a current peer support specialist notes, it is important for peer support specialists "not to be assigned case management tasks that involve doing anything *for* the person rather than with them. For example, I would not set up an intake for an individual on my own accord like a service coordinator might. But as a peer I would sit with the person while they call on speakerphone and give as much support in making that intake as they request" (N. Caruso, personal communication, March 2018).

Agencies must create a structured way to involve individuals in recovery to participate meaningfully in agency operations, such as clinical decision making, staff hiring and training, community education, quality improvement, and oversight. Peer support specialists work together with individuals and families receiving early psychosis services and in a mutually beneficial relationship to give voice to individuals' lived experiences in order to create change within the mental health system. Peer support specialists assist individuals in their recovery by identifying possible barriers to participation and using problem-solving strategies with the individuals and team to address those barriers. Peer support specialists act as a connection for individuals to participate in educational, vocational, or community activities. As noted by a current peer support specialist, "sharing experiences and insights are a fantastic way to learn from one another, and ultimately, progress to advocating together for better mental health services in the future" (N. Cohrs, personal communication, March 2018).

Conclusion

Full integration of peer support specialists into early psychosis intervention treatment teams is based on a clearly defined peer support model. Peer support is a transformative and highly effective strategy for improving engagement, relevance, and outcomes. Peer support is highly aligned with core concepts of first-episode psychosis care, such as resilience, partnership, recovery, and shared decision making. The peer support field continues to grow in available knowledge, training, and effectiveness, and it holds an important key to the future of the early psychosis field.

KEY CONCEPTS

- Peer support is a distinct role with its own history grounded in social justice, intentional community, and belief in recovery.

- Peer support follows the principles of nonhierarchical reciprocity; listening; learning and exploring together; and advocating for the individual's rights, voice, and self-determination. Individual and family peer support emerged through separate but interrelated histories and brings different perspectives to recovery. Professional peer support is increasingly understood as a core element of early psychosis treatment.

- Peer support provides a bridge between the individual and clinical team in all aspects of treatment. Peer support is transformative in nature and, when embraced, may lead to a deep shift in understanding, language, and practice within early psychosis teams as well as the larger organization providing treatment.

- To fully embrace the peer support role, it is important for all members of early psychosis teams to value lived experience as an important source of knowledge and become comfortable with strategic self-disclosure. Teams must intentionally cultivate positive cultural norms that challenge language, assumptions, and practices that are discriminatory and/or negative.

- As with other members of the treatment team, training, supervision, and mentoring, along with pay equity and opportunities for career advancement, are of critical importance to individuals in professional peer support positions.

Discussion Questions

1. How does the concept of peer support services change the conversation around mental health treatment in a broad sense?

2. How does integrating peer support services change the role of clinicians, medical staff, and other treatment team members?

3. How would you collaborate with individual and family peer support specialists in your role as part of a treatment team?

4. What are your ideas about how early psychosis teams can foster nonhierarchical collaborative learning?

5. What do you see as the role of story and self-disclosure in your own practice? How might the context, philosophy, and practices of peer support influence your practice?

Suggested Readings

Caughey M: Creating deep democracy through peer wellness services. Global Journal of Community Psychology Practice 5(1):1–17, 2014

Center for Practice Innovations at Columbia Psychiatry: OnTrackNY Peer Specialist Manual. New York, OnTrackNY, February 2017. www.ontrackny.org/portals/1/Files/Resources/Peer%20Specialist%20Manual%20Final%202_17.17.pdf?ver=2017-04-04-063602-080. Accessed October 10, 2018.

International Association for Peer Supporters: National Practice Guidelines for Peer Supporters. Norton, MA, International Association for Peer Supporters, 2012. Available at: https://na4ps.files.wordpress.com/2012/09/nationalguidelines1.pdf. Accessed February 22, 2019.

Mead S, Hilton D, Curtis L: Peer support: a theoretical perspective. Psychiatric Rehabilitation Journal, 25(2):134–141, 2001 11769979

References

Chinman M, George P, Dougherty RH, et al: Peer support services for individuals with serious mental illnesses: assessing the evidence. Psychiatr Serv 65(4):429–441, 2014 24549400

Davidson L, Bellamy C, Guy K, Miller R: Peer support among persons with severe mental illnesses: a review of evidence and experience. World Psychiatry 11(2):123–128, 2012 22654945

Deegan PE: The independent living movement and people with psychiatric disabilities: taking back control over our own lives. Psychiatr Rehabil J 15(3):3–19, 1992

Frese FJ, Davis WW: The consumer-survivor movement, recovery, and consumer professionals. Prof Psychol Res Pr 28(3):243–245, 1997

Hendry P, Hill T, Rosenthal H: Peer Services Toolkit: A Guide to Advancing and Implementing Peer-Run Behavioral Health Services. Albuquerque, NM, College for Behavioral Health Leadership, 2014

Jones N: Peer Involvement and Leadership in Early Intervention in Psychosis Services: From Planning to Peer Support and Evaluation. Alexandria, VA, National Association of State Mental Health Program Directors, 2015. Available at: www.nasmhpd.org/sites/default/files/Peer-Involvement-Guidance_Manual_Final.pdf. Accessed February 1, 2018.

Kaufman L, Kuhn W, Stevens Manser S: Peer Specialist Training and Certification: A National Overview. Austin, TX, Texas Institute for Excellence in Mental Health, 2016

Mead S: Defining Peer Support. West Chesterfield, NH, Intentional Peer Support, 2003. Available at: https://docs.google.com/document/d/1WG3ul nF6vthAwFZpJxE9rkx6lJzYSX7VX4HprV5EkfY/edit. Accessed February 8, 2018.

Mead S, Hilton D, Curtis L: Peer support: a theoretical perspective. Psychiatr Rehabil J 25(2):134–141, 2001 11769979

Penney D: Defining "Peer Support": Implications for Policy, Practice, and Research. Sudbury, MA, Advocates for Human Potential, 2018. http://ahpnet.com/AHPNet/media/AHPNetMediaLibrary/White%20Papers/DPenney_Defining_peer_support_2018_Final.pdf. Accessed February 22, 2019.

Stastny P, Brown C: Peer specialist: origins, pitfalls and worldwide dissemination [in Spanish]. Vertex 24(112):455–459, 2013 24511563

Tang P: A Brief History of Peer Support: Origins. Chapel Hill, NC, Peers for Progress, 2013. Available at: http://peersforprogress.org/pfp_blog/a-brief-history-of-peer-support origins. Accessed February 8, 2018.

Thurley M, Monson K, Simpson R: Youth Participation in an Early Psychosis Service. Melbourne, Australia, Orygen Youth Health, 2014

CHAPTER 18

Family Intervention and Support in Early Psychosis

Shirley M. Glynn, Ph.D.

A robust body of research suggests that specialized treatment programs for first-episode psychosis (FEP) can improve clinical and functional outcomes (Bird et al. 2010; Kane et al. 2016). These treatment programs typically comprise both pharmacological and psychosocial components, including a family support intervention. Bolstering support for families may be an especially valuable aspect of care in non-affective FEP because the distress, worry, and confusion experienced by the loved ones of an individual with FEP are well documented (Jansen et al. 2015). Furthermore, caregiver burnout may be a particular risk in early psychosis (Onwumere et al. 2018) and can undermine participant support. Unfortunately, lack of family support (Jones et al. 2017) and/or relatives' expression of their distress, concern, and dissatisfaction (high expressed emotion) (Alvarez-Jimenez et al. 2012) are associated with negative early treatment outcomes. In light of these findings, it is perhaps not surprising that there have now been several published reviews and meta-analyses confirming the benefits on the participant and relative FEP outcomes of offering family support and education (Bird et al. 2010).

Because schizophrenia and bipolar illness usually develop during adolescence or young adulthood, many individuals diagnosed with the disorder still rely on their families of origin for their primary social support as they become ill. Young people diagnosed with these disorders often fail to achieve developmental milestones (e.g., graduating from high school or college, getting a first job, moving out of the parental home) in a timely manner. This "offtimedness" often extends the period of the individual's dependence on his or her relatives and places an additional burden and stress on the family. Relatives are often worried and confused by illness-related behavior changes and developmental lags. They may not immediately recognize the presence of a mental illness or may refuse to believe that the illness is present even when it is brought to their attention. Family interventions can play a key role in helping these relatives cope successfully with the illness and support the recovery of their loved one.

It is important to think broadly about family member inclusion in recovery from FEP. Although most FEP materials highlight the involvement of parents or guardians, other kin are also important. Some individuals with psychosis marry or enter conjugal-like relationships, and thus their partners may be the key relatives to engage in the FEP program. Not surprisingly, the stresses of living with a serious psychiatric illness can have a profound impact on a couple, and rates of separation and divorce are higher in couples in which one person has been diagnosed with schizophrenia (Thara and Srinivasan 1997).

The needs and value of including siblings in care should also be considered. The development of a psychosis in a brother or sister can be very troubling. Furthermore, in many families, when the psychosis develops, much (if not all) of the parental nurturance goes into supporting the ill child, and there is less focus on the other children. Sports events are missed; there is less time to help with homework; vacations get canceled. Siblings often experience the loss of the brother or sister as they have known him or her *and* the loss of their parents' attention and guidance. Sibling involvement in an FEP family education program provides a forum for answering siblings' questions, validating their sense of loss, and encouraging their continued development. It can also be a useful tool to engage siblings in supporting the person's recovery.

In this chapter, we present the overall principles and strategies for involving families in FEP treatment. We discuss consent and confidentiality issues first, then review the optimal credentials and characteristics of an effective FEP family clinician. We then discuss the components of a comprehensive FEP family intervention, incorporating a stepped-care approach, and follow with a brief case description. We conclude with a review of key points, relevant questions to consider when developing a local family FEP program, and helpful resources.

Principles and Strategies for Involving Relatives in Treatment of First-Episode Psychosis

There is a robust literature confirming the benefits of involving family members in the care of individuals diagnosed with long-standing psychotic disorders (Lyman et al. 2014), so it is not surprising that many clinical research groups have designed and implemented family intervention programs as part of their FEP programs. Unfortunately, significant design differences across studies render identification of the optimal FEP family program among these variants difficult. For one thing, the centrality of the family intervention to the overall FEP program often determines who actually is enrolled in the program. Participants who do not have consenting family members may not be eligible for an FEP program with a strong family emphasis. In addition, family interventions themselves also often differ substantially in structure. For example, both multifamily and single-family interventions have been offered. In light of these variations, it is currently impossible to conclude that one particular family intervention is preferable to another—the characteristics of the FEP program, as well as the participating individuals' and relatives' needs and preferences, will all likely dictate parameters of the specific family intervention offered at a particular site. *The critical point is that some type of a high-quality family intervention should be available in every FEP program.*

Addressing Consent and Confidentiality Issues

Individuals with FEP are typically young; most programs serve populations ranging from midteenage years to mid to late thirties. These transitional-age individuals may legally be minors or adults, but even those who are adults are often still dependent on their relatives for meeting their instrumental and affiliative needs. A small percentage will be married or in conjugal-like relationships.

Negotiating consent for family involvement in care and establishing guidelines around sharing information among family members is often accomplished easily with individuals with FEP, although it can sometimes become complicated. Some individuals will be minors, and their parents or another responsible adult will be able to consent to their treatment and have access to their medical information. In addition, as will be discussed more fully below, many participants, even those of legal age, are brought to these programs by a family member, often a parent, and the participant will often readily consent to involving his or her family in care.

A small subset of individuals with FEP will be reluctant to have their relatives involved in their care, and some will outright refuse consent to do so. There are many possible reasons for this: the young person may be estranged from his or her relatives or may be suspicious of them, or he or she may want to assert his or her independence. In considering how to proceed, the FEP staff should carefully consider the unique circumstances of the individual and his or her family. There are certainly

understandable and reasonable circumstances that would make someone reluctant to have a family member involved in his or her treatment,
including a history of abuse or neglect. However, barring such negative
factors, particularly if the individual and relative reside together, involving the relative in mental health care can be an invaluable resource
for recovery. If the individual-relative relationship is strong, a good FEP
family education program can render it stronger; if the relationship is
fractious or barely exists, a good FEP family education program can be
a mechanism for healing and bonding. It can be easy for a busy clinician
to immediately accede to a person's reluctance to involve a family
member in care rather than view this as the beginning of a dialogue
about the issue; however, it is important to remember that most often,
the young person will have a relationship (good or bad as it may be)
with that family member long after ending participation in the FEP program. Shoring up the relationship during FEP program participation
can be a critical aspect of recovery.

If the young person expresses reluctance to involve his or her family
in care on entry into an FEP program or if a minor withdraws consent
for family involvement when he or she turns 18 and the treatment team
sees value in encouraging reconsideration of the decision, the following
strategies may prove helpful.

1. Keep the topic open. After an initial refusal, the possibility of family
    involvement can be raised again during treatment team meetings or
    times of transition. An exacerbation of symptoms or a new opportu-
    nity such as a job or return to school sometimes galvanizes people,
    and they become open to trying new strategies; this can be a time of
    family reengagement.
2. Use shared decision making to assure that the person with FEP thor-
    oughly weighs the benefits and risks of family involvement in care.
    Some young people will give an immediate negative response to a
    request for family involvement in care because they want autonomy
    and wish to assert their independence. They may not fully consider
    the benefits of having the treatment team help them enlist their fam-
    ily members in their recovery. Exploring with a trusted clinician the
    potential benefits of family involvement in care can be useful in
    making the decision of whether or not to involve family members.
3. Acquaint the young person with the benefits of family involvement
    in care for the relatives. Some individuals are concerned about bur-
    dening their relatives and thus are hesitant to ask them to come to
    sessions. However, if the clinician describes the benefits for relatives
    (e.g., having the opportunity to have their questions or concerns ad-
    dressed, learning stress management), this sometimes helps the in-
    dividual acquire some perspective on the relative's concerns and
    engenders interest in family involvement.

4. Consider a limited consent for release of medical information. Young people with FEP are often willing to share some information with their relatives (e.g., their treatment plan) but are less willing to have information shared about other topics (e.g., sexual relationships, drug use). As an opening strategy to involve families in care, the FEP team can agree to these restrictions and then work with the individual to modify the rules over time if they seem too constricting. Much of the assessment and initial family illness education can be successfully accomplished without the clinician revealing intimate details of the young person's life.

Who Should Provide First-Episode Psychosis Family Services?

Several members of the team are likely to interact with the relatives of the young person with FEP. For example, relatives may have questions about the young person's medications that warrant a meeting with the prescriber, or they may want to discuss substance abuse issues with whoever on the team is addressing these issues. However, many FEP programs find it most efficient to have the program director also assume the designated role of family clinician. There are several reasons for this delegation of duties. FEP program directors are typically responsible for program recruitment and often have the first contact with the individual's relatives. This early contact can serve as a foundation for later family work. In addition, family work involves integrating aspects of all components of the FEP program, and the program director is uniquely situated to accomplish this task. Finally, the director is often the team member with a more advanced clinical degree—typically at least a master's degree—and is often a licensed clinician. Advanced clinical training is essential because family work can be very complicated. Just having several related individuals in a session makes it more complex. With families, this can be even more thorny because the relationship history preceding the development of the psychosis as well as current stress and symptom levels often color interactions in a negative way; this can require clinical skill to navigate.

Components of a First-Episode Psychosis Family Program

Some families make an accommodation to the development of psychosis in a loved one with grace and acceptance; others struggle and may need more support. A stepped-care approach has been suggested for family work in FEP (Onwumere et al. 2011), and in fact this model was re-flected in the design of the family component in the Recovery After an Initial Schizophrenia Episode Early Treatment Program (RAISE-ETP; Kane et al. 2016). The components of an FEP stepped-care model are presented in Table 18–1.

TABLE 18–1.   Stepped-care model of family intervention for recent-onset psychosis

---

Interventions offered to all individuals with FEP and relatives (with the individual's consent)

   Active engagement

   Individual assessment of relatives

   Brief illness education (group or individual)

   Brief consultation

   Access to the treatment team

   Invitations to relatives to join treatment planning meetings

More intensive optional interventions tailored to specific family need

   Multifamily support groups

   Formal communication and problem-solving skills training

   Referral for individual supportive psychotherapy for relatives

---

Abbreviation.   FEP = first-episode psychosis.

Interventions Offered to Individuals and Relatives

ACTIVE ENGAGEMENT

As described in Chapter 6, "Engaging Families and Individuals in Care," case finding and engagement is often the most challenging task in establishing an FEP program. Some individuals experiencing an FEP may be reluctant or too distressed to seek treatment on their own, and a first contact with a relative, rather than with the person with FEP, is common during engagement in an FEP program. This contact often involves an initial phone call or meeting with family members alone because the individual may still be in the hospital, may feel too ill or distressed to join, or may see little need for help. Accommodating this initial contact with relatives alone often stretches agencies that are used to instituting the informal but frequently used rule "the individual has to want help and must contact the agency himself or herself" as a requirement for service entry. Nevertheless, given the high probability of initial relative-only contact, it is incumbent on the FEP program director or recruiter to become comfortable with discussing services and "pitching" the program to family members first.

In considering strategies for engagement in an FEP program, it is important for the FEP program director or recruiter to consider likely pathways to care. Because some individuals have had mental health challenges long before they developed a psychosis, their family members will already be familiar (at least in broad strokes) with how the mental health system works, may already be clients of the agency, and often comprehend the need for continuity and maintenance of care. Other families will be new to the system and will need an overall orientation on how services are organized and paid for, as well as the importance of sustained care. These families are typically facing an unanticipated psychiatric crisis in their loved one, so they may be understandably distressed themselves and may require repeated exposure to information. Finally, it is important to note that many FEP programs are established in public or nonprofit mental health agencies but will often be recruiting individuals who are younger than age 26 and thus are still covered under their parents' private health insurance. These individuals may have been seeking care in the private sector prior to FEP program entry; they may have little understanding of how the public and/or nonprofit agency works and may have expectations that differ from how the agency conducts business. This transition to a new, often larger, and sometimes seemingly impersonal system needs to be handled with tact and understanding.

Engaging the individual in care involves providing factual information about the program *as well as* using motivational enhancement techniques to counter what may be initial reluctance to enter an intensive FEP program. Many potential program participants and their loved ones may be eager to receive FEP services tailored to their unique needs. Others may be less enthusiastic. Young people may demonstrate reluctance to enter the program, and it is important to recognize that family members may also be hesitant to support their loved one's enrollment; use of motivational enhancement techniques may be important with them as well.

Families may be reluctant to support engagement in an FEP program for many reasons. They may not believe the individual is ill or believe it is a transitory problem that will clear on its own. They may have little concept of how mental health services work and may not immediately see the value of a specialized FEP program. They may have many other burdens in their lives that they judge (often correctly) will interfere with participation in the FEP program, or they may have their own mental health challenges that interfere with help seeking. These are all formidable obstacles to accessing care, and each one will require patience and empathy on the part of the FEP program director or recruiter in these initial conversations.

In every meeting with the family, it is essential that the FEP staff convey an attitude of hope and belief in the possibility of recovery. In initial contacts with family members, the FEP program director or recruiter must be prepared for either an enthusiastic or a more reserved family reaction to the program. He or she must inquire about *and listen carefully* to any concerns raised by either relatives or the person with FEP and be equipped with an array of both practical suggestions and motivational interviewing skills to address the issues raised by the individual and relatives.

Cultural and ethnic considerations also play a role in family engagement. There is a robust literature indicating that stressful life experiences heighten risk for psychosis. Immigration can be a risk factor for some (but by no means all) cultural groups, and institutional racism has also been hypothesized to be a contributing factor. Thus, members of minority groups are often overrepresented in samples of individuals experiencing psychosis, especially nonaffective psychosis (Dealberto 2010). FEP program directors and recruiters must learn to interact effectively with individuals from diverse backgrounds if they are to be successful. This effort can raise many challenges. Language barriers require the use of translators, which can be clinically complicated because of boundary issues if the translator is another member of the family or an unpaid volunteer community member.

Furthermore, psychosis in a child in an immigrant family can be uniquely disruptive. In many immigrant communities, the older children in the family may become the conduits to the new country because they often become more familiarized with the cultural norms through school and social media. These children are often especially valued by the family and are the target of high expectations. Understandably, if one of these children develops a psychotic illness, it can be especially destabilizing for the family. The relatives not only are dealing with unexpected illness but also may have lost their in-house language translator as well as the person who navigates much of the family's interactions with the new society. The situation may be further complicated by the family's cultural beliefs about the causes or treatment of the psychosis, which may conflict with the teaching and practices of the majority culture. Engaging such an individual and his or her relatives in an FEP program can be challenging; it requires the sensitivity and empathy of the FEP program manager or recruiter and perhaps consultation with cultural experts (often a member of a local religious group or another medical professional) to learn enough about the concerns and pressures impinging on the family to interact effectively with them.

Finally, it must be noted that in spite of the best efforts of the care team and the consent of the individual, some families will not become involved in the FEP program, even when the individual consents to their involvement. Often, this absence reflects other pressures in the family, such as complicated work schedules, caretaking for other family members, or mental illness in the relative. Sometimes, the best the team can do is keep the door open, extend an open invitation to the family to engage with the team at a later time, and reach out assertively to the family if circumstances change.

INDIVIDUAL ASSESSMENT OF RELATIVES

Most FEP programs have a standard assessment tool that is used with participants, and responses provide a wealth of information to inform clinicians about how to be helpful to families in their efforts to support the recovery of their loved ones. However, as was discussed in the previous subsection, "Active Engagement," relatives may have their own concerns about their loved one, so it is essential that the family clinician conduct a separate assessment with at least one relative (and more if possible if they intend to participate in the family sessions). This meeting can be vital for alliance building.

Further, integrating the information obtained in the individual and relative assessments is critical to developing an effective treatment team for the individual. Knowing that a family member sees nothing wrong with the individual smoking marijuana and, in fact, smokes it with him or her or that the family member discourages medication adherence can be invaluable in designing a family education program tailored to the unique needs of the participant. Similarly, the family response to the development of psychosis in a loved one may be colored by the fact that either this is a new experience for them or, alternatively, this individual is another in a long line of family members who have serious mental health challenges. This information can be essential to establishing the appropriate affective tone for the sessions. Trying to provide good family education about psychosis without an assessment is like trying to box with one hand tied behind your back.

It is preferable that the family assessment is conducted individually, with just the clinician and the family member present. Although many agencies have a "no secrets" policy and are reluctant to see family members in the absence of the individual with FEP, relatives may be hesitant to share important information in the individual's presence, especially early during FEP treatment, because they fear that sharing information (such as the fact that the individual is aggressive or is not taking his or her medication as prescribed) in front of the individual will create problems at home.

A private meeting can also be invaluable in learning about issues the psychosis has raised for other family members. For example, in a blended family, the behavior and increased dependence resulting from the psychosis often can become a source of friction between the parent and stepparent, causing the parent to have the added burden of trying to protect the young person from the criticism of the stepparent. Although the parent may be unlikely to disclose this situation in a conjoint interview with the individual, he or she may be very willing to discuss it privately with the family clinician. Similarly, parents who have experienced serious mental illness in themselves or in other family members may be especially distressed by the development of psychosis in their child and may need a place to discharge their anxiety or guilt; doing so in front of the child may be counterindicated, but this is still very useful information for the family clinician to have. Although it is optimal to cultivate open sharing of information among all participants in the FEP program, this may take time and should be a goal of the family intervention rather than a prerequisite for entry to the program.

When considering potential topics that may be important to assess when beginning to work with a new family in an FEP program, the items in Table 18–2 can serve as a guideline and can be augmented as needed. The clinician should also be alert to any other needs or concerns the relative raises that might benefit from being addressed in case management. By linking the family with agencies that can assist in meeting these needs, the stress level on the individual can be reduced and a stronger alliance built, to the benefit of all. For example, indigent family members may disclose pressing needs that are not necessarily related to the individual in treatment (e.g.,visa concerns, employment challenges, financial concerns).

BRIEF ILLNESS EDUCATION

The provision of family illness education has several goals: 1) engage and motivate the family in support of the recovery treatment plan; 2) help the family develop hopeful, realistic short-term and long-term expectations for the individual's functioning; 3) assist the family in learning how to be helpful to the individual; and 4) assure that participants have an accurate understanding of factors that improve and hinder good outcomes. Typical topics covered in a brief educational program for psychosis are presented in Table 18–3.

Illness education can often seem like a deceptively easy enterprise— simply providing factual information to individuals to whom it might be important. However, given the complexity of the educational goals, the variation in participants and families, and the uncertainties of early psychosis, the task of providing good illness education to individuals and their loved ones can be more nuanced than it first appears. There are many resources available to facilitate this education (see Suggested Readings at the end of the chapter). Strategies for optimizing brief illness education are presented in the appendix at the end of the chapter.

Brief illness education can be offered in an extended group workshop format or in a series of 5–10 individual sessions. Typically, both the individual and his or her relatives are invited, although if the individual elects not to attend, the relatives can still do so. The benefits of a group

TABLE 18–2.	Assessment probes for relatives supporting an individual in an FEP program

What are the circumstances of the relative's life (e.g., age, marital status, employment, health concerns, kin relation to individual)?

What does the family member understand about the individual's disorder (label, symptoms, treatment, causes)?

Has the family member had prior experience with mental illness in himself or herself or in a loved one?

What factors does the family member think make the symptoms and the individual's situation better?

What factors does the family member think make the symptoms and the individual worse?

What are the individual's strengths?

What does the relative think about the individual's treatment plan? What does he or she like about it? What are his or her concerns? How does he or she feel about the prescribed medication?

What are the main difficulties the relative is having as a result of the psychotic illness? How does he or she cope with them?

Is the individual's illness causing any stress or strain in other family relationships?

Is there an issue about the individual's substance use? How does the relative feel about that?

Is there any concern about safety or aggression in the home? How is the relative managing that?

What are the other significant concerns in the relative's life (e.g., health, job, finances, other family members)?

What strengths does the relative bring to this challenge?

Does the relative have a social network (people on whom he or she can rely)?

Are there any important impending changes coming up for the family?

What additional items (if any) are pertinent to this family?

Abbreviation.   FEP=first-episode psychosis.

educational setting include provision of opportunities for families to learn from each other, the potential for participants to develop a larger social support network, and cost-effectiveness if the group is large enough. The advantages of individual sessions are the ability to hold meetings at the specific time and location most convenient for the participants and the capacity to tailor the information provided to the unique needs of the family. Many agencies do not have sufficient FEP

TABLE 18–3. Topics covered in brief illness education for families of individuals with psychosis

---

Facts about psychosis (e.g., symptoms prevalence, causes, prognosis, treatment)

Medication

Coping with stress

Developing resilience

Relapse prevention planning

Developing a collaboration with mental health professionals

Effective communication

Supporting recovery from psychosis

---

enrollment to cultivate multifamily groups, but these groups can provide some real advantages to participants if they are an option.

BRIEF CONSULTATION

Subsequent to illness education, families often need assistance solving real-world problems, developing plans to meet treatment goals, or accessing resources to support their loved one's recovery. Sometimes there are decisions to be made—such as the individual deciding about applying for disability benefits or returning to school or moving to his or her own place—that may have an impact on relatives. Families can often benefit from expert consultation in these situations, either with the family clinician or with an FEP case manager if the program has one. Typically, a few conjoint sessions to address a specific issue can be useful; often, these sessions can incorporate formal problem solving or use of a pro-and-con decisional balance exercise.

ACCESS TO THE TREATMENT TEAM

Although the family clinician is likely to have the most contact with the participant's relatives, FEP programs rely on interdisciplinary teams to be successful, and family involvement may be important for bolstering medication adherence, practicing skills, and supporting work or school engagement. It is essential that the family clinician have a strong grasp on the individual's treatment program and liaise with other treatment team members when family engagement in other components of the FEP program may be beneficial. Conjoint meetings with the individual, relative(s), family clinician, and other FEP team members can be invaluable in supporting the treatment plan.

INVITATIONS TO RELATIVES TO JOIN TREATMENT PLANNING MEETINGS

Three key aspects of an effective FEP program are instituting an interdisciplinary team, systematically monitoring the individual's progress, and adjusting the treatment plan as needed (White et al. 2015). Typically, treatment planning team meetings are held at least 2–3 times per year for each participant, and encouraging relatives to attend these meetings is an important aspect of an effective family program. Relatives can be an essential source of information about an individual, such as when the person is not taking medication, is aggressive, or is now willingly attending family functions that he or she previously refused to attend. Relatives can also make or break a treatment plan. For example, an individual can articulate a treatment goal of looking for a job and have support from the treatment team, but if a relative discourages the activity because he or she believes that employment may precipitate a relapse or burden the family, there is a high likelihood the goal will not be met. The treatment team meeting also provides a forum for the family to have their concerns addressed. Individuals often spend 2–3 years in an FEP program, but much of the contact with the family is front-loaded. Relatives' ongoing attendance at team meetings can be extremely useful in continuing the alliance with the family as the individual enters the later phases of treatment.

More Intensive Optional Interventions Tailored to Specific Family Need

Indicators of a need for a more intensive level of family services in an FEP program include 1) lack of progress on the individual's goals, 2) high levels of conflict in the family, and/or 3) relatives initiating frequent contact with the clinic with many concerns about treatment and/or the individual. In considering whether to recommend a more intensive family intervention, the treatment team should also take into account 1) family attendance and motivation during early program participation and 2) whether the indicators of a need for intensive services reflect an illness management problem or another concern (e.g., finances, parental marital strife) that might best be handled through accessing another resource. If the problem seems illness related and the family has been attending sessions, then a recommendation for a course of more intensive intervention can be made.

MULTIFAMILY SUPPORT GROUPS

McFarlane et al. (2015) have developed a comprehensive multifamily group intervention for individuals experiencing a very early psychosis (duration less than 30 days) or those at clinical high risk of developing psychosis. The 2-year program is composed of a multiple-family group intervention, assertive case management, medication, and supported employment or education, and it is directed at individuals between ages 15 and 25 years who enroll with their families. The family intervention involves active engagement ("joining"), an educational workshop, and then twice-monthly multifamily problem-solving and support sessions. This intervention has been evaluated in a six-site quasi-experimental trial with very good results (McFarlane et al. 2015).

In some FEP programs that incorporate individual family education, multifamily support groups are offered as a maintenance treatment once individual family work is completed. Group meetings can reduce stigma, encourage positive role-modeling, and increase families' social networks. However, there are obstacles as well. Some individuals do not want their families involved in their care, some individuals' families refuse to be involved or cannot attend regularly, and some FEP programs are too small to recruit enough family members.

FORMAL COMMUNICATION AND PROBLEM-SOLVING SKILLS TRAINING

Evidence-based family programs used with individuals diagnosed with longer-term schizophrenia and bipolar illness typically include formal problem-solving training, and some also offer communication skills instruction (McFarlane 2016) to help families compensate for illness deficits and manage stress more effectively. However, this kind of skills training requires intensive effort across multiple sessions as well as home practice to promote generalization; it follows the core tenets of behavioral interventions, including demonstrations, practice, modeling, coaching, prompting, and rehearsals (see Mueser and Glynn 1999). Although this intensive training will likely be of value to families with clear deficits in these domains, many families entering FEP programs have an adequate level of communication and problem-solving skills and/or benefit sufficiently from the standard family program that additional skills training is not warranted.

REFERRAL FOR INDIVIDUAL SUPPORTIVE PSYCHOTHERAPY FOR RELATIVES

Although many relatives are able to function well and support the individual's recovery with the help of the FEP program, a small subset have a difficult time regaining their equilibrium after the diagnosis of psychosis. These family members often may be struggling with their own mental health challenges, have multiple other stressors in their lives (e.g., health challenges in themselves or another loved one, financial pressures, isolation, family conflict), or find the idea of mental illness in a loved one objectionable. The family clinician may notice that the relative is very agitated or distressed during sessions or makes rejecting statements to the individual; the situation may be so extreme as to interfere with the session agenda. Confronted with such a circumstance, the family clinician can, as an initial intervention, meet separately with the relative for a session or two and provide him or her the opportunity to discharge some of his or her concerns in a reassuring, supportive environment while not exposing the individual to added stress. However, if the relative continues to interact in such a way that the family clinician deems it may be harmful for the individual to continue or it becomes impossible to provide the FEP content, the family clinician may find it useful to refer the family member for separate counseling to provide a forum to explore his or her feelings and attitudes about the individual's psychiatric illness while not derailing the treatment of the individual with FEP.

A Case Description of First-Episode Psychosis Family Intervention

Tanisha, a 39-year-old African American single mother, was referred to the FEP program by the social worker at the hospital where her 17-year-old son, Denzel, was hospitalized for a psychotic episode. Formerly a B student and very active on the basketball team, Denzel started talking about being "punished" by the voices in his head one night and threatened suicide if the voices did not quiet. Tanisha's aunt had struggled with mental illness, and Tanisha recognized that something was very wrong with Denzel. She called 911, and Denzel was admitted to the local county hospital.

Interventions Offered to All Individuals With FEP and Their Relatives

ACTIVE ENGAGEMENT

Denzel was hospitalized for 5 days, and Tanisha was referred to the local FEP program manager and family therapist, Chris. Chris was warm and attentive when Tanisha called to explain her situation and concerns about Denzel. Chris set up an initial appointment for a morning the following week, a few days after Denzel's planned discharge. On the day of the appointment, Denzel said he was "too tired from the medication" and refused to go to the appointment.

Tanisha was not sure what to expect and felt bad that Denzel had not come to the clinic with her, but she was very worried and went to the appointment anyway. Chris agreed to see her and told her that "this happens a lot—family members often come alone at first." He explained about the program, and Tanisha liked what she heard. She was especially interested in helping Denzel graduate from high school—he had only 4 more months. Chris also told Tanisha that there was a family program to help her help Denzel. She was glad of that because she knew she was stressed about Denzel and she thought her older son, Brandon, was, too—he had been angry and was saying that Denzel was just trying to get attention. Chris told Tanisha that Brandon would be welcome to be part of the family sessions, as would Denzel.

Chris spent some time trying to help Tanisha figure out the next step with Denzel—he offered to come to her house or to set up another appointment at the clinic later in the day when Denzel might be more awake. Tanisha decided to set up a late afternoon appointment at the clinic 2 days later and bring only Denzel initially. Denzel was nervous about going back to school and thought he needed some help to figure out what to do, so he reluctantly agreed to go to the appointment with his mother.

Denzel liked Chris when they met—he thought he paid attention and was encouraging, telling Denzel that he still had a chance at going to college if he wanted to down the road. Denzel and Tanisha were introduced to the other FEP team members: the prescriber, supported employment and education (SEE) specialist, therapist, and peer counselor. Denzel agreed to be evaluated for the FEP program, and Tanisha was glad when he was accepted. Although Denzel was a legal minor, Chris made a point of informing him that he needed to consent to having his mother and brother come to family sessions, and that he did not have to attend these sessions if he did not want to do so. Chris asked Denzel what he thought might be the benefits for himself and his family if they learned more about how to help him get back on track and what might be the problems. Denzel did not like the idea of his family meeting with the staff without him, but he knew his mother really wanted to be part of the family program, so he agreed to attend the family meetings with Tanisha and Brandon.

INDIVIDUAL ASSESSMENT OF RELATIVES

Tanisha then began the family part of the program. She completed an interview with Chris, in which they talked about Denzel, but Chris was also interested in her life and what bothered her. She talked about how hard it was to be a working single mom, how she always felt bad about the fact that Denzel and Brandon's father left when Denzel was a baby, and how she was worried about both of the boys—Denzel because of his illness and Brandon because he seemed so angry about it. Tanisha had seen her aunt struggle with homelessness and being in and out of hospitals, and she got tearful when she thought about the same thing happening to Denzel.

Chris also spent time helping Tanisha identify her strengths and support system; afterward, she thought it had been a very long interview, but she felt more hopeful about Denzel. She also encouraged Brandon to meet with Chris; he did not want to go to the individual assessment but agreed to go to the family education session Tanisha had scheduled the next week.

BRIEF ILLNESS EDUCATION

Denzel, Tanisha, and Brandon attended eight family education sessions. The sessions were supposed to be weekly, but because of Tanisha's work schedule as a nurse, sessions were scheduled closer to every 2 weeks. The family covered the topics listed in Table 18–2. Chris made the sessions very conversational and nonstressful and gave everyone useful information sheets to take home. Tanisha liked three things best about the sessions: 1) Chris encouraged Denzel to describe what the voices he heard were like and how he coped with them. She had been afraid to ask Denzel about the voices, but she was curious and was glad he was talking about them. 2) Brandon attended the sessions and seemed to grow calmer and more supportive of Denzel as he learned more about the illness and how Denzel was struggling. He also shared how frightening it was when Denzel got ill and talked about suicide. 3) Tanisha was afraid that Denzel was going to have to go to the hospital again at some point, but she was reluctant to bring up the topic because she thought Denzel would think she did not have confidence in him. She was very relieved Chris had them do planning about relapse prevention.

BRIEF CONSULTATION

By the time the family finished the education sessions, Denzel had been in the FEP program for 4 months. He had worked closely with the SEE specialist, who had been able to help him finish high school by getting tutoring and credit for some FEP activities. Things were going well until Tanisha noticed that Denzel was staying up later and seemed more agitated and irritable. Denzel denied he was hearing voices or felt stressed, but after graduation, he started getting up later and later and staying up until 4 or 5 in the morning. Sleeping problems were one of the relapse warning signs that Chris had identified in the family sessions, so Tanisha called Chris, who suggested a family consultation to address two issues: 1) Was Denzel having a relapse? 2) What was Denzel going to be doing after graduation? Denzel did not want to attend the sessions, but Tanisha was able to convince him to go to at least one meeting with her; Brandon had to work and was unable to attend.

During the session, Denzel had a hard time following the discussion and seemed agitated, although he denied experiencing an increase in symptoms. Chris reviewed the stress management techniques they had covered in the family education and individual therapy sessions and also checked in with Denzel about whether he had missed any medication. Denzel said he hated the medication and was stopping it. Tanisha got very upset. Chris reminded Tanisha that many young people stop taking their medication when they feel better and asked Denzel to come to his next appointment with the prescriber so he could tell him more about his problems with the medication. Tanisha and Chris also encouraged Denzel to meet with the SEE specialist to make a plan to keep busy over the summer.

Chris scheduled a follow-up consultation meeting a week later; only Tanisha attended. She reported that Denzel was doing about the same; he had decided not to take the medication, even after the appointment with the prescriber, and was sill mostly hanging around the house. Chris reviewed the relapse plan so that Tanisha would know how to get help if the situation deteriorated and encouraged her to make sure she continued to take good care of herself, use her coping skills and social supports, and keep in contact with the team. They set up a time for a phone call the following week.

Over the next year, the family had three more rounds of brief consultation to address the following: 1) managing after a relapse (Denzel had been hospitalized again briefly 6 months into the program), 2) helping Brandon and Denzel get along better together (10 months into the program), and 3) helping Denzel figure out if he was ready to move out to live with his girlfriend (13 months into the program).

ACCESS TO THE TREATMENT TEAM

As can be seen, Tanisha had ample opportunity to interact with Chris, the FEP project director and family clinician. She also sat in on several meetings with the SEE specialist and Denzel to discuss how to handle negotiations with the school regarding Denzel's graduation and future plans. She met Denzel's individual therapist and prescriber during the FEP orientation.

INVITATIONS TO RELATIVES TO JOIN TREATMENT PLANNING MEETINGS

Tanisha was invited to Denzel's treatment team meetings quarterly with all the members of the team. This was helpful to Tanisha when Denzel was rehospitalized about 3 months after he stopped taking his medication, and she appreciated the team's guidance and support. By Denzel's second year in the FEP program, he was doing much better. He had a girlfriend and a part-time job as an assistant basketball coach at a local Boys Club and was considering enrolling in community college. He took his medication most days, although he hated the side effects and said he was "not going to take it forever." The primary contact Tanisha had with the treatment team was at these meetings and during occasional phone calls with Chris.

More Intensive Optional Interventions

Chris referred the family to the monthly relative support group after they finished the brief education component of the program, but Tanisha often had to work evenings and was not able to attend. Chris had limited time with the family and knew that mother and son seemed to communicate well, so he incorporated brief communication skills training in the brief consultations for Denzel and Brandon rather than offering more formal sessions. Chris had considered that Tanisha might benefit from her own therapy when she appeared so distraught at the beginning of the program, but she calmed over time and was able to return to more involvement with her church, which seemd to give her support and comfort. Therefore, Chris did not raise the issue of a referral for individual counseling with her.

KEY CONCEPTS

- Family support can play a key role in recovery from psychosis, especially for younger individuals experiencing a first episode.

- Relatives often experience high levels of distress when their loved one develops a psychosis or relapses.

- There is a robust body of literature to suggest that embedding family support within a comprehensive first episode of psychosis (FEP) program offers optimal outcomes.

- There have been many family programs proposed as part of FEP programs, and there is no way to discern at this point if one yields more benefits than another.

- A stepped-care model of increasing family intervention, tailored to individual and family needs, is recommended in order to provide services efficiently.

Discussion Questions

1. What family services does your agency currently offer to all individuals? Should these services be upgraded?

2. Are agency staff skillful in eliciting consent for family involvement in care? Are they competent in shared decision making? Do they know how to discuss limited consent for release of information?

3. Do staff have sufficient information about psychosis to educate families well? Do they need a primer or access to better materials? Who can help them stay current?

Suggested Readings

Bennett M, Drapalski A, Dixon L, et al: Family Treatment and Resources Manual. New York, OnTrackNY, 2018. Available at: www.ontrack ny.org/Portals/1/Files/Resources/Family%20Treatment%20 and%20Resources%20Manual%204.18%20Final.pdf?ver=2018-05-01-120346-543. Accessed December 11, 2018. OnTrackNY also has some great videos of individuals and families presenting issues in FEP recovery that can be accessed at http://practiceinnova-tions.org/Consumers/family and-community-support.

Glynn SM, Cather C, Gingerich S, et al: NAVIGATE Family Education Program (FEP). Bethesda, MD, National Institute of Mental Health, 2014. Available at: http://navigateconsultants.org/manuals. Accessed December 11, 2018. This is the family education manual used in the RAISE-ETP study.

Greenstein, L: Experiencing a Psychotic Break Doesn't Mean You're Broken. Arlington, VA, National Alliance on Mental Illness, March 12, 2018. Available at www.nami.org/Blogs/NAMI-Blog/March-2018/ Experiencing-a-Psychotic-Break-Doesn-t-Mean-You-re. Accessed December 11, 2018.

National Alliance on Mental Illness: What Is Early and First-Episode Psychosis? Arlington, VA, National Alliance on Mental Illness, 2016. Available at: www.nami.org/NAMI/media/NAMI-Media/Images/ FactSheets/What-is-Early-and-First-Episode-Psychosis.pdf. Accessed January 30, 2019.

National Institute of Mental Health: Fact Sheet: First Episode Psychosis. Bethesda, MD, National Institute of Mental Health, 2015. Available at: www.nimh.nih.gov/health/topics/schizophrenia/raise/fact-sheet-first-episode-psychosis.shtml. Accessed December 11, 2018.

Substance Abuse and Mental Health Services Administration: Understanding a First Episode of Psychosis: Caregiver: Get the Facts. Rockville, MD, Substance Abuse and Mental Health Services Administration, 2018. Available at https://store.samhsa.gov/system/ files/sma16-5005.pdf. Accessed January 30, 2019.

References

Alvarez-Jimenez M, Priede A, Hetrick SE, et al: Risk factors for relapse following treatment for first episode psychosis: a systematic review and meta-analysis of longitudinal studies. Schizophr Res 139(1–3):116–128, 2012 22658527

Bird V, Premkumar P, Kendall T, et al: Early intervention services, cognitive-behavioural therapy and family intervention in early psychosis: systematic review. Br J Psychiatry 197(5):350–356, 2010 21037211

Dealberto MJ: Ethnic origin and increased risk for schizophrenia in immigrants to countries of recent and longstanding immigration. Acta Psychiatr Scand 121(5):325–339, 2010 20105146

Jansen JE, Gleeson J, Cotton S: Towards a better understanding of caregiver distress in early psychosis: a systematic review of the psychological factors involved. Clin Psychol Rev 35:56–66, 2015 25531423

Jones N, Godzikovskaya J, Zhao Z, et al: Intersecting disadvantage: unpacking poor outcomes within early intervention in psychosis services. Early Interv Psychiatry October 27, 2017 [Epub ahead of print] 29076244

Kane JM, Robinson DG, Schooler NR, et al: Comprehensive versus usual community care for first-episode psychosis: 2-year outcomes from the NIMH RAISE early treatment program. Am J Psychiatry 173(4):362–372, 2016 26481174

Lyman DR, Braude L, George P, et al: Consumer and family psychoeducation: assessing the evidence. Psychiatr Serv 65(4):416–428, 2014 24445678

McFarlane WR: Family interventions for schizophrenia and the psychoses: a review. Fam Process 55(3):460–482, 2016 27411376

McFarlane WR, Levin B, Travis L, et al: Clinical and functional outcomes after 2 years in the early detection and intervention for the prevention of psychosis multisite effectiveness trial. Schizophr Bull 41(1):30–43, 2015 25065017

Mueser KT, Glynn SM: Behavioral Family Therapy for Psychiatric Disorders. Oakland, CA, New Harbinger, 1999

Onwumere J, Bebbington P, Kuipers E: Family interventions in early psychosis: specificity and effectiveness. Epidemiol Psychiatr Sci 20(2):113–119, 2011 21714356

Onwumere J, Sirykaite S, Schulz J, et al: Understanding the experience of "burnout" in first-episode psychosis carers. Compr Psychiatry 83:19–24, 2018 29505884

Thara R, Srinivasan TN: Outcome of marriage in schizophrenia. Soc Psychiatry Psychiatr Epidemiol 32(7):416–420, 1997 9383973

White DA, Luther L, Bonfils KA, et al: Essential components of early intervention programs for psychosis: available intervention services in the United States. Schizophr Res 168(1–2):79–83, 2015 26307427

APPENDIX

Clinical Strategies for Optimizing Brief Family Education

Help Participants Recognize the Psychiatric Disorder

The symptoms of most nonpsychiatric disorders (e.g., coughing, angina, fever) are easily recognized as being due to physiological problems that are beyond the client's control. In contrast, psychiatric symptoms (e.g., depression, anxiety, social withdrawal) are less readily viewed as reflecting a "disorder" and are more likely assumed to be under the client's voluntary control. One reason why relatives often believe clients have control over their psychiatric symptoms is that many symptoms are defined by the *absence* of particular behaviors or emotions (e.g., negative symptoms in schizophrenia, avoidance in anxiety disorders) rather than the conspicuous *presence* of other behaviors (e.g., bizarre behavior, responding to internal stimuli). A second reason why some psychiatric symptoms may be thought to be under voluntary control is that almost everyone has experienced at least mild levels of depression or anxiety with which they have successfully coped and that they did not allow to interfere much with day-to-day functioning. These experiences can lead to a false impression that psychiatric patients could recover from their problems if only they tried hard enough. The goal of helping the family recognize and accommodate the individual's psychiatric disorder is achieved chiefly through providing information about the causes of the illness and factors that improve or hinder recovery. At the same time, the individual is encouraged to pursue his or her dreams, take responsibility in areas where this seems possible, and avoid assuming the "sick role" and diminishing expectations for a full life. Thus, improving coping, avoiding substance use, and using skills are all important concepts to convey.

Abstracted from Glynn SM, Cather C, Gingerich S, et al: Navigate Family Education Program (FEP). Unpublished manual, 2014.

Manage Initial Diagnostic Uncertainty

First-episode psychosis (FEP) can presage a number of subsequent psychiatric diagnoses (e.g., schizophrenia, schizoaffective disorder, bipolar illness, delusional disorder, psychotic depression) but it can also remit completely. Because the diagnosis is likely to evolve while the individual is in the FEP program, the family clinician must be comfortable with diagnostic and prognostic uncertainty. Some individuals will go on to develop longer-term disorders with poorer functioning, but many will either remit or be able to function well. Thus, the treatment team needs to model (and have) hope, while being honest about issues on which there is uncertainty. Individuals and families may have been given firmer diagnoses by prior treatment teams; the family clinician will need to be adept at discussing the diagnostic uncertainty inherent in early psychosis.

Present Information in an Honest, Direct Manner

Family clinicians sometimes feel uncomfortable when talking with a individual and his or her relatives about the psychosis. All too often, professionals are keenly aware of their own limits in treating serious mental illness, and they recognize the difficult and long struggle many individuals and relatives will face. Nobody likes to be the bearer of bad news. An understandable response of some professionals is to "protect" these participants from what they perceive to be potentially upsetting information about the client's condition. This occurs particularly in FEP, when there may still be some doubt about the accuracy of the client's diagnosis and the client and relatives may seem overwhelmed and/or fragile.

The common, but often erroneous, assumption is that individuals and relatives will be shocked and dismayed to learn that the client has a specific psychiatric disorder. The opposite is often true. Participants frequently express gratitude to professionals who are direct in educating them about their disorder, even when it is a serious one. A vital principle of illness education is that the family clinician always strives to provide participants directly and honestly with the most accurate facts available about the disorder, while never deliberately withholding information. Through direct communication about the individual's disorder, the family clinician creates a supportive and collaborative working relationship with the whole family that will endure throughout the course of therapy.

Avoid Making Assumptions About Participants' Beliefs

Individuals and relatives come to the experience of a psychosis with a whole life history learning about psychiatric illness through the media, their social networks, and (possibly) personal experiences. The family clinician can have no way of knowing in advance what beliefs participants are bringing to the work. Religious beliefs may color how individuals conceptualize the illness, and even medical and mental health professionals may have ideas that are inconsistent with optimal recovery strategies as supported by research. Thus, the family clinician should not make any assumptions about a shared knowledge and attitude base among participants. Rather, he or she should always ask questions to discern how the participants understand topics prior to presenting educational materials and tailor discussions to accommodate unusual beliefs.

Make Sessions Lively and Interactive

The family clinician cannot rely solely on didactic teaching methods but must strive to make the educational sessions as interactive as possible. Successful educational sessions require that the family clinician continually elicit the individual's and relatives' experiences with the disorder. The family clinician must probe the participants regarding their knowledge about educational topics to be covered, including what they have heard about the disorder (e.g., myths, readings they have done). There are check-ins with participants throughout the sessions regarding the information presented and the pace of the presentation. Clinician stories and experiences can be invaluable in making critical educational points. The family clinician should ask frequent questions to elicit the participants' understanding of the material presented. By adopting an interactive approach to education, the family clinician is able to evaluate the participants' acquisition of basic information about the disorder, identify any misinformation they hold about the disorder, and pace the presentation of new material accordingly. Furthermore, by continually seeking feedback and input, the family clinician avoids the pitfalls of overloading participants with information, resulting in boredom and disengagement.

The information is summarized using visual aids, such as blackboards and handouts. Videos (often from YouTube or trusted resources) can be very helpful but should be screened by the clinician for accuracy. The teaching format resembles a cross between a classroom, with the family clinician assuming the role of the teacher, and a discussion, with the family clinician acting as a facilitator. The conversation is guided by the family clinician so as to cover the curriculum as planned while soliciting the experiences and understanding of participants and their comments and questions throughout the session.

One useful strategy for keeping the sessions lively to elicit the individual's personal experiences when discussing symptoms and making these the focus of conversation. The individual can be connoted as "the expert" and given an opportunity to expand on his or her experiences. Many families may have discussed psychosis in general or may have read it about it on the Internet but have not actually discussed what the individual is living and how it impacts him or her. This conversation can help engender empathy and understanding in relatives.

CHAPTER 19

Suicide Risk, Assessment, and Intervention in Early Psychosis

Jill Harkavy-Friedman, Ph.D.

APPROXIMATELY 15% of people who die by suicide are psychotic at the time of their death. In the United States in 2017, 47,173 people died by suicide (Centers for Disease Control and Prevention 2018), and so it can be estimated that 7,076 people with psychosis died by suicide that year. Many of those who died by suicide may have been in their first psychotic episode because the risk is 1.6–2.0 times higher in the first few years than in later years, although the suicide risk remains increased throughout the lifespan when psychosis is present. The good news is that most people with psychosis do not die by suicide, and early identification (Melle et al. 2006) and treatment can help reduce the risk of suicide attempts (Fedyszyn et al. 2014).

Suicidal Ideation and Behavior

When suicide is being discussed, it is important to be specific about whether suicidal ideation, suicide attempts, or death by suicide is the focus. Suicidal ideation is relatively frequent, particularly among people with psychosis, and has been found to be present among 20%–40% of individuals early in the course of psychotic disorders. Most people with suicidal ideation do not engage in suicidal behavior. Studies have shown that the rate of suicide attempts during the first few years of psychosis is around 10%, with the first attempt often occurring before any treatment contact. Death by suicide in the first 3 years ranges from 1.9% to 3% (Nordentoft et al. 2015). Compared with the general population, in which the age-adjusted rate is 14 per 100,000 (Centers for Disease Control and Prevention 2018), the rate for those with early psychosis is significantly high. One can see that suicidal ideation is a warning sign for suicide; however, suicide risk can be understood only by considering a host of biological, psychological, social, and environmental factors that contribute to risk. It is also important to remember that many people who die by suicide die on their first attempt, so assessing for risk and having conversations about distress and suicidal ideation are important components of clinical care.

Although there has been little research regarding risk factors for suicide among individuals with early psychosis, several factors emerge consistently (Nordentoft et al. 2015). These factors include previous suicide attempt, prior or comorbid major depression, alcohol and other substance use, and poor premorbid problem solving. Longer duration of untreated psychosis and more severe psychotic symptoms have also been associated with suicide attempts. A study by Melle et al. (2006) demonstrated that a public information campaign about early signs of psychosis decreased the time between first symptoms and first mental health contact and resulted in fewer people experiencing suicidal ideation as assessed at clinical intake.

Long-term factors that have been found to be associated with suicide risk across mental health conditions include early abuse, neglect or trauma, family history of mental health conditions or suicide, chronic physical health conditions or pain, head trauma, and genetics associated with sensitivity to stress and resilience. Shorter-term environmental and social factors that can precipitate suicidal behavior include prolonged stress such as that caused by ongoing harassment, bullying, or relationship problems; stressful life events such as divorce or financial problems; exposure to suicide; and access to lethal means (Figure 19–1). Many contributors must be present before any individual is at risk for suicide, and there is no single cause. Like people without psychosis, individuals with psychosis report that suicide attempts may be precipitated by loss of a love relationship or another significant social stressor. Among people with psychosis, it is often reported that being bothered by psychotic symptoms and depression each served as a precipitant.

Case Example 1: "Not Right in My Head"

Sue was 15 years old when she made her first of four suicide attempts. The year prior to her first attempt, she had dropped out of high school because of poor grades and difficulty functioning. For a year, she would not come out of her room in her mother's house and suffered from severe self-neglect, unable to engage in activities of daily living. She had

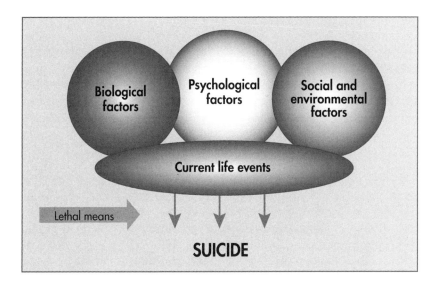

FIGURE 19–1. A conceptual model for understanding suicide: interaction of risk and protective factors.

Source. American Foundation for Suicide Prevention.

referential delusions, engaged in limited communication, and had avolition and affective blunting. Prior to her psychosis, she experienced two major depressive episodes lasting 2–3 months each. In the past, she had been physically abused by her mother, who had an alcohol use disorder. Her father had two brief psychotic episodes during cannabis use. Sue made her first attempt because "My mind was not working right and I was not right in my head—probably because I didn't get enough sleep." After an overdose, she was admitted to a medical unit at a local hospital, where she stayed for a few days before being transferred to a psychiatric inpatient unit.

The case of Sue demonstrates the multiple factors that contribute to suicidal behavior. She had experienced previous depressions, was likely psychotic when hiding in her room for a year, functioned poorly premorbidly, had a history of being abused, and had a family history of mental illness and substance use. Early intervention could have been helpful in preventing her suicidal behavior.

Warning Signs for Suicidal Behavior

Suicidal ideation is not static; it often comes and goes, such that a person is not always acutely suicidal or even thinking about suicide. Although this makes it difficult to detect more immediate risk, it does mean that in-

terventions can be implemented to help individuals learn to manage suicidal ideation and prevent suicidal behavior. The key is to identify
warning signs, which may be long-standing or may be brief or fleeting
(Figure 19–2). Warning signs do not always include suicidal ideation,
however. Sometimes in the months and weeks before an attempt, individuals may speak about killing themselves and express feelings of
hopelessness, entrapment, and being a burden to others. They may talk
about having no reason to live or note that family and friends will not
miss them after they are gone. These individuals may often feel depressed or anxious, or they may appear to lack interest. They may be easily agitated or irritable, or recently may have experienced something that
led him to feel humiliated. Behaviorally, they may increase use of alcohol
or drugs, withdraw from activities, and isolate themselves from family
and friends. They may sleep too much or too little or have insomnia.
Sometimes, people visit or call friends and family to "say good-bye" or
give away possessions. Not all warning signs will be present, but some
will, and it is easy to write them off as unimportant, as part of a phase or
as a form of attention seeking. It is important to keep in mind that suicidal individuals, at least in their suicidal crisis, lose access to their usual
problem-solving and coping abilities. They experience cognitive inflexi-
bility and believe that nothing will end their pain (American Foundation
for Suicide Prevention 2019). If they are able to get through the crisis, it
is possible that they may never engage in suicidal behavior.

For people with psychosis, command auditory hallucinations may
or may not result in suicidal behavior. Some people resist acting on
voices telling them to kill themselves, whereas others respond to their
voice(s) and engage in suicidal behavior. There are no data providing
information about who will or will not act in response to command auditory hallucinations. In fact, a person may not engage in suicidal behavior related to command auditory hallucinations at one point in his
or her illness but may respond at another time. Therefore, command auditory hallucinations always need to be taken seriously, and a person
experiencing such voices can develop tools for coping and managing
rather than reacting in response.

Case Example 2: Thought to Action

Ted was 28 years old and had a history of alcohol use disorder that was
in remission when his psychotic symptoms began. He did not receive
treatment even though he had been experiencing delusions and hallucinations for a couple of years and his functioning was declining. He
heard voices berating him and had paranoid and referential delusions
that people were talking about him and accusing him of malevolent behavior. He had periods of depressed mood, but his symptoms never met
the criteria for major depression. One day, in a matter of minutes, Ted
quickly picked up a razor and made cuts on his arm, saying that he
thought someone in Spain wanted to kill him. He had considerable

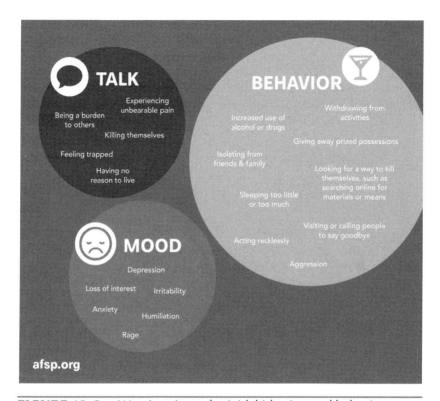

FIGURE 19–2. Warning signs of suicidal ideation and behavior.
Source. American Foundation for Suicide Prevention.

bleeding and was brought by a family member to the local emergency department, where he received wound care and antibiotics but no stitches. He was admitted to the inpatient psychiatric unit.

In Ted's case, there were many notable risk factors for suicide, and he was hearing berating voices that made him uncomfortable and also had frightening paranoid delusions. He was experiencing significant distress because he had never received treatment. Members of his support system were not aware of the process that was unfolding, and his suicide risk was not detected. This highlights the need for public education about psychosis and suicide.

Assessment of Suicide Risk

The goal of a suicide risk assessment is to gather information to gain knowledge about the individual's potential suicide contributors and protective factors. The assessment provides the foundation for ongoing assessment and understanding of the person's suicide risk over time. A suicide risk assessment includes obtaining a full description of past and present suicidal ideation and behavior as well as an evaluation of the previously noted risk factors, including mental health conditions, health history, premorbid adjustment, family history of mental health conditions and suicidal behaviors, history of trauma or abuse, impulsiveness and aggressive behavior, current levels of pain, and general sense of health and well-being. Substance use, including its impact on mood and behavior, is often a factor in suicidal behavior. It is important to note any changes in patterns and consequences of use and other potentially risky behavior. It is also important to gain a sense of the person's usual level of optimism and pessimism and his or her hopes and aspirations for the future.

All of this information is relevant for foreseeing both longer-term and short-term risk. Such an evaluation serves as a barometer for ongoing assessment of risk and provides a context for risk considerations throughout treatment. Even with the best assessment, however, suicidal behavior may be sustained over months and years, or the time between thought and action can be minutes to hours, and intervention is not always possible. This highlights the need for ongoing assessment and inclusion of how to address suicide risk as part of an intervention plan.

Clinicians should ask directly about suicidal ideation and behavior. This will not make the person suicidal, and it may bring relief. When assessing an individual for past and current suicidal ideation and behavior, it is important to ask about ideation and behavior separately. With regard to ideation, it is critical to ask the individual to describe his or her thoughts and their frequency and persistence, as well as planfulness and intent to die. Suicide is often an ambivalent act, so any intent is of concern. The clinician should gather a thorough history of the method used or being considered, what occurred or might occur as a result of applying the method, and any medical damage and intervention from previous attempts. In addition, the clinician should explore the individual's understanding of lethality. People are not necessarily knowledgeable about lethality, so the individual's perception of lethality provides insight into his or her thinking.

It is important to understand the circumstances, including thoughts and feelings, that surrounded previous attempts because such understanding is a window into future risk and intervention. A clinician cannot make assumptions about what the person is thinking and feeling. If risk factors and warning signs emerge, it is important ask about them. However, just because a person does not have a past attempt or past suicidal behavior does not mean that he or she is not at risk; 60% of suicide deaths occur on the first attempt (Bostwick et al. 2016). Ongoing consideration of risk factors over the course of treatment can save a life.

Assessment of acute risk also involves identifying current psychiatric and medical conditions and the effectiveness and side effects associated with current treatment. Because life stress can serve as a precipitant of suicidal behavior, the clinician should become knowledgeable about any stressors or changes that may be current or pending in the near future. If the individual is taking medications, a review of medications, including effectiveness, adherence, and side effects, is essential. The person's report, as well as information from previous clinicians and the availability of social support for adherence, should be considered.

Case Example 3: "You Don't Look Psychotic"

Ramon was entering college when he began hearing voices, and months later he experienced his first episode of major depression. He had never experienced any suicidal ideation and had no history of suicide attempt. He was hospitalized to treat his psychotic symptoms and depression. Once stabilized, he was discharged to outpatient treatment, continuing to take risperidone and venlafaxine. He looked good physically and was functioning well. He returned to school and felt well for the next 8 months. The clinician felt that given Ramon's return to full functioning, he probably had never been psychotic and suffered only from depression. Shortly thereafter, Ramon began hearing voices again, and his thoughts became more paranoid. Distressed at the return of his symptoms, he killed himself.

This case highlights the importance of keeping in mind individuals' self-reported symptom history, their medical records, their feelings about their psychotic illness, their adherence to and benefit from medication, and their sense of well-being, especially when a medication change is being considered. It also serves as a reminder that effective treatment is possible and that people with psychosis can have full and enriching lives. With appropriate medication, Ramon was able to return to his premorbid level of functioning. His family was aware of the resurgence of his psychotic symptoms during the medication change and believed that the treating clinician was monitoring him closely.

Brief Interventions to Prevent Suicidal Behavior

The months and weeks before and after the first treatment contact are critical when working with someone in the early phase of psychosis (Ayesa-Arriola et al. 2015). The individual is facing a major life change. Supports may be weakened because of recent isolation or behavior. The individual is likely to be having difficulty processing current information and may generally be quite uncomfortable. New medications may be on the horizon, and they may take time to become effective and may induce unwanted side effects. Most often, the clinician has never seen the person at his or her best and most functional level, and it may be difficult to imagine that the individual has ever been different from his or her current clinical presentation. For these reasons, it is useful to include family and other social supports in the process of early intervention.

The first and most immediate interventions depend on the level of suicide risk, stability of thought and behavior, and available resources. Concern about immediate risk, based on the person's presentation, may warrant constant observation and extended stay in an emergency department, crisis center, or inpatient hospital. Just because someone is thinking about suicide does not mean that he or she is at imminent risk and needs to be hospitalized. Partial hospitalization, rapid referral, brief intervention in the emergency department, and/or safety planning with follow-up may be effective interventions.

Regardless of the clinical intervention, from the outset, it is essential to limit access to lethal means and provide lethal means counseling to available supports about how to safely store or remove potential means. Suicide can occur only when there is access to lethal means, and removal of access is one of the most effective interventions in the suicidal crisis. Suicidal individuals who are in crisis are lacking cognitive flexibility, and their rigid and limited thinking makes it difficult for them to generate alternative methods if their primary plan is thwarted. By limiting access to lethal means, there is time for the situation and person to de-escalate and increases the likelihood of intervention.

Developing a crisis or safety plan has been found to be effective for suicidal individuals with psychosis (Fedyszyn et al. 2014; Nordentoft et al. 2002). The value of such plans is that they provide a set of tools for the individual to use when heading toward a suicidal crisis. These plans include specifying distracting activities that can be engaged in alone or with others and identifying family and friends or community members who can be contacted when the person is experiencing distress. The individual should also be provided with names of professionals who can be reached out to during emergencies and numbers for crisis hotlines, textlines, or other services that are available 24/7. Personal warning signs and reasons for living are also identified, as are steps to be taken to eliminate access to lethal means. Throughout treatment, the plan can be updated and revised. The safety plan needs to be developed collaboratively on the basis of what the person can and will do. It should be written down, and it needs to be feasible and accessible. It is also helpful to include family members or other close contacts in the development of the plan. Smartphone apps for safety planning, such as SafetyNet and MY3, are available so that the plan can be easily accessible and revised as needed.

During the crisis, evaluation of physical health is often not undertaken, yet we know that delirium or other mental status changes can be accompanied by psychosis, agitation, and/or mood alterations, sometimes initially in the absence of altered sensorium. Further, some psychotic and mood disorders can be precipitated by brain trauma, infection, or metabolite imbalance. The individual should undergo a medical workup, including neuroimaging to rule out brain injury, stroke, or tumor, and the clinician should consider a range of possible factors, including infection; hypoxia; hyperthyroidism or hypothyroidism; substance intoxication or withdrawal; heavy metal poisoning; vitamin B_{12}, thiamine, or folate deficiencies; seizures; encephalopathy; and renal, hepatic, or cardiac failure. Much suffering can be avoided by identifying physical health conditions that can lead to disruption of mental status and brain functioning, both abruptly and gradually. At the outset of treatment, it is essential to have a thorough workup that includes blood tests, possible neuroimaging, lumbar puncture, and/or electroencephalography, and in some circumstances consideration of metabolomics and genetic anomalies can prove fruitful.

Case Example 4: "Where's My Cortisol?"

Meredith is a 20-year-old college student who was doing well in school her first semester. In the middle of her second semester, she became extremely depressed and unable to leave her room. She became paranoid about her peers and was grandiose about her importance and abilities. She stopped going to class and avoided other people. As she began failing classes, she became more distressed. One day Meredith decided it was time to end it all, and she made a very serious suicide attempt, causing multiple knife wounds. She was hospitalized psychiatrically and sent home with a medical leave of absence. Her anxiety often made it impossible for her to leave her house, and her family did not understand and viewed her as lazy. She began psychotherapy, and the therapist requested that she have a complete physical. Ultimately, after Meredith spent months in this condition, a cousin agreed to accompany her to a primary care physician. A simple blood test revealed that she had literally no cortisol, and her physician conducted follow-up tests, determining that the cause was Addison's disease. Cortisol replacement therapy was started. Meredith's mood immediately improved and her anxiety decreased, although it remained to some degree. She spoke about her suicide attempt, saying, "That wasn't me, and I see that now that I feel back to myself." In retrospect, Meredith realized that her decline was more gradual and occurred over an extended time. Given how terrible she felt before being diagnosed, she is motivated to manage her Addison's disease to avoid the mental health and physical symptoms.

Meredith's case emphasizes the importance of treating the whole person, mind and body. Without the physical evaluation, she would have suffered much longer and might have died by suicide.

Clinical Treatment to Reduce Suicide Risk

Evaluation for medication or adherence to an already prescribed medication regimen is a vital component for early intervention. Researchers have demonstrated that as psychotic symptoms improve, risk is decreased, although risk remains because of the multidetermined nature of suicide (Riesselman et al. 2015). Clozapine and lithium have been found to decrease suicide risk. Treatment with the goal of eliminating psychotic and affective symptoms while minimizing side effects is a process that takes time. Collaboration between the clinician, the person experiencing psychotic symptoms, and his or her family is critical. Psychotic symptoms can be very distressing, so careful attention to maximizing benefits obtained from medication through ongoing discussions about symptoms is critical. Recall how the lack of communication and close monitoring of Ramon contributed to his death by suicide.

Medication alone, however, is not enough, and the combination of medication and psychotherapy has been found to be more effective than medication alone. Psychotherapies such as cognitive-behavioral therapy (CBT) or interpersonal therapy can be helpful to the person with respect to managing his or her thoughts and feelings and improving social connections. When it comes to reducing suicide risk, developing tools the individual can use to manage his or her suicidal behavior directly have been shown to be effective (Kasckow et al. 2011). Therapies such as CBT–suicide prevention (CBT-SP), dialectical behavior therapy, attachment-based family therapy, and collaborative assessment and management of suicidality have all been found to reduce suicidal behavior, although not all have been evaluated specifically for people with early psychosis. Each of these therapies provides a theoretical framework for understanding how to approach the management of suicidal ideation so that the suicidal thought does not translate into action. In general, these approaches aim to identify proximal risk factors and stressors, consider negative thoughts and feelings, improve emotion regulation and behavioral control, and develop effective problem-solving skills.

Enlisting the support of family and friends is an essential component of living with mental health conditions and suicide risk. Obtaining consent in the first session to be able to contact at least one person in the individual's life is important. It can be explained that this contact is for emergencies if the person is a danger to self or others and to locate the individual if he or she is not responding. In addition, the clinician can suggest that this emergency contact and other friends and family members can be helpful in treatment because they can observe changes in thought and behavior that could be essential for assessing risk. Many suicide loss survivors report that they were excluded from therapy, and we have learned that their input is critical and potentially life-saving. In addition to addressing suicide risk, engaging supports in treatment with people with early psychosis has been found to be beneficial for treatment implementation and effectiveness (Nordentoft et al. 2002).

Conclusion

Suicide risk in early psychosis is a concern. Suicide is complex, with many health, historical, social, and environmental factors converging in the context of life stress and accessibility of lethal means. Early identification of psychosis can reduce suicide risk. A comprehensive evaluation of suicidal ideation and behavior and contributors to suicide risk is the first component of an effective treatment plan. Interventions that reduce psychotic and mood symptoms are essential but not sufficient for managing suicide risk, and suicidal ideation and suicidal behavior must be addressed directly. Enlisting supports and developing a well-rounded treatment plan can provide the opportunity for people with early psychosis to develop a life worth living.

KEY CONCEPTS

- Suicide is complex, and there is no single cause but rather a confluence of risk factors, including life stress and access to lethal means.

- A full assessment of suicidal ideation and behavior and potential contributors and protective factors at the beginning of treatment, and continued assessment and monitoring throughout treatment, are critical.

- In addition to reducing symptoms and improving functioning, tools to manage suicidal ideation and behavior reduce the transition from suicidal thought to suicidal behavior.

- Inclusion of supports and continuity of care are key factors for suicide reduction.

Discussion Questions

1. Do you spend time with your clients discussing current and past suicidal ideation and factors that contribute to suicide

risk and prevention? How can you facilitate such conversations so that clients do not act on these thoughts?

2. Have you developed a suicide prevention plan for your clinical practice?

3. Would you think that your thoughts and feelings about suicide and suicidal clients might contribute to their comfort discussing suicidal ideas and concerns about their life?

4. How would you ask a client if he or she has lethal means at home, and how would you ask him or her to remove them from the home or limit access?

Suggested Readings

American Foundation for Suicide Prevention: www.afsp.org
Galynker I: The Suicidal Crisis. New York, Oxford University Press, 2017
Jamison KR: An Unquiet Mind: A Memoir of Moods and Madness. New York, Knopf, 1995
Nordentoft M, Madsen T, Fedyszyn I: Suicidal behavior and mortality in first-episode psychosis. J Nerv Ment Dis 203(5):387–392, 2015 25919385

References

American Foundation for Suicide Prevention: Suicide statistics. 2019. Available at: https://afsp.org/about-suicide/suicide-statistics. Accessed January 30, 2019.
Ayesa-Arriola R, Garcia Alcaraz E, Hernández BV, et al: Suicidal behaviour in first-episode non-affective psychosis: specific risk periods and stage-related factors. Eur Neuropsychopharmacol 25(12):2278–2288, 2015 26475577
Bostwick JM, Pabbati C, Geske JR, McKean AJ: Suicide attempt as a risk factor for completed suicide: even more lethal than we knew. Am J Psychiatry 173(11):1094–1100, 2016 27523496
Centers for Disease Control and Prevention: Fatal Injury Reports, National, Regioal and State, 1981fl2017. Atlanta, GA, Centers for Disease Control and Prevention, 2018. Available at https://webappa.cdc.gov/sasweb/ncipc/mortrate.html. Accessed January 30, 2019.
Fedyszyn IE, Robinson J, Harris MG, et al: Suicidal behaviours during treatment for first-episode psychosis: towards a comprehensive approach to service-based prevention. Early Interv Psychiatry 8(4):387–395, 2014 23964750
Kasckow J, Felmet K, Zisook S: Managing suicide risk in patients with schizophrenia. CNS Drugs 25(2):129–143, 2011 21254789

Melle I, Johannesen JO, Friis S, et al: Early detection of the first episode of schizophrenia and suicidal behavior. Am J Psychiatry 163(5):800–804, 2006 16648319

Nordentoft M, Jeppesen P, Abel M, et al: OPUS study: suicidal behaviour, suicidal ideation and hopelessness among patients with first-episode psychosis: one-year follow-up of a randomised controlled trial. Br J Psychiatry 181(suppl 43):s98–s106, 2002 12271808

Nordentoft M, Madsen T, Fedyszyn I: Suicidal behavior and mortality in first-episode psychosis. J Nerv Ment Dis 203(5):387–392, 2015 25919385

Riesselman A, Johnson E, Palmer E: Lithium and clozapine in suicidality: shedding some light to get out of the dark. Mental Health Clinician 5(5):237–243, 2015

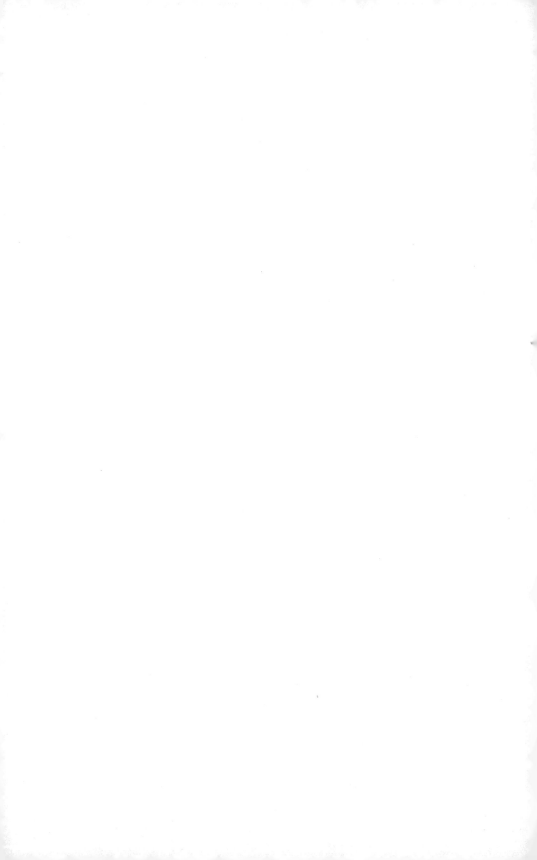

CHAPTER 20

Using Technology to Advance Early Psychosis Intervention

Benjamin Buck, Ph.D.
Dror Ben-Zeev, Ph.D.

YOUNG people experiencing first-episode psychosis (FEP) are members of a so-called *digital native* generation and express strong interest in the delivery of mental health services via the Internet, social media, and mobile devices (Lal et al. 2015). Interventions and service-delivery strategies that leverage technology may also be particularly well suited to addressing already identified service gaps in FEP care. As noted by Lal and colleagues (2015), technology-enhanced interventions have the potential to be convenient, accessible, and consistent. They also allow individuals with FEP to remain anonymous and thus circumvent barriers posed by stigma. Finally, the reduced burden on individuals, their families, and clinics to meet staffing needs is reduced when people can reach evidence-based services without having to go to a brick-and-mortar clinic.

When an individual with FEP initiates contact with a provider, there are myriad moments in which the use of innovative technologies could enhance the quality of detection, intervention, and maintenance of gains from treatment. First, early-phase psychosis intervention requires assessment to appropriately identify individuals who might be at risk for future chronic mental illness; existing tools are limited in their ability to accurately predict who will convert to chronic and persistent psychotic illness.

Second, interventions best suited for FEP (i.e., coordinated specialty care; Kane et al. 2016) are still widely underused, even after individuals experience a first episode. Approximately half of individuals who experience FEP do not receive either psychosocial or pharmaceutical treatment in the first year, and following that episode, 12-month mortality is 24 times higher than in an age-matched comparison sample (Schoenbaum et al. 2017). Technology-enhanced interventions may provide lower-cost standardized options for delivery of care that are flexible, consistently available, and convenient.

Third, a persisting challenge in FEP intervention pertains to maintenance of treatment gains. Although FEP programs have demonstrated short-term efficacy, some chart review studies demonstrate reduced sustained impact over time (Gafoor et al. 2010). Online or mobile approaches provide ample options for stepped-down services that might maintain gains generated by intensive first-episode interventions in a less restrictive setting.

A growing body of evidence suggests that individuals with severe mental illnesses seek support online—from support groups, chat rooms, message boards, and online gaming communities (Highton-Williamson et al. 2015). Previous research has demonstrated that this is a common practice in efforts to connect with others with similar experiences and to receive support for progress toward one's recovery goals (Naslund et al. 2014). It remains to be seen whether these novel technologies can effectively address the needs of individuals in the midst of a first episode. Their ubiquity, however, underscores the need for researchers and providers to develop their understanding of these resources and how they can be adapted to address service gaps. In this chapter we provide several prototypes of innovations in the application of technology to first-episode intervention that show potential to improve care in three areas: (1) detection (i.e., assessment of risk and selection of treatment course), (2) intervention (i.e., delivery of treatments themselves), and (3) maintenance of treatment gains (i.e., stepped-down services). Finally, we use a brief clinical vignette to highlight opportunities for technology to address limitations and gaps in care in the treatment of individuals with FEP.

Detection: Clinical Decision Support and Risk Prediction

Early intervention can reduce the long-term impact of a psychotic episode; its effectiveness, however, is dependent on valid early detection. An array of instruments have been used to identify individuals at risk for conversion to an episode of psychosis (Rotondi et al. 2005), including the Structured Interview for Psychosis-Risk Syndromes (SIPS; Miller et al. 2003) and the Comprehensive Assessment of At-Risk Mental States (CAARMS; Yung et al. 2005), as well as traditional symptom severity interviews such as the Brief Psychiatric Rating Scale (BPRS; Overall and Gorham 1988) and the Positive and Negative Syndrome Scale (PANSS; Kay et al. 1987). These instruments typically contain some combined examination of family history of psychotic disorder and the severity of positive, negative, and general psychopathology symptoms. Meta-analytic estimates (Fusar-Poli et al. 2012) suggest that once young people are identified with one of these instruments as being at high risk, they have an 18% risk of transition after 6 months, 22% after 1 year, 29% after 2 years, and 36% after 3 years.

Determining risk involves a complex Bayesian calculation that combines multiple factors concurrently. Technologies that automate this process could facilitate such calculations, thus making them more common in regular practice. Cannon and colleagues (2016) piloted the use of a *psychosis risk calculator* built on clinical, cognitive, and demographic characteristics, including select SIPS items, cognitive skill in symbol coding, a brief general cognitive assessment, a recent decline in functioning, the experience of trauma, male gender, and a history of psychosis. This calculator was later validated by a second research group (Carrión et al. 2016), providing strong predictions of conversion that improved on existing instruments (area under the curve 0.790: 95% confidence interval 0.644–0.937). Predictions are represented in two plots that symbolize the 1- and 2-year risk of conversion to psychosis based on a sample of 596 clinical high-risk participants from the North American Prodrome Longitudinal Study (Figure 20–1).

Cannon and colleagues' risk calculator is comparable to extant risk calculators for other chronic medical conditions, including heart disease and cancer. However, given the paucity of published studies demonstrating effective use of the risk calculator in treatment settings, the impact on long-term outcomes of having access to such a calculator is unknown. It is also unclear whether such tools are best suited for primary care or general mental health clinics rather than those dedicated to specialized care for FEP. Regardless, providers who use calculators that easily and concisely summarize risk estimates may be empowered to better identify and triage individuals with greater needs, share these estimates with clients and their families to engage them in care, and use such estimates to inform treatment selection.

One limitation of automated risk calculation is its dependence on factors that are already identified or assessed by clinicians. Other technologies go a step further by attempting to identify risk factors that are undetectable to typical clinical interviews. One prototype of such a tool is in the automated analysis of free speech. Bedi and colleagues (2015) assessed 34 clinical high-risk individuals on a quarterly basis after com-

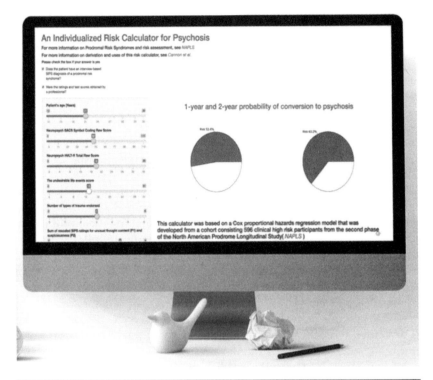

FIGURE 20–1.   Screenshot of the North American Prodrome Longitudinal Study individualized risk calculator.

Source.   Cannon et al. 2016; http://riskcalc.org/napls. The photos of computing devices were downloaded from the PEXELS database (www.pexels.com). Used with permission of the developers.

pleting open-ended, 1-hour qualitative interviews at a baseline visit. Of this initial sample of 34 participants, 5 individuals converted to schizophrenia. The speech patterns of these 5 were compared with the nonconverters according to their internal coherence using latent semantic analysis (LSA). LSA estimates the coherence of a speech sample by assessing the extent to which each utterance relates to the content of speech that preceded that utterance. The strongest predictors that distinguished converters from nonconverters was the minimum coherence (or maximum discontinuity) during the interview, as well as use of *determiners* (e.g., that, what, whatever) and maximum phrase length. With these characteristics, a machine-trained algorithm was able to use baseline speech data to successfully predict conversion with 100% accuracy relative to SIPS predictions at the same points, which were significantly less accurate.

This methodology was later validated with multiple forms of speech elicitation in a second sample of 59 individuals at clinical high risk (Corcoran et al. 2018). This study demonstrated consistent accuracy (72%) in the ability of the LSA algorithm to distinguish the speech of individuals with recent-onset psychosis from that of nonclinical controls. Although all of these technologies are in their infancy, they show remarkable promise in improving quality and dissemination of tools aiming to predict an individual's future conversion to psychosis. Between computerized risk calculators and automated analysis of speech, a 2- to 3-hour assessment could considerably improve the quality of such predictions, whether specifically in FEP clinics or in settings where staff are likely to encounter individuals at potential risk (i.e., schools, community mental health centers, or primary care clinics).

Mobile Interventions: A Therapist in Your Pocket

Although assessment and risk calculators provide useful tools for identifying individuals broadly at risk (or in need of treatment), there is additional utility for individuals in identifying their high-risk *moments*. There is increasing evidence that psychotic symptoms are not static but, rather, that episodes emerge when an individual is faced with environmental stressors. Individuals in the midst of a first episode demonstrate increased sensitivity to stressful events, ascribe aberrant salience to otherwise neutral stimuli (Reininghaus et al. 2016a), and tend to anticipate threat at greater levels than do control subjects (Reininghaus et al. 2016b).

These findings have bolstered extant theories of psychosis, such as the cognitive model of positive symptoms (Garety et al. 2001), which argues that psychotic symptoms emerge from aberrant cognitive processes in response to stress (i.e., the stress-vulnerability model) (Zubin and Spring 1977). Advances in mobile health (mHealth) technologies allow assessment at these critical moments and opportunities to disrupt the means through which symptoms impact functioning. Ecological momentary assessment (EMA) involves a device (usually a smartphone) that prompts an individual to complete brief assessments in day-to-day life. Sudden changes in presentation or symptom exacerbation might identify a relapse; when these changes occur, brief interventions could help prevent psychosis.

The FOCUS smartphone intervention system (Figure 20–2) prompts users to complete brief (i.e., two-item) assessments of changes in a number of domains, including sleep quality, auditory hallucinations, mood, and social engagement (Ben-Zeev et al. 2013). FOCUS was developed by researchers, clinicians, and individuals with schizophrenia and is designed to assess current symptoms and deliver brief interventions that are well suited to address those changes. In pilot studies of persons with chronic schizophrenia (Ben-Zeev et al. 2014), individuals were prompted five times per day (in addition to having ongoing access to the app as desired). On the basis of responses to brief assessments of changes in the clinical areas of interest, the app provides brief interventions with illustrative images (in text, audio, or video) derived from various evidence-based approaches in the treatment of psychosis: cognitive restructuring, behavioral activation, illness management and recovery, social skills training, and sleep hygiene. Pilot research has demonstrated FOCUS to be acceptable to patients, and over a study period of 1 month, a sample of 33 individuals with schizophrenia or schizoaffective disorder experienced significant reductions in positive symptoms of psychosis, general psychopathology, and depression, mood, and anxiety symptoms that were significantly correlated with the number of contacts recorded by the FOCUS system (Ben-Zeev et al. 2014).

Beyond delivering illness management tools in real time, mHealth systems can also be used to facilitate ongoing assessment and coordination with the clinic. Providers can view securely delivered FOCUS data shortly after they are collected and, in response, contact individuals directly to conduct additional assessment or provide support. These assessments can also be used in in-person sessions to generate insight or facilitate changes in treatment plan. A provider and client can reflect together on changes throughout the week; examine relationships between cognitive, emotional, and behavioral factors; and build a coping strategy accordingly.

Measurement-based care (MBC), which incorporates frequent assessment into the course of individual psychiatric treatment to facilitate clinical decision making, is demonstrated to consistently improve outcomes across a range of conditions (Fortney et al. 2017), but few studies have examined the impact of implementation of MBC in FEP treatment settings. Case studies have been reported that outline the roles of mHealth support specialists as providers who check, interpret, and follow up on EMA data. With improved access to day-to-day functioning, the mHealth support specialist is empowered to provide personalized interventions (e.g., sleep hygiene support, cognitive restructuring) by phone or video conferencing, depending on need in a time-sensitive manner (Jonathan et al. 2017).

Niendam and colleagues (2018) provided an example of mobile MBC in their description of Ginger.io, an app that prompts individuals to respond to daily and weekly surveys of medication adherence, mood, and social activities and weekly surveys of symptoms. The results of these surveys are provided to clinicians via a simple dashboard. Additionally, clinicians are provided with alerts and warnings if patients report significant changes via the app. Clinicians are then in-

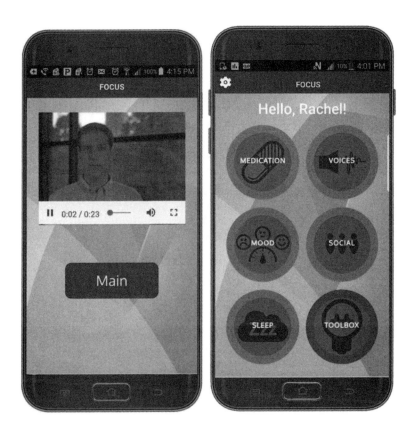

FIGURE 20–2.   Example screenshots of FOCUS (Ben-Zeev et al. 2013) video (left) and text-only interventions (right).
Source.   iStockPhoto. Posed by model.

structed to review survey responses with clients during their regularly scheduled sessions. Participant retention in the Ginger.io study was high (66% of enrolled individuals remained for at least 6 months), and people consistently completed the weekly (77%) and daily (69%) surveys. Almost half (40%) of individuals reported that the app helped them remember to take medication. The daily and weekly assessments of mood and positive symptoms were highly correlated to clinician-rated symptoms, suggesting that these tools provide valid estimates of symptom levels.

A similar system, LifeData, conducts daily and weekly surveys related to similar key recovery outcomes and shares them with providers (Kumar et al. 2018). More than half (56%) of all eligible clients across four community outpatient early psychosis clinics enrolled, and, of this sample, a majority reported that sharing daily and weekly surveys with their treatment team improved the quality of their treatment services, their relationship to the treatment team, and their motivation to maintain medication and symptom management routines.

Although EMA might improve assessment by providing access to clients in the moment and in their daily lives, other limitations remain. EMA is still susceptible to social desirability or minimization and can be perceived as burdensome or disruptive to clients. To address these limitations, systems have been developed to collect data to generate estimates of risk using existing sensors in smartphones. Passive sensing using existing mobile phone sensors—including cameras, microphones, accelerometers, and GPS—has been piloted in general undergraduate samples to predict relevant psychological domains. In these pilot studies, sensor-generated estimates of physical activity, sleep duration, and geospatial locations were associated with daily stress (Ben-Zeev et al. 2015). More recently, these methods have been piloted in samples of individuals with schizophrenia. Although full study results are forthcoming, five individuals' data streams over the course of 1 year have been published to demonstrate the wide range of *relapse signatures* that precede a psychiatric hospitalization in both sensing and EMA data. For example, individuals from this sample produced data suggesting different indicators, including a significant physical activity drop-off, sleep disruptions, atypical device activities, and exacerbation of symptoms recorded via EMA (Ben-Zeev et al. 2017).

Combined with a clinician review mechanism (i.e., a dashboard), if signs of relapse can be identified and relayed to treatment teams, interventions can be provided much more efficiently and effectively to prevent significant functional disruption. Although these are exciting developments, empirical work examining these technologies is scant, and future study and validation will define the specific uses of these tools. Nonetheless, at present, a number of potentially useful technologies have demonstrated feasibility and acceptability in the population with severe mental illness.

Online Interventions and Telehealth: A Clinic on Your Desktop

Mental health systems that leverage mobile devices often provide so-called "just-in-time" interventions, or brief strategies that are designed to provide support in the moment as a supplement to usual care. Additional advancements using technology go beyond such brief services to provide prolonged access to services, including evidence-based therapy modules, online social communities, and contact with clinical providers. The delivery of integrated services online circumvents a number of ongoing barriers in the treatment of FEP. These systems are proposed to require fewer individual providers per client and therefore could be more affordable to clinics. They are also designed to increase availability because they can be accessed at any time and do not require the individual to leave home. This ease of access and anonymity could reduce barriers instituted by the perceived stigma of regularly attending a psychiatric clinic in person. Further, if online interventions are able to engage clients who have completed a course of treatment in a first-episode clinic, they could reduce the drop-off in treatment benefits that tends to occur after individuals terminate these services (Gafoor et al. 2010). Online intervention services could be a proper strategy for delivering anonymous "booster" sessions after the completion of more intensive services. In this manner, online and mobile interventions provide a potential critical answer to the extant gap in stepped-down care for individuals with FEP.

One example is HORYZONS (Alvarez-Jimenez et al. 2013), an online system that integrates peer-to-peer social networking, individualized psychosocial interventions, and contact with providers as online facilitators (Figure 20–3). HORYZONS was based on positive psychology principles and self-determination theory, with a particular focus on generating autonomy, mastery, and a sense of social connection. Given the particular disruption to one's social network that often occurs because of a psychotic episode, HORYZONS is centered on the social community. It is designed to provide a Facebook news feed–style update stream, where users can share their experiences and perspectives with one another. Further, participants can propose and complete specific behavioral challenges and solicit suggestions and feedback through a "talk it out" forum. In addition to the social community, HORYZONS provides psychoeducation and interactive therapy modules in line with mindfulness-based intervention, positive psychology techniques, and facilitated social connections. The system is designed for a provider to function in the role of facilitator; the facilitator can suggest content to individual clients, monitor site content for safety, and contact individuals to provide additional support should the need arise.

Pilot data for HORYZONS (Alvarez-Jimenez et al. 2013) included 20 individuals who had experienced a recent FEP, and results demonstrated that individuals used the system frequently (log-ins $M=13.50$, standard deviation=11.95) and on a consistent basis (70% for at least 3 of 4 weeks). Participants found it to be useful, and 90% said they would recommend it to others. In particular, social networking features were popular (95% of participants used these features), and usability statistics compared favorably with existing short-term open-access Internet-based mental health programs. Over the 1-month study period, users also demonstrated a significant drop ($d=0.60$) in depressive symptoms.

Web-based interventions have also been applied to address barriers that emerge in the application of family-based therapies and psychoed-

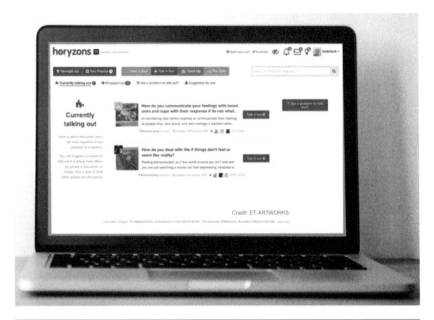

FIGURE 20–3.   Screenshot of HORYZONS, a platform designed for individualized positive psychology interventions and peer support for individuals with first episode of psychosis.

Source.   Alvarez-Jimenez et al. 2013; rawpixel.com via PEXELS. The photo of the computing device was downloaded from the PEXELS database (www.pexels.com).

ucation for the loved ones of an individual with FEP. Rotondi and colleagues (2005, 2010) designed an online psychoeducation intervention for both individuals with schizophrenia (not exclusively FEP) and a support person involving a website that provides psychoeducation, online therapy group bulletin boards, an opportunity to ask experts questions, and relevant community news. Studies examining this intervention randomly assigned people with schizophrenia and family supports (preserving dyads) to treatment as usual or an enhanced treatment condition that involved access to the online intervention. Across studies, this approach appeared to be feasible and acceptable to participants. Three-month outcomes revealed that individuals with schizophrenia with access to the intervention reported lower perceived stress and higher social support relative to the treatment-as-usual condition (Rotondi et al. 2005). Follow-up studies examining one-year outcomes (Rotondi et al. 2010) revealed a significant decrease in positive symptoms and an increase in knowledge of illness among individuals with schizophrenia. Support persons similarly experienced an increase in knowledge about the illness relative to usual care.

Conclusion

There are ample opportunities for digital health technologies to enhance the delivery services for individuals with FEP. We provide a demonstrative example of how these approaches may be integrated in a technology-enhanced coordinated care clinic (TECCC) for FEP.

Case Example

Eric is an 18-year-old high school senior. At the behest of his parents and friends, Eric presented to his primary care provider, reporting to her that he has felt "down, tired, and worn down" for several months. What Eric did not report was that he has also experienced consistent auditory hallucinations that comment on his daily activities. He has also stopped attending extracurricular activities, and his grades have dropped from a 3.0 GPA to a semester GPA of 1.0. Noting that Eric reported that his mother has bipolar disorder and a paternal uncle had schizophrenia, Eric's primary care physician referred him to a TECCC for FEP. On arrival at the TECCC, Eric completed a 2-hour baseline assessment, including cognitive assessments, a prodromal symptom interview, and an open-ended speech sample, which was automatically transcribed and run through machine-learning algorithms. Eric's risk of conversion probability was calculated by the prodromal risk calculator, and he was scheduled for a series of appointments with individual and family providers, as well as medication management with the clinic psychiatrist.

Partially as a result of these services, Eric's functioning stabilizes. He began scheduling get-togethers with old friends and engaging with his parents and siblings. Eric's interpersonal style in treatment, however, is somewhat guarded. He is quiet, shy, and sometimes reluctant to share his difficulties and stressors with his individual providers. Eric does not tell his treatment team that he has been experiencing increased distress during evenings in the last several weeks as he anticipates final exams, the end of high school, and the departure of close friends for college. As he ruminates, particularly after dark, he notices that he starts to feel as though his neighbors are watching his computer monitor, a suspicion that is fostered by his continued auditory hallucinations.

Thankfully, Eric has access to an mHealth app after hours. On this app Eric reports that he has been experiencing increased auditory hallucinations in the evenings. When his ratings of depressive or positive symptoms spike, Eric's mobile app provides brief suggestions of interventions to try, including cognitive restructuring exercises that challenge his beliefs about the power and uncontrollability of his voices. The app also provides him with reminders to continue taking his medication. Together with passive sensing of changes in behavior (i.e., Eric's late hours and increased phone activity into the late hours), these EMA ratings are transmitted to Eric's individual provider at TECCC. This leads to an open conversation at the clinic about recent changes in Eric's presentation. Eric is relieved to able to discuss these stressors with his provider.

After several months of active treatment, Eric demonstrates significant changes since he first engaged with his primary care provider. He
is open with friends and family members about his psychotic symptoms, and he has a well-crafted relapse prevention plan. He plans to attend a local college and is working part time at a nearby coffee shop. He
also is interested in providing peer support to other individuals receiving care at TECCC. Because of his improved functioning and busy
schedule, he realizes he is unlikely to be able to attend twice-weekly sessions at the TECCC. As his providers prepare for the end of their regularly scheduled visits, they introduce him to the online recovery
community through TECCC. In this online recovery community, Eric
has ongoing access to continuously updated evidence-based therapy
modules. He is particularly interested in those centered on a new interest of his, meditation. He also appreciates that the online community
has a base of users who are open about their own experiences with psychosis. Eric has time to come back to the clinic only once every month or
two, but he logs on to the online community frequently, particularly
when he is more distressed.

Eric's parents are also involved in the stepped-down relapse prevention plan. They are given access to a companion online community
for the loved ones of individuals with psychosis. This is particularly
useful as Eric's parents prepare for his move to his own apartment. They
seek support not only from clinic facilitators but also from fellow family
members of young people with FEP who have dealt with the stress of
watching their loved one recover. Eric and his family members learn
new skills to support him as he recovers, moves away from home, and
eventually graduates from college with a degree in computer science.

Eric's story demonstrates that technology-enhanced interventions do
not have to revolutionize existing treatment practices; rather, they can
have a significant impact on the effectiveness and accessibility of treatment through addressing existing gaps in care. None of these technologies are proposed at present to replace existing in-person mental health
services; rather, they are proposed to supplement and improve existing
care to amplify its potential impact. Although available tools provide exciting developments in ideal conditions, this area is a nascent one.

Many health technologies reviewed in this chapter demonstrate im-
pressive findings in pilot trials and feasibility studies; however, fewer
have been well validated in large-scale randomized trials. Further, a
number of the interventions described in this chapter have promising
results with samples of individuals with chronic schizophrenia but not
persons in the midst of FEP. Although large-scale demonstrations of effectiveness of the newest technologies in FEP are few, their feasibility is
clear and their potential is notable. As these tools and systems evolve,
the number of clinical uses that could be addressed by them will only
grow. If the development of FEP services mirrors development of numerous areas in health services, or even the development of business or

transportation, technology will play a significant role in expansion and sustainability of effective interventions for this population.

KEY CONCEPTS

- Several technology-enhanced assessments and interventions show promise in the treatment of first-episode psychosis (FEP); these tools apply across detection, intervention, and maintenance of treatment gains.

- Technology-enhanced interventions may be particularly well suited to address challenges that are specific to FEP care, including individual engagement, cost, and step-down care services.

- Prototype digital health resources have limitations. They lack large-scale empirical validation, and many have been examined only in a chronic psychosis population.

Discussion Questions

1. What existing service gaps or weaknesses in your particular clinic are best addressed with technology?

2. What is the degree of comfort of your clinical staff with using technology in FEP treatment? How does this comfort level compare with that of the typical individual?

3. What is the current role of the Internet and mobile devices in the lives of individuals at your clinic? How might any existing enthusiasm in this area be leveraged in the service of recovery?

Suggested Readings

Alvarez-Jimenez M, Alcazar-Corcoles MA, González-Blanch C, et al: Online, social media and mobile technologies for psychosis treatment: a systematic review on novel user-led intervention. Schizophr Res 156(1):96–106, 2014 24746468

Ben-Zeev D, Drake RE, Corrigan PW, et al: Using contemporary technologies in the assessment and treatment of serious mental illness. Am J Psychiatr Rehabil 15(4):357–376, 2012

O'Hanlon P, Aref-Adib G, Fonseca A, et al: Tomorrow's world: current developments in the therapeutic use of technology for psychosis. BJPsych Advances 22:301–310, 2016)

References

Alvarez-Jimenez M, Bendall S, Lederman R, et al: On the HORYZON: moderated online social therapy for long-term recovery in first episode psychosis. Schizophr Res 143(1):143–149, 2013 23146146

Bedi G, Carrillo F, Cecchi GA, et al: Automated analysis of free speech predicts psychosis onset in high-risk youths. NPJ Schizophr 1(1):15030, 2015 27336038

Ben-Zeev D, Kaiser SM, Brenner CJ, et al: Development and usability testing of FOCUS: a smartphone system for self-management of schizophrenia. Psychiatr Rehabil J 36(4):289–296, 2013 24015913

Ben-Zeev D, Brenner CJ, Begale M, et al: Feasibility, acceptability, and preliminary efficacy of a smartphone intervention for schizophrenia. Schizophr Bull 40(6):1244–1253, 2014 24609454

Ben-Zeev D, Scherer EA, Wang R, et al: Next-generation psychiatric assessment: using smartphone sensors to monitor behavior and mental health. Psychiatr Rehabil J 38(3):218–226, 2015 25844912

Ben-Zeev D, Brian R, Wang R, et al: CrossCheck: integrating self-report, behavioral sensing, and smartphone use to identify digital indicators of psychotic relapse. Psychiatr Rehabil J 40(3):266–275, 2017 28368138

Cannon TD, Yu C, Addington J, et al: An individualized risk calculator for research in prodromal psychosis. Am J Psychiatry 173(10):980–988, 2016 27363508

Carrión RE, Cornblatt BA, Burton CZ, et al: Personalized prediction of psychosis: external validation of the NAPLS-2 psychosis risk calculator with the EDIPPP project. Am J Psychiatry 173(10):989–996, 2016 27363511

Corcoran CM, Carrillo F, Fernández-Slezak D, et al: Prediction of psychosis across protocols and risk cohorts using automated language analysis. World Psychiatry 17(1):67–75, 2018 29352548

Fortney JC, Unützer J, Wrenn G, et al: A tipping point for measurement-based care. Psychiatr Serv 68(2):179–188, 2017 27582237

Fusar-Poli P, Bonoldi I, Yung AR, et al: Predicting psychosis: meta-analysis of transition outcomes in individuals at high clinical risk. Arch Gen Psychiatry 69(3):220–229, 2012 22393215

Gafoor R, Nitsch D, McCrone P, et al: Effect of early intervention on 5-year outcome in non-affective psychosis. Br J Psychiatry 196(5):372–376, 2010 20435962

Garety PA, Kuipers E, Fowler D, et al: A cognitive model of the positive symptoms of psychosis. Psychol Med 31(2):189–195, 2001 11232907

Highton-Williamson E, Priebe S, Giacco D: Online social networking in people with psychosis: a systematic review. Int J Soc Psychiatry 61(1):92–101, 2015 25381145

Jonathan GK, Pivaral L, Ben-Zeev D: Augmenting mHealth with human support: notes from community care of people with serious mental illnesses. Psychiatr Rehabil J 40(3):336–338, 2017 28891660

Kane JM, Robinson DG, Schooler NR, et al: Comprehensive versus usual community care for first-episode psychosis: 2-year outcomes from the NIMH RAISE early treatment program. Am J Psychiatry 173(4):362–372, 2016 26481174

Kay SR, Fiszbein A, Opler LA: The Positive and Negative Syndrome Scale (PANSS) for schizophrenia. Schizophr Bull 13(2):261–276, 1987 3616518

Kumar D, Tully LM, Iosif A-M, et al: A mobile health platform for clinical monitoring in early psychosis: implementation in community-based outpatient early psychosis care. JMIR Ment Health 5(1):e15, 2018 29487044

Lal S, Dell'Elce J, Tucci N, et al: Preferences of young adults with first-episode psychosis for receiving specialized mental health services using technology: a survey study. JMIR Ment Health 2(2):e18, 2015 26543922

Miller TJ, McGlashan TH, Rosen JL, et al: Prodromal assessment with the Structured Interview for Prodromal Syndromes and the Scale of Prodromal Symptoms: predictive validity, interrater reliability, and training to reliability. Schizophr Bull 29(4):703–715, 2003 14989408

Naslund JA, Grande SW, Aschbrenner KA, et al: Naturally occurring peer support through social media: the experiences of individuals with severe mental illness using YouTube. PLoS One 9(10):e110171, 2014 25333470

Niendam TA, Tully LM, Iosif AM, et al: Enhancing early psychosis treatment using smartphone technology: a longitudinal feasibility and validity study. J Psychiatr Res 96:239–246, 2018 29126059

Overall JE, Gorham DR: The Brief Psychiatric Rating Scale (BPRS): recent developments in ascertainment and scaling. Psychopharm Bull 24(1):97–99, 1988

Reininghaus U, Gayer-Anderson C, Valmaggia L, et al: Psychological processes underlying the association between childhood trauma and psychosis in daily life: an experience sampling study. Psychol Med 46(13):2799–2813, 2016a 27400863

Reininghaus U, Kempton MJ, Valmaggia L, et al: Stress sensitivity, aberrant salience, and threat anticipation in early psychosis: an experience sampling study. Schizophr Bull 42(3):712–722, 2016b 26834027

Rotondi AJ, Haas GL, Anderson CM, et al: A clinical trial to test the feasibility of a telehealth psychoeducational intervention for persons with schizophrenia and their families: intervention and 3-month findings. Rehabil Psychol 50(4):325–336, 2005 26321774

Rotondi AJ, Anderson CM, Haas GL, et al: Web-based psychoeducational intervention for persons with schizophrenia and their supporters: one-year outcomes. Psychiatr Serv 61(11):1099–1105, 2010 21041348

Schoenbaum M, Sutherland JM, Chappel A, et al: Twelve-month health care use and mortality in commercially insured young people with incident psychosis in the United States. Schizophr Bull 43(6):1262–1272, 2017 28398566

Yung AR, Yuen HP, McGorry PD, et al: Mapping the onset of psychosis: the Comprehensive Assessment of At-Risk Mental States. Aust N Z J Psychiatry 39(11-12):964–971, 2005 16343296

Zubin J, Spring B: Vulnerability—a new view of schizophrenia. J Abnorm Psychol 86(2):103–126, 1977 858828

CHAPTER 21

Inpatient Care for Early Psychosis

A RECOVERY-ORIENTED PERSPECTIVE

Zheala Qayyum, M.D.
Kristen Sayles, M.S., R.N.
Hyun Jung Kim, M.D.
Gerrit Van Schalkwyk, M.B., Ch.B.

INDIVIDUALS in the early stages of psychosis may require hospitalization for a variety of reasons. Symptoms may be severe to the point of impairing functioning. Individuals' thoughts, speech, and behavior may be a source of concern to themselves or others, leading to contact with mental health providers and, potentially, inpatient treatment. In some cases, individuals may come into contact with law enforcement owing to behaviors that are a consequence of their mental illness. Unfortunately, hospitalization is frequently the result of a concern that is held by family, legal, or medical systems, and patients may not always understand the process as a therapeutic intervention (Van Schalkwyk et al. 2015a). Inpatient hospitalization may involve direct or observed exposure to emergency medication administration, restraint, or seclusion, and patients who do not have an explicit understanding of the purpose

of the inpatient setting may form negative impressions of it being a restrictive environment in which they find themselves contained against
their will.

Despite this potential disconnect, hospitalization is also an opportunity to develop shared treatment goals, clarify diagnosis, and engage
the patient's family in a critical process of ongoing psychoeducation. In
this chapter, we present a recovery-oriented approach to inpatient treatment for people in early psychosis in which we aim to shift the focus
from rapid symptom reduction and medication toward a consideration
of how evidence-based treatment can be best provided in a way that is
responsive to the patient's own agenda. It is our view that although
such an approach expands the task of the initial hospital stay, it has the
potential to promote better overall engagement with services and lead
to improved treatment outcomes in terms of both symptom relief and
psychosocial aspects of recovery.

Developing Shared Treatment Goals

The goals of hospitalization may appear obvious when considered from
a purely biomedical framework—from this perspective, the goal is to
make an accurate diagnosis and initiate treatment that will reduce
symptoms. Although this is an important goal, it is seldom the only
goal and may at times be in conflict with the patient's perspective on the
key issues he or she is facing. In a qualitative study of 11 individuals
who spoke about their experience of initial treatment for psychotic
symptoms, participants described a disconnect between their major
concerns—everyday challenges such as getting along with family and
doing well at work and school—and the issues that appeared to be the
focus of their treatment, such as safety, medication adherence, and
symptom reduction (Van Schalkwyk et al. 2015a). Ironically, in some
cases it appeared that a treatment approach that overemphasized these
aspects ultimately undermined treatment engagement and thus worsened, rather than improved, adherence to recommended treatment.

The experience of individuals in the first episode of psychosis has
been the subject of a number of qualitative studies (Boydell et al. 2010),
and a key finding is the importance of developing shared priorities for
treatment. In an optimal setting, this should not lead to the development of conflict. If patients receive detailed education about their diagnosis, the likely clinical course, and the potential utility of a range of
treatments, it is likely that they, too, will prioritize treatment that seeks
to minimize their symptoms. Challenges arise when these treatment
goals are imposed in a noncollaborative manner.

Even in instances where clinical teams are motivated to develop
shared treatment goals, there may be challenges when patients do not

experience their current situation as indicative of a treatable illness. In these cases, a number of strategies are possible. First, it is critical to explore whether there are any issues in the patient's life around which he or she would like to receive support. In our clinical experience, individuals in the early stages of psychosis often have prominent concerns around issues such as identity formation, mood symptoms, and social functioning. Empirical research exploring treatment priorities has also identified the importance of general and physical wellness for many patients (Ramsay et al. 2011). By identifying and including these goals in the overall treatment approach, it is more likely that a collaborative treatment relationship will emerge from which ongoing discussions can be had around aspects of treatment that patients may consider to be of lesser importance.

It is important to recognize that patients may decide not to take medication and that having a diagnosis of a psychotic disorder does not imply that a patient is unable to exercise choices as a health care consumer. Patients may believe that the side effects of medication will outweigh the benefit or that they are not experiencing sufficient impairment from their symptoms to warrant medication in the first place. In inpatient settings, our experience is that power struggles and paternalistic approaches are for the most part ineffective and may in some instances lead to only short-term treatment adherence that falls apart after the patient returns home. Rather, an ongoing dialogue is indicated, in which trust is built over time and an effort is made to understand in better detail the patient's own vision for his or her life. This may include frank feedback from the provider on how the patient's symptoms could obstruct these goals but should also include support and suggestions for other practical strategies for how such challenges can be overcome. In a recent clinical example, a patient who was refusing medication frequently became paranoid during group therapy and would shout at other patients and then run to her room. In the course of a therapeutic encounter, it was suggested to the patient that the way she was responding to these situations put her at risk of being targeted in her community and that she might benefit from learning some new coping skills for managing these uncomfortable feelings.

There may be instances when patients continue to avoid medication despite efforts at collaborative treatment engagement, and clinical teams become concerned as to the patients' safety and ability to achieve a meaningful recovery. A range of approaches to this problem exists. Some jurisdictions will support the involuntary administration of medication, but in our view, this approach has significant limitations, and when it is used, it should not replace ongoing efforts at developing a shared treatment plan. At times, it may be appropriate to allow a patient to reenter his or her community even if he or she is experiencing a high degree of symptoms, while ensuring the ongoing availability of

treatment and engaging family to the maximum extent possible to ensure the patient's safety. This experience of allowing the patient to have
a chance to succeed may serve to greatly advance a treatment alliance,
provided necessary safety planning is in place—this includes ensuring
that a clinical team will be available to check in on the patient and that
family feels empowered to bring the patient back to the hospital if
safety concerns arise. Patients may end up doing well despite the concerns of the clinical team. And when patients do return to the hospital,
they may immediately have a greater degree of trust in a clinical team
that did not coerce them into treatment but remains available to provide
support in helping them return to their communities more successfully.

Milieu Considerations

A well-managed therapeutic inpatient environment can set the stage for
effective treatment engagement, but considerable effort is required to
achieve this aim. Teenagers and young adults experiencing early psychosis require several milieu considerations in order to decrease their
distress, facilitate optimal functioning, and provide an environment
that supports recovery. Critical to this aim is an environment that provides evidence-based care that is free of coercion, provides appropriate
interventions to decrease anxiety, and instills hope and a sense of empowerment for both the patient and his or her family.

The inpatient environment has the potential to generate anxiety, being an unfamiliar space where individuals do not have access to com-
forts and supports that may have been available at home. Further,
anxiety symptoms have been clearly linked with psychosis (Achim et
al. 2011; Addington et al. 2011; Yun et al. 2011). A study of at-risk adolescents described the profile of an individual at high risk for psychosis
as being characterized by high levels of anxiety symptoms, particularly
cognitive anxiety (Granö et al. 2014). As such, it is of primary importance that efforts are taken to reduce sources of anxiety and provide
necessary structure that can reduce risks for thought and behavioral
disorganization. Cognitive-behavioral therapy and psychoeducational
groups designed to decrease anxiety and increase problem-solving
skills for both the patient and the family are linked to decreased emergency department visits and decreased negative symptoms (Calvo et al.
2014). Other non-medication-based interventions to aid in this endeavor include yoga, sensory interventions, art therapy, music therapy,
and problem-solving groups. Such interventions may both directly help
symptoms and increase resilience by imbuing a sense of self-efficacy
and capacity for positive, prosocial engagement.

The use of sensory rooms is a proactive prevention tool that helps to
maintain a noncoercive therapeutic environment while providing a

calm and quiet space where a person with psychotic symptoms can feel safe. Sensory rooms are generally a well-soundproofed space that contains a range of items that can either increase sensory stimulation (e.g., music players, deep and soft chairs, scented oils) or decrease stimulation by providing an escape from the regular milieu environment. Sensory rooms allow staff to build rapport and remain present with the patient during times of distress but also remain open to continued expression of emotions in a safe space (Seckman et al. 2017). In addition, the use of sensory room tools ensures optimal sensory modulation tailored to individual preferences and needs, which allows the patient to practice self-regulation during times of distress (Sutton et al. 2013). This in turn increases resiliency and autonomy and decreases risk for relapse.

Studies suggest that yoga is effective in decreasing anxiety and increasing self-efficacy (Kwasky and Serowoky 2018). In addition, yoga has the potential to help young people learn to self-soothe, regulate emotional responses, and decrease distress from anxiety-producing situations such as hospitalization and family conflict (Re et al. 2014). Use of art, in particular mandala art therapy, can increase a sense of hope and potentially increase subjective well-being and resilience (Kim et al. 2018).

It is important that staff supporting the milieu are involved with regular discussions regarding the patient's diagnosis and clinical needs. A daily "huddle" may be helpful in order to review each case in detail, from initial presentation to the last 24 hours of each patient's response to interventions. At our program at Butler Hospital, we use a range of additional mechanisms for improving dissemination of the clinical formulation and treatment plan. Key techniques include the following:

- Biweekly walking rounds with the patient and entire treatment team to increase knowledge and communication from a patient-inclusive perspective, which serves to get everyone on the same page, including the adolescent or young adult patient
- Weekly case studies to learn from and increase future skillful interventions
- Monthly educational meetings designed to teach staff new skills, such as mindfulness, cognitive-behavioral therapy, and general group leadership
- Biannual team building exercises to increase trust, communication, and active listening skills
- Leading by example and providing in-the-moment feedback for staff during their care of a patient with psychosis, which leads to increased competency and tolerance when intervening with an agitated or paranoid patient
- Leadership that validates staff and encourages them to use intervention tools that empower the patient during times of stress or impulsive behaviors rather than coercive interventions to maintain safety

Youth in their first episode may experience both short- and long-term fear if exposed to other patients who have significant issues around aggression or appear disengaged from treatment or whose behavior otherwise suggests that mental illness is a chronic and debilitating condition. In this context, we find it optimal to place patients experiencing their first episode of psychosis on our adolescent unit, where they can experience support and hope by observing similar-age peers who may have less chronic or serious mental health concerns.

Supporting youth in the first episode of psychosis during hospitalization is not without challenges. There are financial challenges, with limited resources available to support education and training of staff and to purchase necessary equipment for therapeutic interventions. The short length of stay that is typical in modern hospitals may make it difficult to achieve adequate stabilization and illness education. A short length of stay may also contribute to an ever-changing milieu dynamic (given rapid patient turnover), which can cause an increase in psychotic symptoms and anxiety despite the therapeutic environment.

Family Engagement

The involvement and engagement of the family in the treatment of patients with early psychosis cannot be emphasized enough, particularly in the inpatient setting. Family engagement has consistently been associated with better outcomes and can influence both treatment adherence and the course of the illness (Del Vecchio et al. 2015; Doyle et al. 2014; Knock et al. 2011). It is important to bear in mind that because the onset of psychotic symptoms can begin in adolescence, the patient may still be embedded within the family and thus may be subject to the attitudes, beliefs, and help-seeking behaviors of the family. The family's concerns can include worry about isolative behaviors or social and emotional withdrawal, fear of stigma, fear of loss, and parental guilt (Connor et al. 2016). Understanding that family systems can be complex can be helpful in identifying the key members who provide support and are trusted by the patient. In the case of minors, clarification of legal custody status and authority for medical decision making is important to obtain, as well as supporting documents when necessary.

During an inpatient hospitalization, it can be distressing for family members to relinquish the care of a loved one to the inpatient treatment team while facing unanswered questions and uncertainty. Some families may have uncertainty about how to discuss their concerns with the mental health team and can benefit from clear and repeated information and an invitation to engage (Lucksted et al. 2016). Establishing contact with the family at the onset of the hospitalization and involving them in treatment planning by arranging formal family meetings can help mitigate some of this expected anxiety.

Family meetings provide an opportunity to synthesize input from family members, outpatient providers, school systems, pediatricians or primary care physicians, and social services when involved. It is often helpful to gather the key players, especially those who have established a trusted relationship with the patient and family prior to the hospitalization. Our experience from collaborating with the Specialized Treatment Early in Psychosis (STEP) program at Yale University has illustrated that such collaboration allows for a smoother transition from outpatient care to a shorter, better-coordinated inpatient hospital stay when needed and vice versa. This also allows both inpatient and outpatient teams to address the family's uncertainty about the course of treatment following the acute hospitalization and to establish direct engagement.

One of the most important goals of having a family meeting is to foster engagement and provide thorough psychoeducation. The diagnosis, including genetic and environmental risks such as substance abuse and trauma, should be discussed while providing a scaffolding to facilitate appropriate interpretation of the information provided. It is also important to address diagnostic uncertainty when present. The uncertainty may be due in part to ambiguity in clinical presentation, prominent confounding factors, or lack of data to ascertain with clarity the onset of an early psychotic episode. Education about symptoms such as hallucinations and paranoia should be presented in a way that minimizes stigma about psychiatric illness and medical jargon. This makes symptoms—such as an exaggeration of the normal fear response—more relatable and understandable. Although it is necessary to explain the roles of stress and individual coping responses in the illness, it is also important to highlight the role of family support and resilience. which may instill hope and promote a sense of agency in the family. At times, family members may be overwhelmed with all the information and details of the discussion, so it is appropriate to provide informational materials to support the data reviewed that family can refer to at a later time.

Families may benefit from therapeutic support of their own in order to find guidance in dealing with stressful situations, gain a better understanding of the illness, and improve familial communication. This can help reduce such emotions as criticism, hostility, enmeshment, and conflict. Families also have their own beliefs about psychopharmacological interventions that are important to explore because they will influence patient and family engagement. This may be especially pertinent to treatment adherence once the patient transitions out of the inpatient setting and even more so depending on the severity of the illness. Family members are often ideally suited to provide medication monitoring and to ensure the patient's adherence to treatment recommendations.

Often, family members will ask for guidance about how to navigate the youth's independence while needing to provide supervision, especially in the critical period following discharge. It is helpful to identify shared goals with the patient that can be worked toward with family support. Emphasis should be placed on focusing on health and wellness as the path to enable attainment of social and academic engagement or employment while recruiting the family's support in fostering a sense of agency in the youth. At times, it can be difficult to foretell the pace of these next steps; often, they require a slow and deliberate reassessment of the patient's progress and stress tolerance. Here again, if possible, introduction and involvement of the outpatient treatment team while the patient is hospitalized can be extremely helpful.

Family engagement is also essential in safety planning for discharge. Although the risk of violence due to psychiatric illness is low, there is a relatively elevated risk of violence toward self and others associated with early psychosis, compounded by impulsivity and substance use, particularly in those who are not taking antipsychotic medications (Moulin et al. 2018; Nielssen et al. 2012). Ensuring that the medications are securely stored and appropriately administered and that the patient does not have access to weapons is crucial.

If there are significant deficits in independent functioning, necessitating greater supervision, support, and monitoring, an assessment of the patient's decisional capacity for the short term may be required. The inpatient hospitalization may be the time to introduce the family to pursuing conservatorship of the patient for medical decision making if necessary. This should be considered only when attempts at fostering patient autonomy and decision making have failed, when ongoing nonadherence to treatment recommendations have evidently placed and continue to place the patient at higher than acceptable risk of unsafe behaviors, or when the patient is no longer capable of taking care of himself or herself even with the supports provided. It is important to approach this as a last resort and on a temporary basis, with the plan to reevaluate the conservatorship while working to enhance the patient's ability to regain independent functioning.

Making and Communicating a Diagnosis

A thorough biopsychosocial formulation can be a valuable tool in making a developmentally informed assessment of early psychosis. Often, the inpatient hospitalization is the first contact the patient and the family has with the mental health system. It is therefore critical that they experience the diagnostic process as thorough and trustworthy and that the diagnosis is communicated in a thoughtful and convincing manner.

A comprehensive diagnostic approach should involve the exclusion of drugs of abuse or medical illness as contributing to the presenting symptoms (Gray et al. 2016). When presentations are atypical, additional workup may include electroencephalography and magnetic resonance imaging to exclude less common neurological disorders (Dalmau et al. 2008). A developmentally informed perspective is also valuable in placing the symptoms in context—early trauma or signs of developmental delay may speak to the potential for a distinct underlying diagnosis. Autism spectrum disorders are a particularly important consideration to explore because there can be significant overlap in clinical presentation (Van Schalkwyk et al. 2015b).

Hearing the diagnosis of a psychotic disorder can be difficult for a family, especially because in early psychosis many patients are navigating school and beginning to separate and individuate from their parents, which the illness can disrupt. There may also have been symptoms preceding the onset of frank psychotic symptoms that were more consistent with anxiety, depression, or obsessive-compulsive disorder, leading to diagnostic confusion. It is often helpful to emphasize that mental illness is something the patient has and does not define the patient. Supporting the identity of the patient is paramount, and this is often lost in the context of the patient and family members feeling helpless in the confines of an inpatient unit.

For some patients and families, the biological model of explaining the illness may provide a framework for understanding what to expect. For many other patients, however, the explanation of psychiatric symptoms as understandable psychological and emotional responses to life events can help reduce fear and stigma (Read et al. 2006). The continued support of the inpatient and outpatient teams should be emphasized, and the diagnosis should be communicated in an optimistic, nonlabeling manner. The treatment team must model and convey hope in a manner that is believable to the patient.

If there is inadequate evidence to support that what the patient is experiencing is truly a first psychotic episode, then it is prudent to highlight the diagnostic uncertainty and hold off until there is further information. Often, the diagnosis becomes clearer over the course of time, sometimes over a few inpatient encounters. The initial presentation may resemble or be confounded by other variables such as concurrent substance use, anxiety, or affective disorders. A thorough discussion of the possible trajectories of the current presentation can function as a starting point for ongoing evaluation and conversation, acting as a bridge until diagnostic certainty is attained.

Approaching Medication

Patients presenting for inpatient hospitalization for early psychosis range from those who are medication naïve to those who have been started on antipsychotic medications as outpatients prior to their hospitalization and those who have been treated for depressive or anxiety disorders previously. It is important to consider that the biological model encapsulates the assumption that medications are the primary means through which the absence of symptoms can be achieved. With a recovery-oriented approach, however, we hope to facilitate patient engagement, integration, and meaningful functioning even if complete remission is not achieved. Therefore, medications are only part of the comprehensive biopsychosocial treatment plan that is to be developed for the patient.

Evidence-based practices should guide the selection of a suitable antipsychotic agent. Findings from the Treatment of Early Onset Schizophrenia Spectrum Disorders (TEOSS) study indicated treatment response in the first 2 weeks of treatment for both first- and second-generation antipsychotics (Sikich et al. 2008). This is closely reflected in what we have found to be the average length of stay for patients with early psychosis, although some patients may need a longer inpatient stay, especially if the first trial of medication does not result in an adequate clinical response and medications need to be switched. The TEOSS study also showed no signifsicant differences in efficacy between first- and second-generation antipsychotic agents, although the side effects were different. Risperidone was associated with greater weight gain, and olanzapine was associated with significantly higher weight and increases in fasting cholesterol, low-density lipoprotein, insulin, and liver transaminase levels when compared with molindone. Akathisia was more prominent in patients who received molindone, whereas prolactin elevation was greatest in the risperidone group.

Research has identified no significant differences in discontinuation rates or symptom control between first- and second-generation antipsychotic medications (Crossley et al. 2010). There is also no clear evidence to suggest the superiority of one particular second-generation antipsychotic over another. Aripiprazole tends not be associated with dyslipidemia or hyperprolactinemia, although it is still associated with weight gain in youth. Younger patients and adolescents may also respond to standard doses of risperidone, whereas ziprasidone and aripiprazole may be effective at lower doses (Datta et al. 2012). Therefore, the selection of antipsychotic medications requires a thoughtful discussion with the patient, led in part by the side effect profiles of these agents and patient preference.

The inpatient setting presents the unique challenge of ensuring that treatment response is observed with appropriate symptom reduction in a short period of time. This often requires starting at a low dose followed by aggressive medication titration. The antipsychotic agent should be titrated to the usual effective dose and observed for response for at least a few days unless limited by side effects, in which case the medication should be switched to a different agent that has lower probability of the adverse effects experienced. For more treatment-refractory illness or in severe cases with profound negative symptoms, medications such as clozapine may also need to be considered (Veerman et al. 2017). In psychotic patients who present with malignant catatonia or catatonia that is nonresponsive to benzodiazepine treatment, electroconvulsive therapy should be used (Benarous et al. 2018). Electroconvulsive therapy may also be a treatment consideration if the patient's medical status or medical history precludes treatment with antipsychotic medications (Flamarique et al. 2017).

Starting any antipsychotic medication requires obtaining informed consent from the patient. In the case of minors, their guardians can provide permission to start psychopharmacological treatment, but an adolescent patient's own engagement and assent are very important because involuntary treatment has been shown to negatively impact medication adherence (Timlin et al. 2015). Patients older than 18 years are required to provide autonomous informed consent. This can pose a challenge if the patient is reluctant to initiate a medication trial, which often may be because of his or her psychotic state or paranoid ideation regarding medications rather than being an indicator of autonomous functioning or beliefs about medications (Schwartz et al. 1988). In such cases, involuntary medications may need to be pursued to minimize the untreated duration of psychotic illness.

Rarely, the patient may be agitated or combative, in which case emergent use of antipsychotic medications may be warranted because not using involuntary medications at this time in particular can result in increased risk of seclusion and restraint or violent episodes (Flammer and Steinert 2016). However, it is important to retain the therapeutic alliance and reestablish the patient's role in leading decisions about his or her own treatment as soon as is safely possible. In such instances, discussing the temporary nature of the intervention, emphasizing the positive effects of the medications to alleviate the symptoms that the patient finds particularly bothersome, and, most importantly, recruiting family support are often helpful.

Even in cases where the patient is older than 18 years, it is important to have the family involved, engaged, and on board with the need for psychopharmacological intervention because improved familial relational functioning closely correlates with medication adherence for the youth (Timlin et al. 2015). There may be hesitancy to initiate an antipsychotic medication, particularly if negative symptoms are predominant or psychotic symptoms are not overt or because of familial concerns about the stigma surrounding mental illness. Previous experience with side effects may also fuel reluctance, especially around sensitivity to weight gain, extrapyramidal symptoms, or dystonic reactions, which can be acutely distressing for the patient. In this situation, any history of a positive antipsychotic response for a family member might be helpful, although this course must be taken with caution so as not to perpetuate any negative identification with a family member who has chronic psychotic illness. Additional caution is warranted in the use of antipsychotic medications in patients with neurodevelopmental disorders because they may demonstrate greater sensitivity to adverse effects.

It is helpful to have the patient's recovery goals be as closely aligned to treatment goals as possible, with pharmacological treatment being a vehicle to facilitate this onward journey. Youth taking antipsychotic medications have reported benefits such as better concentration and academic performance, improved relationships with others, and improved self-control. Reasons for disliking medications include feeling different, fear of social stigma, and concerns about long-term effects. In adolescent patients, it was also found that good familial support and lack of perceived coercion to take medication result in improved medication adherence (Moses 2011).

During the hospitalization, close assessment of antipsychotic response and careful monitoring for side effects are required. Obtaining laboratory tests to establish the baseline metabolic and hepatic function is important, along with electrolytes and complete blood counts. There may be underlying baseline risk factors for metabolic syndrome in medication-naïve patients that should be identified (Fleischhacker et al. 2013). Laboratory tests ideally should be repeated periodically during the inpatient admission because transient transaminitis and neutropenia can occur. Electrocardiographic monitoring is also important because patients with early psychosis are at an elevated risk for QTc prolongation during even a relatively short period (2–4 weeks) of treatment with antipsychotic medications (Zhai et al. 2017). Additionally, assessment for extrapyramidal symptoms and involuntary movements should be incorporated into the daily examination of the patient. Clinicians also should hold a high suspicion for catatonia in patients with significant social withdrawal and slowing or unusual excitation. Using scales such as the Abnormal Involuntary Movement Scale (AIMS; Guy 1976) or the Catatonia Rating Scale (CRS; Bräunig et al. 2000) is often helpful in tracking the severity of symptoms.

Successful Transitioning

A successful hospitalization should include a positive transition back to the community along with outpatient care. Building a collaborative therapeutic alliance with patients and families is critical for this goal (Bonnie et al. 2015). Although some youth develop insight into their mental health difficulties, others do not and may deny that they have treatment needs at all. Engaging the family is a key strategy in supporting such youth—even for the patients who have reached the age of majority. It is important to respect patients' autonomy while reassuring them that family involvement can be extremely helpful to increase the chance of successful transition back to the community.

If the patient is still in school, coordination of transition planning with the school is necessary. The capacity of individual schools to address student mental health concerns is vastly varied, especially as it relates to severe mental health concerns such as psychotic disorders. Many schools and colleges do not have relevant protocols or resources in place and may need guidance from the treatment team on how to support the student's successful transition back to the learning environment. Educators and support staff are typically eager to receive recommendations provided by the inpatient team, although available resources may limit their capacity to implement all the recommendations provided.

Providing a comprehensive sign-out to the outpatient treatment team when the patient is discharged from the inpatient service should be considered the standard of care. In addition to basic information about the patient's diagnosis, hospital course, discharge medications, and plans, further in-depth discussion regarding recommendations for future treatment and foreseeable challenges can be extremely valuable information to the outpatient team for a successful transition of care. If available, referrals to specialized outpatient programs (such as CSC model clinics) should be considered. These programs may deliver comprehensive care involving pharmacological treatment, individual therapy, family interventions, and case management. Some of these programs are even able to provide inpatient outreach services to engage with patients and begin the process of developing a treatment alliance while the patients are still in the hospital.

In the year following a new psychosis diagnosis, the death rate for young people is 24 times higher than for young people without psychosis (Schoenbaum et al. 2017). Thorough safety plans, including storage of medications, supervision, and removal of potential weapons, should be explicitly discussed with patients and, if possible, with family. If relevant, psychoeducation regarding substance use and its impact on psychotic disorders should be provided along with motivational interventions promoting abstinence.

Conclusion

Inpatient hospitalizations may often be the first time a patient with early psychosis makes contact with the mental health system or health care in general. At other times, this may be a recurrent experience over a prolonged clinical course. Regardless, it is important to create a therapeutic alliance in the inpatient setting that moves away from solely emphasizing psychopharmacological treatment and instead steps toward integrating what is important to the patient and his or her family.

The inpatient setting is ideally suited to providing a safe physical space that allows for close monitoring and observation, but it is also confining and can make the patient feel more helpless. This is important to consider because patients may respond to these feelings with anger or increasing isolation. The clinical team is responsible for creating an environment where the patient can safely explore these issues and find greater understanding of how the treatment recommendations presented will align with his or her own goals.

The team should also conduct thorough diagnostic evaluations, formulate a comprehensive treatment plan, and facilitate coordination of care. It is paramount to engage the patient's family and other social support systems involved to facilitate a smooth transition from the hospital. The hospitalization should not only focus on reduction of symptoms so as to successfully and safely transition patients back to care in the community but also support patients in finding hope and what gives meaning to their life, help reestablish their identity, and allow them to take responsibility for their own recovery.

KEY CONCEPTS

- There are multiple specific considerations that may help support individuals in the early stages of psychosis during their hospitalization.

- The impulse to prioritize starting antipsychotic medication may prove counterproductive if a treatment alliance is not fostered.

- Family engagement and collaboration with outpatient services is critical in ensuring that gains made during hospitalization are sustained and built on.

Discussion Questions

1. How might an inpatient unit strive to create a positive environment for a patient in the early stage of psychosis?

2. What steps can be taken to foster a treatment alliance?

3. What are some options when patients are not interested in taking medications?

Suggested Readings

Hayes D, Kyriakopoulos M: Dilemmas in the treatment of early-onset first-episode psychosis. Ther Adv Psychopharmacol 8(8):231–239, 2018 30065814

Hickman G, Newton E, Fenton K, et al: The experiential impact of hospitalisation: parents' accounts of caring for young people with early psychosis. Clin Child Psychol Psychiatry 21(1):145–155, 2016 25926618

Kline E, Thompson E, Schimunek C, et al: Parent-adolescent agreement on psychosis risk symptoms. Schizophr Res 147(1):147–152, 2013 23570897

Mayer N, Petrovic BR, Grah M, et al: Treatment of patients in early phase of psychosis on psychotherapeutic inpatient unit—presentation of the therapeutic programme and evaluation of some aspects. Psychiatr Danub 29(suppl 3):447–451, 2017 28953806

Reynolds N, Desai R, Zhou Z, et al: Psychological interventions on a specialist early intervention inpatient unit: an opportunity to engage? Early Interv Psychiatry 12(6):1094–1099, 2018 28664646

References

Achim AM, Maziade M, Raymond E, et al: How prevalent are anxiety disorders in schizophrenia? A meta-analysis and critical review on a significant association. Schizophr Bull 37(4):811–821, 2011 19959704

Addington J, Epstein I, Liu L, et al: A randomized controlled trial of cognitive behavioral therapy for individuals at clinical high risk of psychosis. Schizophr Res 125(1):54–61, 2011 21074974

Benarous X, Raffin M, Ferrafiat V, et al: Catatonia in children and adolescents: new perspectives. Schizophr Res 200:56–67, 2018 28754582

Bonnie RJ, Stroud C, Breiner H (eds): Investing in the Health and Well-Being of Young Adults. Washington, DC, National Academies Press, 2015

Boydell KM, Stasiulis E, Volpe T, Gladstone B: A descriptive review of qualitative studies in first episode psychosis. Early Interv Psychiatry 4(1):7–24, 2010 20199476

Bräunig P, Krüger S, Shugar G, et al: The Catatonia Rating Scale I—development, reliability, and use. Compr Psychiatry 41(2):147–158, 2000 10741894

Calvo A, Moreno M, Ruiz-Sancho A, et al: Intervention for adolescents with early onset psychosis and their families: a randomized controlled trial. J Am Acad Child Adolesc Psychiatry 53(6):688–696, 2014 24839887

Connor C, Greenfield S, Lester H, et al: Seeking help for first-episode psychosis: a family narrative. Early Interv Psychiatry 10(4):334–345, 2016 25303624

Crossley NA, Constante M, McGuire P, et al: Efficacy of atypical v. typical antipsychotics in the treatment of early psychosis: meta-analysis. Br J Psychiatry 196(6):434–439, 2010 20513851

Dalmau J, Gleichman AJ, Hughes EG, et al: Anti-NMDA-receptor encephalitis: case series and analysis of the effects of antibodies. Lancet Neurol 7(12):1091–1098, 2008 18851928

Datta SS, Kumar A, Wright SD, et al: Atypical antipsychotics for psychosis in adolescents. Cochrane Database Syst Rev (10):CD009582, 2012 24129841

Del Vecchio V, Luciano M, Sampogna G, et al: The role of relatives in pathways to care of patients with a first episode of psychosis. Int J Soc Psychiatry 61(7):631–637, 2015 25614470

Doyle R, Turner N, Fanning F, et al: First-episode psychosis and disengagement from treatment: a systematic review. Psychiatr Serv 65(5):603–611, 2014 24535333

Flamarique I, Baeza I, de la Serna E, et al: Thinking about electroconvulsive therapy: the opinions of parents of adolescents with schizophrenia spectrum disorders. J Child Adolesc Psychopharmacol 27(1):75–82, 2017 26983067

Flammer E, Steinert T: Association between restriction of involuntary medication and frequency of coercive measures and violent incidents. Psychiatr Serv 67(12):1315–1320, 2016 27476807

Fleischhacker WW, Siu CO, Bodén R, et al; EUFEST study group: Metabolic risk factors in first-episode schizophrenia: baseline prevalence and course analysed from the European First-Episode Schizophrenia Trial. Int J Neuropsychopharmacol 16(5):987–995, 2013 23253821

Granö N, Karjalainen M, Edlund V, et al: Anxiety symptoms in adolescents at risk for psychosis: a comparison among help seekers. Child and Adolescent Mental Health 19(2):97–101, 2014

Gray R, Bressington D, Hughes E, et al: A systematic review of the effects of novel psychoactive substances "legal highs" on people with severe mental illness. J Psychiatr Ment Health Nurs 23(5):267–281, 2016 27037639

Guy WA: Abnormal Involuntary Movement Scale (AIMS), in ECDEU Assessment Manual for Psychopharmacology. Washington, DC, U.S. Department of Health, Education, and Welfare, 1976, pp 534–537

Kim H, Kim S, Choe K, et al: Effects of mandala art therapy on subjective well-being, resilience, and hope in psychiatric inpatients. Arch Psychiatr Nurs 32(2):167–173, 2018 29579508

Knock J, Kline E, Schiffman J, et al: Burdens and difficulties experienced by caregivers of children and adolescents with schizophrenia-spectrum disorders: a qualitative study. Early Interv Psychiatry 5(4):349–354, 2011 22032549

Kwasky AN, Serowoky ML: Yoga to enhance self efficacy: an intervention for at-risk youth. Arch Psychiatr Nurs 32(1):82–85, 2018 29413079

Lucksted A, Stevenson J, Nossel I, et al: Family member engagement with early psychosis specialty care. Early Interv Psychiatry 12(5):922–927, 2016 27863039

Moses T: Adolescents' commitment to continuing psychotropic medication: a preliminary investigation of considerations, contradictions, and correlates. Child Psychiatry Hum Dev 42(1):93–117, 2011 20953829

Moulin V, Golay P, Palix J, et al: Impulsivity in early psychosis: a complex link with violent behaviour and a target for intervention. Eur Psychiatry 49:30–36, 2018 29353178

Nielssen OB, Malhi GS, McGorry PD, et al: Overview of violence to self and others during the first episode of psychosis. J Clin Psychiatry 73(5):e580–e587, 2012 22697204

Ramsay CE, Broussard B, Goulding SM, et al: Life and treatment goals of individuals hospitalized for first-episode nonaffective psychosis. Psychiatry Res 189(3):344–348, 2011 21708410

Re P, McConnell JW, Reidinger G, et al: Effects of yoga on patients in an adolescent mental health hospital and the relationship between those effects and the patients' sensory-processing patterns. J Child Adolesc Psychiatr Nurs 27(4):175–182, 2014 25327305

Read J, Haslam N, Sayce L, et al: Prejudice and schizophrenia: a review of the 'mental illness is an illness like any other' approach. Acta Psychiatr Scand 114(5):303–318, 2006 17022790

Schoenbaum M, Sutherland JM, Chappel A, et al: Twelve-month health care use and mortality in commercially insured young people with incident psychosis in the United States. Schizophr Bull 43(6):1262–1272, 2017 28398566

Schwartz HI, Vingiano W, Perez CB: Autonomy and the right to refuse treatment: patients' attitudes after involuntary medication. Hosp Community Psychiatry 39(10):1049–1054, 1988 3229738

Seckman A, Paun O, Heipp B, et al: Evaluation of the use of a sensory room on an adolescent inpatient unit and its impact on restraint and seclusion prevention. J Child Adolesc Psychiatr Nurs 30(2):90–97, 2017 28653508

Sikich L, Frazier JA, McClellan J, et al: Double-blind comparison of first- and second-generation antipsychotics in early onset schizophrenia and schizoaffective disorder: findings from the treatment of early onset schizophrenia spectrum disorders (TEOSS) study. Am J Psychiatry 165(11):1420–1431, 2008 18794207

Sutton D, Wilson M, Van Kessel K, et al: Optimizing arousal to manage aggression: a pilot study of sensory modulation. Int J Ment Health Nurs 22(6):500–511, 2013 23374543

Timlin U, Hakko H, Riala K, et al: Adherence of 13–17 year old adolescents to medicinal and non-pharmacological treatment in psychiatric inpatient care: special focus on relative clinical and family factors. Child Psychiatry Hum Dev 46(5):725–735, 2015 25307994

Van Schalkwyk GI, Davidson L, Srihari V: Too late and too little: narratives of treatment disconnect in early psychosis. Psychiatr Q 86(4):521–532, 2015a 25663602

Van Schalkwyk GI, Peluso F, Qayyum Z, et al: Varieties of misdiagnosis in ASD: an illustrative case series. J Autism Dev Disord 45(4):911–918, 2015b 25218849

Veerman SR, Schulte PF, de Haan L: Treatment for negative symptoms in schizophrenia: a comprehensive review. Drugs 77(13):1423–1459, 2017 28776162

Yun DY, Hwang SS, Kim Y, et al: Impairments in executive functioning in patients with remitted and non-remitted schizophrenia. Prog Neuropsychopharmacol Biol Psychiatry 35(4):1148–1154, 2011 21466833

Zhai D, Lang Y, Dong G, et al: QTc interval lengthening in first-episode schizophrenia (FES) patients in the earliest stages of antipsychotic treatment. Schizophr Res 179:70–74, 2017 27727006

CHAPTER 22

Care for Adolescents on the First-Episode Psychosis Continuum

Rhoshel K. Lenroot, M.D.
Tresha A. Gibbs, M.D.

ALTHOUGH the peak age of onset of psychotic disorders is in late adolescence and early adulthood, a substantial number of individuals first experience psychotic symptoms during adolescence (here defined as ages 13–17 years). Adolescence is also a particularly important time for identifying individuals who may be at clinical high risk for psychosis because this is the developmental stage when the majority of individuals who ultimately transition to a psychotic disorder will experience their first prodromal symptoms. In samples of help-seeking adolescents at clinical high risk, approximately 25% transition to a full psychotic disorder over 2 years. Even in those who do not transition, the presence of attenuated psychotic experiences is associated with general psychopathology and impairment in social functioning (Fusar-Poli et al. 2017).

Recognition of the importance of adolescence in early intervention efforts has resulted in most clinical services for early psychosis spanning an age range that begins at around 13–15 years and extends into the mid-twenties. Structuring services to cross the transition from adolescence into adulthood has many benefits, including the ability to maintain continuity of care during the period of greatest vulnerability for onset of psychotic disorders. However, it also requires that the services staff be able to work effectively with young people who are in different developmental stages.

Adolescence, by definition, is the period of transition between childhood and adulthood. Sexual maturation is one of the defining factors, which may occur relatively early during adolescence, whereas neurodevelopment continues well into early adulthood. The social environment and accompanying expectations also change during this period, typically shifting from being largely oriented to and determined by the family environment and structured educational settings to having more emphasis on developing and sustaining social relationships in the larger community. These changes occur within the context of the increasing latitude and responsibility in decision making that are associated with adult status.

The onset of psychosis during this critical period can adversely affect an adolescent's ability to navigate these developmental tasks, with potentially long-term adverse effects beyond the functional impact of the symptoms themselves. Participating with same-age peers in the tasks of establishing social networks and sexual relationships can be particularly challenging if adolescents' ability to interpret social cues is limited or if they are socially withdrawn because of anxiety or paranoia. Cognitive difficulties such as poor concentration and working memory not only impact scholastic performance but can also specifically impact the ability to manage competing demands and complex decisions needed to develop independence. Establishing a sense of identity can be particularly difficult for young people if they or those around them have become unsure whether they can trust their beliefs and perceptions about the world.

Developmental characteristics thus need to be taken into account when caring for adolescents and their families. Although data are sparse, there is some evidence that a younger age of onset of psychotic symptoms may be associated with particular clinical and biological characteristics and risk factors. Psychosocial interventions that are effective in adults may not be suitable for the level of cognitive development of an adolescent, and although the indications for psychopharmacological treatments are similar in adolescents and adults, the small amount of research available suggests some additional specific considerations to take into account when working with adolescents. However, despite the challenges of working with adolescents, there may also be an increased potential for positive outcomes. One of the few outcome studies of intervention programs for first-episode psychosis that examined age effects found more robust functional improvements in individuals who presented before the age of 18, suggesting that these younger individuals may also be more able to respond to appropriate intervention (Amminger et al. 2011).

Extensive reviews of diagnosis and treatment of individuals with first-episode psychosis or who are considered to be at clinical high risk for psychosis are provided in Chapter 8, "Assessment and Targeted Intervention in Individuals at Clinical High Risk for Psychosis," and Chapter 9, "Medical Workup for First-Episode Psychosis." In this chapter, we focus on aspects of these conditions specifically relevant to adolescents presenting before age 18.

Developmental Considerations in the Presentation of Early Psychosis

There is extensive evidence that young people who go on to develop a psychotic disorder often have early evidence of social, motor, and language problems. In the Avon Longitudinal Study of Parents and Children, individuals in England were evaluated at multiple time points from infancy to young adulthood, and these evaluations identified progressive deficits in functional IQ over the lifespan for those who developed psychosis by late adolescence (Mollon et al. 2018). In addition to functional IQ, lags in working memory, attention, visuospatial functioning, and language were noted throughout development. These dramatic signs were not seen in the young people who developed affective disorders. Adolescents who have transitioned to primary psychotic disorders are consistently found to have impairments in cognitive functions such as social cognition, verbal fluency, and memory, which likely contribute to the functional deterioration characteristic of these disorders. Although adolescents at clinical high risk are also more likely on average to have difficulty with cognition, particularly in domains of attention, memory, visuospatial ability, and processing speed, recent findings have suggested that these deficits are more severe in the subset of individuals who eventually develop psychosis and remain relatively mild in those who do not (Seidman et al. 2016).

Generally and historically, the data have supported the finding that onset of schizophrenia before age 18 is associated with worse cognitive function. In a meta-analysis that compared cognitive assessment findings in persons with schizophrenia before age 19, onset after 19, and onset after age 40, younger individuals had significant deficits compared with older ones (Rajji et al. 2009). These included deficits in full-scale IQ, processing speed, verbal and working memory, and executive function. A study of the 20-year course of schizophrenia found social functioning to be relatively preserved from the beginning of the disorder, suggesting that the highest level of functioning prior to the disorder tends to be retained (Velthorst et al. 2017). This is consistent with a recent meta-analysis of longitudinal changes in cognition in early psychosis, which did not find evidence of further cognitive decline in either clinical at-risk subjects or those with a first episode of psychosis (Bora and Murray 2014). However, despite the substantial evidence of earlier onset being associated with worse cognitive function at presentation, an early psychosis intervention program that looked at relative outcomes of individuals who presented before age 18 found that they had greater functional improvements, raising the question of whether the greater plasticity of the adolescent brain could be an advantage when provided with appropriate intervention (Amminger et al. 2011).

Longitudinal brain imaging studies suggest that the progressive brain changes observed in adolescent-onset psychosis converge on similar findings as seen in imaging studies of adults with chronic psychosis, specifically decrease in frontal and temporal gray matter volumes, increase in lateral ventricular volume, and decrease in cerebellar volume. What appears unique to those who develop psychotic disorders at a younger age is more rapid loss of frontal cortical regions, particularly over the first few years of their illness (Fraguas et al. 2016).

A number of risk factors have been associated with the development of psychosis, including biological factors (e.g., male gender, family history of psychosis, obstetric complications) and environmental factors (e.g., urbanicity), coming from a minority population, exposure to early life stressors, and cannabis use (van Os et al. 2010). The risk factors that appear to be most strongly associated with an earlier age of onset include male gender, obstetric complications, family history of psychosis, and cannabis use, although there is some evidence that the accumulation of several factors, including migration status and social class at birth, that are not individually predictive may together increase the likelihood of developing psychosis earlier in life (O'Donoghue et al. 2015).

A history of childhood trauma is relatively common in adolescents at clinical high risk, appears to predict risk of transition to psychotic disorder, and has been associated with severity of psychotic symptoms (Mayo et al. 2017). Whether the vulnerable individual is more likely to be traumatized or whether trauma is causally related to psychosis is currently unclear. In addition to exposure to potentially traumatic events such as domestic or community violence or sexual abuse, an often underrecognized source of traumatic interpersonal experiences that may have an adverse effect on development and is relatively common in adolescents is bullying in schools and on social media. Screening for traumatic experiences and for symptoms of posttraumatic stress in children requires a developmental approach, and the use of adolescent-specific screening tools for posttraumatic stress disorder (PTSD) is encouraged. Treatment of PTSD, if present, is essential (Mayo et al. 2017).

For some people, adolescence includes experimentation with a variety of substances, including tobacco, alcohol, and cannabis, and there is strong evidence that cannabis is a dose-dependent risk factor for chronic psychotic disorder. Data suggest that adolescence is a period in which the developing brain is particularly sensitive to effects of cannabis, such that heavy cannabis exposure is associated with earlier onset of emotional, behavioral, and/or cognitive symptoms and greater risk of developing psychosis (Ongür et al. 2009). Exposure to highly potent tetrahydrocannabinol (THC) in particular is associated with behavioral disturbances. The growing legalization of marijuana means increased access; according to the Youth Risk Behavior Surveillance Data from 2017, 20% of high school students had used cannabis in the preceding month (Kann et al. 2018). The proportion of adolescents who view marijuana use as potentially harmful has been dropping steadily, with a 2017 U.S. national survey finding that only 34% of eighth graders and 14% of twelfth graders felt that occasional use was risky (Johnston et al. 2018).

In addition to effects of age, studies suggest that genetic risk factors may interact with cannabis exposure. Several studies have found that individuals with a family history of psychosis are more sensitive to becoming psychotic after cannabis use. Potential specific genetic risk factors have also been identified. One is the gene encoding catechol-*O*-methyltransferase (COMT), an enzyme that plays a key role in the breakdown of dopamine in the prefrontal cortex. Several studies reported that individuals with the genetic variant of COMT that breaks down dopamine more quickly have an increased risk of developing psychosis following exposure to cannabis (Arendt et al. 2008; Kahn et al. 2011), although other studies did not find such an association (Boydell et al. 2007). A second gene, *AKT1*, encodes an enzyme that interacts with glycogen synthase kinase during cell processes such as transcription, apoptosis, and proliferation. *AKT1* is stimulated by cannabinoids, and cannabis users with a specific polymorphism in *AKT1* have been found to have a significantly higher (twofold to sevenfold) risk of developing psychosis. Other genetic factors that have been linked to risk for psychosis in cannabis users with less evidence thus far include *DAT1*, neuregulin 1, and brain-derived neurotrophic factor (Radhakrishnan et al. 2014).

Differential Diagnosis

The clinical differential diagnosis of an adolescent presenting with positive symptoms of hallucinations, paranoia, or other delusions or disorganized thought is broad and may include affective disorders, anxiety disorders, obsessive-compulsive disorder, trauma- or stressor-related conditions, substance use disorders, personality disorders, and neurodevelopmental disorders. Clinicians should maintain a developmental perspective when interviewing, assessing, and diagnosing adolescents. Adolescents are likely to present for evaluation after referral by a school official, pediatrician, primary care provider, or family member. Adolescents are more likely than adults to present with negative symptoms and flat affect (Ballageer et al. 2005).

The clinician may face a diagnostic challenge because suspicion of a psychotic disorder may not be the anticipated focus of the initial presentation. Often, the presenting complaints described by the adolescent or referrer may be mood, social, and cognitive functioning problems, including irritability, depression, social withdrawal, or difficulties with attention. The adolescent may be experiencing failure to progress as expected in coursework because of inattention or lack of motivation. He or she may avoid social contact and be notably paranoid in the school social setting. The adolescent may not reveal the presence of hallucinations or delusions unless directly questioned. Questionnaires such as the 21-item Prodromal Questionnaire (PQ-B) developed by Cannon and Loewy (Loewy et al. 2011); the Early Psychosis Screener (EPS; Brodey et al. 2017); and the Yale University Prevention through Risk Identification, Management, and Education (PRIME) Screen (Miller et al. 2004) may help elucidate symptoms.

An additional consideration is that it is not uncommon for children and adolescents to have psychotic experiences, although most of them do not progress to a psychotic disorder as they age. The prevalence of hallucinations among adolescents ages 13–18 is approximately 7.5% (Sikich 2013). Symptoms that are termed *psychotic experiences* versus a *disorder* are usually transient hallucinations, mostly stress induced, and are not associated with functional impairment or abnormal social cognition and insight. Signs of apparent paranoid ideation may overlap with adolescent self-consciousness, and signs perceived as thought process and thought content abnormalities on mental status examination may be due to learning or neurodevelopmental disorders, some of which may affect expressive language skills in affected adolescents. Psychotic symptoms are more common in adolescents with trauma-related disorders, and a unique aspect of assessing the trauma experience in adolescents is that they may not yet have a narrative or labels for their experience. A trauma-informed approach to assessment is essential.

Whereas adults may commonly obtain mental health care through acute care settings because of active and impairing positive symptoms, adolescents can present earlier because of their immersion in the family, school, and community systems. This provides an opportunity for close assessment earlier in the course of the illness and the opportunity to intervene before the potentially steep decline in social functioning that has been observed in both affective psychosis and schizophrenia-related disorders. The positive effects of early intervention on symptom, cognitive, and functional outcomes have now been well demonstrated, supporting the value of early recognition and diagnosis (Amminger et al. 2011).

Considering relevant genetic, acute, or chronic medical or neurological disorders is essential in the initial assessment. This process includes assessing for symptoms to suggest a genetic syndrome, epilepsy, tumor, metabolic disorders, autoimmune illness, substance use, or traumatic brain injury. For adolescents with a history of childhood deviations in physical, neurological, psychological, or social development or marked difficulties in academic achievement, a more detailed developmental history and assessment are needed to contextualize any current signs and symptoms.

Neuropsychological testing can identify the degree and domains of cognitive impairment, and projective testing can elaborate on psychotic thoughts or identify more subtle levels of thought disorder, which may be helpful for understanding the client and obtaining rehabilitative supports. Neuropsychological testing is less likely to be helpful in diagnosing individuals at high risk or in predicting long-term course.

For adolescents, it is important to assess the family structure and functioning as a routine part of the evaluation. It is not uncommon for family relationships to undergo a period of strain during the period of individuation and related changes in expectations that are part of normal maturation. When there are worries that a young person is developing a mental illness, these strains can become more severe.

The prodromal stage of schizophrenia has been associated with negative experiences in the parent-caregiver relationship (Tomlinson et al. 2014). Family members may struggle during the prodromal phase with uncertainty about their adolescent and with how to obtain help. The experience of feeling "criticized" by parents and caregivers is a common experience in adolescents who are developing their unique identity. In the context of a new onset mental illness, high expressed emotion can worsen anxiety and social functioning (Onwumere et al. 2009). For adolescents who have transitioned to schizophrenia, a family with high expressed emotion puts them at increased risk of relapse. On the other hand, healthy parent-child relationships in adolescents can decrease adolescent risk behaviors such as drinking and substance use. The struggles with external and internal conflicts that adolescents may be having in negotiating changing relationships with authority figures within their family system may also affect their relationships with clinicians, and this can become particularly challenging when the experience of family relationships has been problematic because of loss, abuse, or neglect.

Cultural factors are important to consider in interacting with adolescents and their families. The meaning of specific symptoms commonly associated with psychosis may be different across cultures. For example, in some cultures, seeing or hearing loved ones who have died is accepted as part of the grieving process. Auditory hallucinations of helpful voices or other unusual perceptions may be considered by adolescents or their family as a special ability, sometimes inherited, rather than a sign of pathology. However, international studies have found that most cultures do identify a pathological state associated with the disordered thoughts and behavior of chronic psychosis. Being attentive to the meanings of the symptoms for an individual adolescent and family while remaining alert to evidence of functional impairment or distress can help to guide assessment. Focusing on the presence of distress associated with unusual perceptions, rather than on how they should be interpreted, can help to support the therapeutic alliance by identifying common treatment goals around improving function.

Suicide risk among adolescents with psychosis is a serious concern, and there is strong evidence that these adolescents are more likely to die by suicide, particularly in the first 3 years after diagnosis, compared with the general population (Simon et al. 2018). Clinicians should screen for depressed mood and a significant decline in role functioning, both of which may lead to hopelessness and self-harm. Suicidal ideation is common among young people at clinical high risk for psychosis. A study by Gill et al. (2015) suggested that suicidal ideation in adolescents may not come to light unless there is active screening for passive suicidal ideation and intensity of suicidal thoughts. They suggested using the Columbia Suicide Severity Rating Scale to accurately characterize the presence of suicidality in these adolescents on a spectrum of thoughts and behaviors. Negative symptoms may obscure the evaluation, but screening for passive suicidal ideation in particular in this population is encouraged (Gill et al. 2015; Taylor et al. 2015).

Identification and Engagement

Despite the accumulating evidence that early intervention in psychosis is associated with better long-term outcomes, duration of untreated psychosis is often still prolonged. Some studies have found that duration of untreated psychosis is longer in adolescents than adults. As discussed in the section on developmental considerations above, a variety of factors may make it more difficult to identify at-risk adolescents and engage them in treatment, and these will differ for each child and family system. Predominant negative symptoms can delay initial diagnosis until onset of either frank psychosis or bizarre behavior. The level of family engagement may impact time to treatment referral because the meaning of the behavioral change is often seen from the lens of the family's cultural, medical, and social history or circumstances. Stigma, particularly the idea that people with mental illness are "crazy," is still common and may add to reluctance to seek help. Parents' fears that they may potentially be blamed can also impede engagement with services. Schools with many high-risk youth may struggle to identify and meet the needs of adolescents with prodromal symptoms. In some school systems, the adolescent experiencing prodromal symptoms is more likely to drop out of school than receive a clinical referral for behavioral change. The frequent ambiguity of clinical presentations in adolescents may also delay accurate diagnosis.

As discussed in more detail in Chapter 4, "Early Intervention and Policy," and Chapter 11, "Intervening Early," over the past 20 years there has been increasing support for specialized multidisciplinary early psychosis services. These services aim to decrease duration of untreated psychosis through early identification and rapid access to appropriate interventions for young people with first-episode psychosis and those who are at clinical high risk (Lloyd-Evans et al. 2011; Tiffin and Welsh 2013). Case identification is facilitated through intensive outreach to families and community organizations, paired with rapid access to assessment and treatment.

Schools are a particularly important partner for services working with adolescents because teachers, advisors, coaches, or other school personnel may be the first to notice that an adolescent is struggling. Building partnerships with schools can also facilitate obtaining educational support for adolescents in order to minimize academic disruption. Schizophrenia is one of the conditions covered under the Individuals with Disabilities Education Act (IDEA) under the category of serious emotional disturbance. Adolescents with psychosis may also be eligible for 504 plans, which provide support based on Section 504 of the federal Rehabilitation Act of 1973. Opportunities to explore supported employment should also be considered with youth.

The coordinated specialty care approach for individuals identified in the earliest phases of their illness has been shown to lead to better long-term outcomes, including less cognitive deterioration and improved social and vocational functioning (Albert et al. 2017; Amminger et al. 2011). For adolescents, willingness to engage with services may be enhanced by creating a youth-friendly space that is more congruent with young people's developmental needs than is commonly found in either pediatric or adult settings and that explicitly involves families while also recognizing that the young person is on the path to adulthood. Maintaining a recovery-based orientation that can support adolescents in identifying strengths and learning to manage symptoms in the context of navigating toward developmentally appropriate social, educational, and vocational goals is critical. Involving trained youth peer specialists may be a particularly effective intervention for helping to establish engagement because it meshes with adolescents' developmentally normal tendency to seek out peers rather than adults. Peer specialists can be an important source of social connection in the presence of a psychiatric disorder typically associated with increasing isolation.

Psychosocial Interventions

Current clinical guidelines concur that psychosocial interventions are an essential component of treatment for adolescents with first-episode psychosis and are the recommended first-line intervention for those at clinical high risk (Addington et al. 2017; Crockford and Addington 2017; Early Psychosis Guidelines Writing Group and EPPIC National Support Program 2016; UK National Institute for Health and Care Excellence 2013). There is as yet relatively little research regarding specific effects of psychosocial treatments in adolescents or of interventions developed specifically for this population, highlighting a critical gap in the evidence base. The discussion that follows therefore relies primarily on data available from adult populations.

Family interventions have been associated with stabilization of symptoms, improved general function, and decreased risk of relapse and are included within current clinical guidelines as an essential part of effective treatment. Family interventions may be particularly important for adolescents because they are more likely to be living within a family system. Although different models for family intervention have been studied, most combine psychoeducation with therapeutic interventions to facilitate problem solving, stress management, and communication skills within the family (Tiffin and Welsh 2013).

Family interventions can be carried out either with a single family or in a group of several families, who meet regularly for up to 2 years. Although multifamily group models include the same components as other family interventions, they have the potential for the added benefit of the creation of a support network among the participating families, which can enhance each family's sense of agency and decrease the stigma and social isolation experienced by many families. However, it is important to determine with each family whether they prefer a single or group format because cultural or other considerations may affect their level of comfort in participating in either model.

Individual therapies for adolescents with first-episode psychosis typically include psychoeducation, relapse prevention, and stress management, in addition to other components as indicated such as social skills and life skills training. At present, cognitive-behavioral therapy for psychosis (CBTp) has been recommended by the National Institute for Health and Care Excellence in the United Kingdom for use in adolescents on the basis of the relatively robust evidence base for its positive effects in adults. However, it is not clear whether adolescents have the same level of benefit from this specialist intervention. One study comparing CBTp with supportive counseling in both adolescents and young adults found that the younger group benefited more from the supportive therapy, whereas the older group benefited from CBTp (Haddock et al. 2006). This result may speak to the need to modify CBTp for the different level of cognitive maturity in adolescents, or it may support the positive effects of a less specific supportive intervention in younger individuals.

The increasing recognition of the potential impact of exposure to stressful life events during development on the risk for psychosis, clinical course, and response to treatment is also raising questions about how best to modify psychotherapeutic interventions to address trauma-related symptoms in individuals with early psychosis. Although there is not yet sufficient evidence to support a specific model, the integration of components from therapies such as trauma-focused cognitive-behavioral therapy (TF-CBT) are currently being considered. TF-CBT is a model that has been well validated in adolescents and may hold promise in this population as well (Mayo et al. 2017).

Recognition of the central role of cognitive deficits in determining functional capacity of individuals with psychosis has stimulated efforts to develop interventions for cognitive remediation. Cognitive remediation therapy consists of behavioral training techniques targeting cognitive processes such as memory, attention, executive function, and social cognition or meta-cognition. The goal of cognitive remedial therapy is for gains in these areas to generalize to daily living and to persist over time (Wykes et al. 2011). There has been sufficient evidence for the positive effects of cognitive remediation therapy for adults with schizophrenia that it has now been incorporated into several guidelines for treatment (Wykes et al. 2011). There is as yet much less known about effectiveness in adolescents, although preliminary reports have shown beneficial effects of cognitive remediation therapy for adolescents with first-episode psychosis (Puig et al. 2014) and for young people who are at clinical high risk (Loewy et al. 2016). Much work remains to be done to determine what the optimal cognitive remediation strategy may be for this age group, but the potential benefits of addressing cognitive deficits during adolescence and decreasing adverse effects on educational and vocational trajectories suggest that developments in this area should be watched closely.

Pharmacological Interventions for Adolescents With First-Episode Psychosis

Antipsychotics effectively decrease positive psychotic symptoms for most individuals with first-episode psychosis, resulting in relief of distress and improvement in social functioning. Several of these medications have been approved by the U.S. Food and Drug Administration for this indication and are considered safe with known side effects. Studies among adolescents have shown modest response rates, such as 34%–50% in the Treatment of Early Onset Schizophrenia Study (TEOSS; Sikich et al. 2008). In this study, 119 adolescents with schizophrenia were randomly assigned to treatment with atypical antipsychotics risperidone or olanzapine or the typical antipsychotic molindone. Over the 8 weeks of the study, symptoms declined 21%–47% for participants in all groups, with peak response rate in 2 weeks and no significant difference between typical versus atypical antipsychotics (Sikich et al. 2008). In another study based on a network meta-analysis of data of adolescents with psychosis, Pagsberg et al. (2017) found that there was equivalence in Positive and Negative Syndrome Scale score reduction with aripiprazole, asenapine, paliperidone, risperidone, quetiapine, and molindone. The response for ziprasidone was not as strong, suggesting it may not be the ideal first-line agent.

The role of long-acting injectables is particularly pertinent to adolescents with first-break psychosis. In this population, adherence and insight may be influenced both by the disorder and by the adolescent's developmental stage. The clinician may thus need to consider long-acting injectables very early on. Although research on long-acting injectables in adolescents is sparse, an observational study comparing effects of three available long-acting formulations (risperidone, aripiprazole, and paliperidone palmitate) in 30 adolescents found that all three medications were largely well tolerated and resulted in similar levels of improvement as measured by the Children's Global Assessment Scale (Fortea et al. 2018). These adolescents had a combination of a psychotic disorder with high levels of comorbid disruptive behavior and substance use and were prescribed an injectable drug because of a history of low adherence and poor insight.

Clozapine has been found to be effective in adolescents with early-onset schizophrenia (Schneider et al. 2014). Benefits include its efficacy in treatment-resistant cases and its low risk of movement-related extrapyramidal symptoms. However, the side-effect profile includes symptoms that may be particularly difficult for adolescents to tolerate, such as weight gain, metabolic changes, drowsiness, salivation, and possible increased seizure risk. The required clozapine protocol of repeat blood draws to monitor for agranulocytosis may be inconvenient and possibly aversive to some adolescents. Nonetheless, it serves an important role in the clinical toolbox for select populations.

Adverse effects are an aspect of treatment with all medications. Informed consent procedures with adequate information on risks and benefits and guideline-based monitoring and intervention for adverse long-term impacts facilitate safe prescribing. Consideration of the metabolic risk profile when selecting an antipsychotic medication is an essential aspect of harm mitigation for adolescents for whom long-term, possibly lifetime, treatment is the expectation. Although efficacy of antipsychotic medications is similar to what is seen in adults, younger people are more likely than adults to respond to lower doses. They may also be more sensitive to weight gain and movement side effects. For these reasons, a "start low, go slow" approach is highly recommended. Detailed comparative data can be found in the 2017 Association for Healthcare Research and Quality comparative effectiveness publication (Pillay et al. 2017).

Treating affective symptoms in this population can improve the treatment course and minimize risk of harm to self or others. In adolescents with first-episode psychosis, onset of depressive symptoms may be an indication for initiation of a first-line agent, typically a selective serotonin reuptake inhibitor, with close monitoring for onset of any change in behavior. New-onset impulsivity, psychomotor activity, or aggressive or hostile behavior may require diagnostic reassessment and consideration of mood-stabilizing treatment for what may be a developing bipolar spectrum illness.

Often, adolescents and their families will inquire about the long-term plan for treatment after the stabilization or even remission of positive psychotic symptoms. Unfortunately, at present there are limited empirical data on the best course. The plan should be individualized for each individual, and it may be necessary to observe an adolescent over time to confirm a definitive diagnosis. Providers should consider using a shared decision-making approach with the adolescent and family in order to maintain engagement and allow for ongoing candid discussions about treatment priorities as the course of the disorder unfolds.

A diagnosis of first-episode schizophrenia tends to remain stable, whereas individuals with schizophreniform disorder, major depressive disorder with psychotic features, or substance-induced psychosis are more likely to receive an alternative diagnosis at follow-up points. For individuals with schizophrenia experiencing their first episode of psychosis, the most conservative recommendation to date is to avoid discontinuation because it leads to relapse. A recent systematic review of studies reporting recurrence rates following medication discontinuation estimated that symptoms recurred in 77% of patients after 1 year and in more than 90% of patients by 2 years (Zipursky et al. 2014). Advising families of this data can assist in decision making. Clinical signs that a psychotic experience is not a chronic psychotic disorder and thus that the adolescent may be a good candidate for discontinuation of treatment after remission of positive symptoms include a sudden onset of symptoms, rapid resolution of symptoms with treatment, and no significant loss in function. For an adolescent with schizophrenia who wishes to discontinue treatment, provider and family should have an open discussion about risks and benefits of this decision. Particularly among adolescents, it is important to validate individuals' attempts at understanding their illness and its treatment, to engage them respectfully in a developmentally appropriate way, and to aim for an overall positive treatment experience.

Pharmacological Interventions for Adolescents at Clinical High Risk

It would be ideal to have an intervention that could prevent transition to psychosis in at-risk adolescents, and efforts to identify such treatments are under way. Studies to date have not supported the use of antipsychotics for prevention of psychosis because they have not shown evidence of sustained differences in transition rates, and side effects such as weight gain are considerable (Stafford et al. 2015). Existing guidelines generally also do not recommend use of antipsychotics for attenuated psychosis symptoms unless there is significant clinical distress that cannot be adequately addressed by first-line psychosocial treatments such as CBTp (Addington et al. 2017; Early Psychosis Guidelines Writing Group and EPPIC National Support Program 2016; UK National Institute for Health and Care Excellence 2013). There has been some evidence that antidepressants may have an impact on the rate of transition to psychosis (Cornblatt et al. 2007). Fatty acids such as eicosapentaenoic acid demonstrate some promise as well (McGorry et al. 2017). Psychotropic medications do play a clear role in treating the co-occurring conditions that are common in clinical high-risk adolescents, such as depression and anxiety, when individuals with these conditions have not responded to psychosocial interventions.

Conclusion

Working with adolescents who are learning to manage symptoms of psychosis requires that the clinician be willing to adapt to meet developmental needs of young people who may be at very different places along the road to adulthood. One of the hardest tasks for both the clinician and the young person and his or her family can be the willingness to tolerate uncertainty. Although the body of knowledge about diagnosis and intervention for adolescents who are experiencing first-episode psychosis or who are at clinical high risk for psychosis has been growing rapidly, we still lack the means to predict accurately what the clinical course is likely to be for an adolescent who has just started having symptoms. Therefore, a critical aspect of treatment is maintaining a recovery-oriented framework that includes attention to preserving engagement through potentially changing clinical states and the flexibility to adjust approaches as needed. Although adolescence can add challenges for clinicians, it also is a time when effective intervention can make an enormous difference in the course of a life.

KEY CONCEPTS

- Thirty percent of individuals with a psychotic disorder have their first episode during adolescence.

- Developmental differences should be kept in mind during assessment and diagnosis of adolescents with psychosis.

- Assessment of family function and inclusion of the family in the treatment process is particularly important in adolescents, who are likely to be living with their family.

Discussion Questions

1. What might the differences be in processes around informed consent and confidentiality when working with youth younger than age 18?

2. How might a clinician approach or partner with schools in communicating with youth and families about mental health concerns?

3. Given that hallucinations are more common in younger teens but often resolve, how might clinicians determine when hallucinations indicate clinical high risk or first-episode psychosis?

4. What are some strategies for supporting secondary school youth in interacting with their peers and discussing what is happening to them?

Suggested Readings

Fusar-Poli P, McGorry PD, Kane JM: Improving outcomes of first-episode psychosis: an overview. World Psychiatry 16(3):251–265, 2017 28941089

Pagsberg AK, Tarp S, Glintborg D, et al: Acute antipsychotic treatment of children and adolescents with schizophrenia-spectrum disorders: a systematic review and network meta-analysis. J Am Acad Child Adolesc Psychiatry 56(3):191–202, 2017 28219485

Sikich L: Diagnosis and evaluation of hallucinations and other psychotic symptoms in children and adolescents. Child Adolesc Psychiatr Clin N Am 22(4):655–673, 2013 24012079

Tiffin PA, Welsh P: Practitioner review: schizophrenia spectrum disorders and the at-risk mental state for psychosis in children and adolescents—evidence-based management approaches. J Child Psychol Psychiatry 54(11):1155–1175, 2013 24102356

References

Addington J, Addington D, Abidi S, et al: Canadian Treatment Guidelines for Individuals at Clinical High Risk of Psychosis. Can J Psychiatry 62(9):656–661, 2017 28730848

Albert N, Melau M, Jensen H, et al: The effect of duration of untreated psychosis and treatment delay on the outcomes of prolonged early intervention in psychotic disorders. NPJ Schizophr 3(1):34, 2017 28951544

Amminger GP, Henry LP, Harrigan SM, et al: Outcome in early onset schizophrenia revisited: findings from the Early Psychosis Prevention and Intervention Centre long-term follow-up study. Schizophr Res 131(1–3):112–119, 2011 21741219

Arendt M, Mortensen PB, Rosenberg R: Familial predisposition for psychiatric disorder: comparison of subjects treated for cannabis-induced psychosis and schizophrenia. Arch Gen Psychiatry 65(11):1269–1274, 2008 18981338

Ballageer T, Malla A, Manchanda R, et al: Is adolescent-onset first-episode psychosis different from adult onset? J Am Acad Child Adolesc Psychiatry 44(8):782–789, 2005 16034280

Bora E, Murray RM: Meta-analysis of cognitive deficits in ultra-high risk to psychosis and first-episode psychosis: do the cognitive deficits progress over, or after, the onset of psychosis? Schizophr Bull 40(4):744–755, 2014 23770934

Boydell J, Dean K, Dutta R: A comparison of symptoms and family history in schizophrenia with and without prior cannabis use: implications for the concept of cannabis psychosis. Schizophr Res 93(1–3):203–210, 2007 17462864

Brodey BB, Addington J, First MB, et al: The Early Psychosis Screener (EPS): item development and qualitative validation. Schizophr Res Dec 15, 2017 [Epub ahead of print] 29254878

Cornblatt BA, Lencz T, Smith CW, et al: Can antidepressants be used to treat the schizophrenia prodrome? Results of a prospective, naturalistic treatment study of adolescents. J Clin Psychiatry 68(4):546–557, 2007 17474810

Crockford D, Addington D: Canadian schizophrenia guidelines: schizophrenia and other psychotic disorders with coexisting substance use disorders. Can J Psychiatry 62(9):624–634, 2017 28886671

Early Psychosis Guidelines Writing Group, EPPIC National Support Program: Australian Clinical Guidelines for Early Psychosis, 2nd Edition Update. Melbourne, VIC, Australia, Orygen, 2016

Fortea A, Ilzarbe D, Espinosa L, et al: Long-acting injectable atypical antipsychotic use in adolescents: an observational study. J Child Adolesc Psychopharmacol 28(4):252–257, 2018 29381388

Fraguas D, Díaz-Caneja CM, Pina-Camacho L, et al: Progressive brain changes in children and adolescents with early onset psychosis: a meta-analysis of longitudinal MRI studies. Schizophr Res 173(3):132–139, 2016 25556081

Fusar-Poli P, McGorry PD, Kane JM: Improving outcomes of first-episode psychosis: an overview. World Psychiatry 16(3):251–265, 2017 28941089

Gill KE, Quintero JM, Poe SL, et al: Assessing suicidal ideation in individuals at clinical high risk for psychosis. Schizophr Res 165(2–3):152–156, 2015 25960038

Haddock G, Lewis S, Bentall R, et al: Influence of age on outcome of psychological treatments in first-episode psychosis. Br J Psychiatry 188:250–254, 2006 16507967

Johnston LD, Miech RA, O'Malley PM, et al: Monitoring the Future: National Survey Results on Drug Use—2017 Overview, Key Findings on Adolescent Drug Use. Bethesda MD, Institute for Social Research, 2018. Available at: www.monitoringthefuture.org/pubs/monographs/mtf-overview2017.pdf. Accessed September 27, 2018.

Kahn RS, Linszen DH, van Os J: Evidence that familial liability for psychosis is expressed as differential sensitivity to cannabis: an analysis of patient-sibing and sibling-control pairs. Arch Gen Psychiatry 68(2):138–147, 2011 20921112

Kann L, McManus T, Harris WA, et al: Youth risk behavior surveillance— United States, 2017. MMWR Surveill Summ 67(8):1–114, 2018 29902162

Lloyd-Evans B, Crosby M, Stockton S, et al: Initiatives to shorten duration of untreated psychosis: systematic review. Br J Psychiatry 198(4):256–263, 2011 21972275

Loewy RL, Pearson R, Vinogradov S, et al: Psychosis risk screening with the Prodromal Questionnaire—brief version (PQ-B). Schizophr Res 129(1):42–46, 2011 21511440

Loewy R, Fisher M, Schlosser DA, et al: Intensive auditory cognitive training improves verbal memory in adolescents and young adults at clinical high risk for psychosis. Schizophr Bull 42(Suppl 1):S118–S126, 2016 26903238

Mayo D, Corey S, Kelly LH, et al: The role of trauma and stressful life events among individuals at clinical high risk for psychosis: a review. Front Psychiatry 8:55, 2017 28473776

McGorry PD, Nelson B, Markulev C, et al: Effect of omega-3 polyunsaturated fatty acids in young people at ultrahigh risk for psychotic disorders: the NEURAPRO randomized clinical trial. JAMA Psychiatry 74(1):19–27, 2017 27893018

Miller TJ, Chicchetti D, Markovich PJ, et al: The SIPS Screen: a brief self-report screen to detect the schizophrenia prodrome. Schizophr Res 70(suppl 1):78, 2004

Mollon J, David AS, Zammit S, et al: Course of cognitive development from infancy to early adulthood in the psychosis spectrum. JAMA Psychiatry 75(3):270–279, 2018 29387877

O'Donoghue B, Lyne J, Madigan K, et al: Environmental factors and the age at onset in first episode psychosis. Schizophr Res 168(1–2):106–112, 2015 26232243

Ongür D, Lin L, Cohen BM: Clinical characteristics influencing age at onset in psychotic disorders. Compr Psychiatry 50(1):13–19, 2009 19059508

Onwumere J, Kuipers E, Bebbington P, et al: Patient perceptions of caregiver criticism in psychosis: links with patient and caregiver functioning. J Nerv Ment Dis 197(2):85–91, 2009 19214042

Pagsberg AK, Tarp S, Glintborg D, et al: Acute antipsychotic treatment of children and adolescents with schizophrenia-spectrum disorders: a systematic review and network meta-analysis. J Am Acad Child Adolesc Psychiatry 56(3):191–202, 2017 28219485

Pillay J, Boylan K, Carrey N, et al: First- and Second-Generation Antipsychotics in Children and Young Adults: Systematic Review Update (Comparative Effectiveness Reviews No 184). Rockville, MD, Agency for Healthcare Research and Quality, 2017

Puig O, Penadés R, Baeza I, et al: Cognitive remediation therapy in adolescents with early onset schizophrenia: a randomized controlled trial. J Am Acad Child Adolesc Psychiatry 53(8):859–868, 2014 25062593

Radhakrishnan R, Wilkinson ST, D'Souza DC: Gone to pot—a review of the association between cannabis and psychosis. Front Psychiatry 5:54, 2014 24904437

Rajji TK, Ismail Z, Mulsant BH: Age at onset and cognition in schizophrenia: meta-analysis. Br J Psychiatry 195(4):286–293, 2009 19794194

Schneider C, Corrigall R, Hayes D, et al: Systematic review of the efficacy and tolerability of clozapine in the treatment of youth with early onset schizophrenia. Eur Psychiatry 29(1):1–10, 2014 24119631

Seidman LJ, Shapiro DI, Stone WS, et al: Association of neurocognition with transition to psychosis: baseline functioning in the second phase of the North American Prodrome Longitudinal Study. JAMA Psychiatry 73(12):1239–1248, 2016 27806157

Sikich L: Diagnosis and evaluation of hallucinations and other psychotic symptoms in children and adolescents. Child Adolesc Psychiatr Clin N Am 22(4):655–673, 2013 24012079

Sikich L, Frazier JA, McClellan J, et al: Double-blind comparison of first- and second-generation antipsychotics in early onset schizophrenia and schizoaffective disorder: findings from the Treatment of Early Onset Schizophrenia Spectrum Disorders (TEOSS) study. Am J Psychiatry 165(11):1420–1431, 2008 18794207

Simon GE, Stewart C, Yarborough BJ, et al: Mortality rates after the first diagnosis of psychotic disorder in adolescents and young adults. JAMA Psychiatry 75(3):254–260, 2018 29387876

Stafford MR, Mayo-Wilson E, Loucas CE: Efficacy and safety of pharmacological and psychological interventions for the treatment of psychosis and schizophrenia in children, adolescents and young adults: a systematic review and meta-analysis. PLoS One 10(2):e0117166, 2015 25671707

Taylor PJ, Hutton P, Wood L: Are people at risk of psychosis also at risk of suicide and self-harm? A systematic review and meta-analysis. Psychol Med 45(5):911–926, 2015 25298008

Tiffin PA, Welsh P: Practitioner review: schizophrenia spectrum disorders and the at-risk mental state for psychosis in children and adolescents—evidence-based management approaches. J Child Psychol Psychiatry 54(11):1155–1175, 2013 24102356

Tomlinson E, Onwumere J, Kuipers E: Distress and negative experiences of the caregiving relationship in early psychosis: does social cognition play a role? Early Interv Psychiatry 8(3):253–260, 2014 23489370

UK National Institute for Health and Care Excellence: Psychosis and Schizophrenia in Children and Young People: Recognition and Management (Clinical Guideline 155). London, UK National Institute for Health and Care Excellence, 2013

van Os J, Kenis G, Rutten BP: The environment and schizophrenia. Nature 468(7321):203–212, 2010 21068828

Velthorst E, Fett AJ, Reichenberg A, et al: The 20-year longitudinal trajectories of social functioning in individuals with psychotic disorders. Am J Psychiatry 174(11):1075–1085, 2017 27978770

Wykes T, Huddy V, Cellard C, et al: A meta-analysis of cognitive remediation for schizophrenia: methodology and effect sizes. Am J Psychiatry 168(5):472–485, 2011 21406461

Zipursky RB, Menezes NM, Streiner DL: Risk of symptom recurrence with medication discontinuation in first-episode psychosis: a systematic review. Schizophr Res 152(2–3):408–414, 2014 23972821

CHAPTER
23

Special Populations: College and University Students

Kate V. Hardy, Clin.Psych.D.
Jacob S. Ballon, M.D., M.P.H.
Mehak Chopra, D.O.
Douglas L. Noordsy, M.D.

THE college or university setting presents many challenges for young people—particularly those with an emerging illness. Psychotic symptoms are generally still developing in college students, resulting in diagnostic uncertainty at the initial point of identification and treatment. Students presenting with first-onset of psychotic symptoms may go on to develop a schizophrenia spectrum disorder, but their symptoms could also be due to substance use, mood disorders, trauma, or certain medical conditions. Because the etiology of psychosis can vary, a comprehensive assessment is essential.

This chapter is presented as an update to Hardy KV, Gonzalez-Flores B, Ballon JS: "Intervening Early in First-Episode Psychosis in a College Setting," in *University Student Mental Health: A Guide for Psychiatrists, Psychologists, and Leaders Serving in Higher Education*. Edited by Roberts LW. Washington, DC, American Psychiatric Association Publishing, 2018, pp. 285–298. Copyright © 2018 American Psychiatric Association Publishing. Used with permission.

Universities often struggle with how to respond ethically and legally to students presenting in crisis with psychosis (Hardy et al. 2018a). Although college is an exciting time for students, it is a major life transition with numerous demands and challenges. Academic stress, social pressures, continuous sleep disruptions, separation from family, and an increase in responsibilities can leave students more vulnerable to substance use and other mental health problems. Given these demands, college students may experience their first onset or exacerbation of mental health problems. Consider the following example.

Case Example 1

Sam is an 18-year-old student athlete on the tennis team who spends many hours practicing his sport. After a successful high school career, he enrolled in an elite university as a pre-med student. Over the course of his freshman year, Sam started to feel sad and more irritable, frustrated, and anxious. He was having difficulty sleeping and noticed it was challenging to pay attention in class and during practice. His coach and teammates also noticed that he wasn't playing tennis as well as in the past. Sam confided in a friend that he was hearing the voices of an angel and a demon in his head. He felt that his mind was torn between the good and evil of these spirits, and this interrupted his concentration in other tasks. Sam presented to his student health center reluctantly. He did not say he was hearing voices, but he did mention that he felt as if things were not going well for him in his mind. Sam was referred for supportive psychotherapy, and he told his counselor that his parents would not approve of him being on medication. After building rapport with his therapist, he revealed that he felt that taking medication was a sign of weakness. Despite a robust coordinated specialty care (CSC) service located in his county, Sam was not referred for specialized early psychosis treatment. He began to speak more openly with his counselor about auditory hallucinations and referential ideas. At the end of the quarter, Sam expressed to his brother that he was having thoughts of suicide. He was taken to a local hospital and admitted to an inpatient unit. He was put on medical leave from school, and he stopped playing competitive tennis. After his hospitalization, Sam was sent home, and it is unclear if he will ever be able to reenroll at his university.

Unfortunately, this case presents a common description of how the onset of psychosis, and access to treatment, occurs for thousands of young adults in the United States each year. Symptoms of psychosis typically emerge in late adolescence and early adulthood, mapping onto the period when young people are starting college or university. Nearly 70% of U.S. high school students enrolled in college in 2017 (U.S. Bureau of Labor Statistics 2018). With 100,000 new cases of psychosis occurring each year in the United States, it can be expected that a significant number of students will experience their first episode of psychosis while on a college campus.

Specialized early psychosis services are now more broadly available in the United States. However, to provide early intervention, there must first be effective early identification. Research has demonstrated that the duration of untreated psychosis (DUP) is an important factor in the long-term prognosis of individuals experiencing a first episode of psychosis. Although college-age individuals who engage in higher education may have a shorter mean DUP, the DUP still exceeds optimal for most (Hardy et al. 2018b). Early psychosis studies consistently find that shorter DUP is associated with better symptom and functional outcomes, but no research has addressed an optimal DUP for return to full academic and occupational functioning. Clinical experience and extrapolation from existing evidence suggest that a DUP less than 12 weeks may be most likely to achieve this high bar.

Challenges in the identification of psychosis exist in all settings but may be particularly acute in a college setting, where students present with a range of mental health problems. Young people experience increased autonomy and decreased oversight as they transition to a college campus and spend less time with family members while engaging in education and work activities. Increased anonymity can result in mental health difficulties going unrecognized and untreated. Broadly speaking, symptoms are considered to cross the threshold to full psychosis when they are experienced with 100% conviction and have an impact on the behavior or functioning of the individual. However, psychotic disorders often have a prodromal period, or a time preceding the onset of full psychosis when attenuated symptoms may occur. During this stage, symptoms are often nonspecific and may be ascribed to other diagnoses, including depression, anxiety, or attention-deficit/hyperactivity disorder, or simply may be considered a normative reaction to the stressors of college life. However, a deeper look will often reveal accompanying attenuated (or subthreshold) symptoms or even brief, full psychotic symptoms that may indicate high risk for developing full psychosis. Early symptoms often include distressing and impairing perceptual disturbances such as hearing or seeing things that other people do not experience, unusual thoughts, or suspiciousness. It is important to assess for signs of psychosis because early identification will shorten DUP and help to identify the most appropriate treatment plan for the young person. The Prodromal Questionnaire-Brief (PQ-B) is a simple self-report screening tool that can assist with identification of early psychosis (Loewy et al. 2011).

One of the first signs that a student is struggling with a mental health problem is a change in academic performance. Faced with possible hallucinations or preoccupying thoughts in the form of delusions, as well as possible cognitive symptoms, a student struggling with psychosis may have decreased grades, turn in incomplete assignments, or miss classes. Additionally, there are often observable changes in behavior atypical for the young person. However, when examining behavior, it is important to consider the cultural and environmental context. Case Example 1 describes a spiritual battle that Sam was experiencing between an angel and a demon, but this would not be clearly indicative of a potential problem if this type of language is normative for a person's religious background.

Studies have demonstrated the impact of psychosis on cognitive functioning, which may consequently have an effect on academic functioning. In the North American Prodromal Longitudinal Study (NAPLS), people at clinical high risk for schizophrenia were compared with healthy control subjects and people diagnosed with schizophrenia. Cognitive changes were seen in the high-risk group and are a key component of the composite risk score that has been developed from this work (Cannon et al. 2016). Cognitive changes in early psychosis typically relate to processing speed, verbal learning, and working memory. Deficits in these areas put students at a great disadvantage compared with their peers. Further, many students look to psychoactive substances, including psychostimulants—prescribed or not—to help improve these deficits. These medications unfortunately can worsen nascent psychotic symptoms.

Beyond cognitive changes, social changes are also typically seen at the onset of psychosis. Many students will become withdrawn and begin to isolate themselves socially. Withdrawing into their own thoughts often further separates students from peers, making detection more difficult. However, this also presents an opportunity for early detection because behavior that is atypical for the student may be a red flag for further investigation. Residential college settings surround students with a range of roommates, resident advisors, and deans who may notice changes in behavior and encourage evaluation. When the student presents for evaluation, screening tools for early signs of psychosis may aid in the detection of symptoms indicative of a risk of developing psychosis (Loewy et al. 2005).

The college setting provides some advantages for early identification. Students expose their thinking in assignments and classroom discussion. They have committed to a course schedule, and deviations from that schedule may highlight onset of behavioral change. Similarly, they are engaged in social networks with peers and resident advisors who may also notice changes in thought or behavior. Compared with same-age peers who are not employed or in school, opportunities for identification of changes in cognition and behavior are extensive.

In addition to the college years being a vital time period for early detection of psychosis, it is also important to keep in mind that high school students may present with prodromal symptoms. Data from a study in Australia showed that nearly one-third of people diagnosed with a psychotic illness are diagnosed between ages 15 and 19 (Amminger et al.

2006). High school is an important time in a youth's life when he or she is experiencing many transitions. It is a time of both social stressors and academic challenges. In this setting, it is important for school staff to be vigilant for persistent changes in the mood or demeanor of a student.

Barriers to Treatment Among College Students With Serious Mental Illness

Individuals with serious mental illness are often challenged by stereotypes, prejudice, and discrimination from the general public and even from health care professionals. They are often depicted as dangerous, violent, and unreliable in media reports and popular culture. These stigmatizing attitudes delay help seeking and are a significant barrier to initiating treatment. There are three distinct forms of stigma: 1) public stigma, 2) perceived stigma, and 3) personal stigma. Public stigma is defined as the collective negative views about mental illness held by a community; perceived stigma refers to one's beliefs regarding how society views individuals with mental illness; and personal stigma includes one's self-directed negative thoughts and beliefs about mental illness and how they impact one's ability to succeed (Kosyluk et al. 2016).

Stigma impacts a person at multiple levels, including academic performance and retention, self-esteem, job occupation, housing retention, and overall quality of life. Feelings of guilt and shame are often associated with stigma. Because of the fears of being labeled as "mentally ill," many people with serious mental illness withdraw from their inner social circles, especially during the early stages of psychosis when unchallenged delusions begin to become concrete. Furthermore, students who isolate themselves have lower levels of community engagement and social relationships. Withdrawal from social networks may make identification even more challenging.

Research has found that unfamiliarity with serious mental illness is a strong predictor of stigmatizing attitudes. A major obstacle in connecting students with mental health services is the lack of familiarity of the symptoms and early warning signs of psychosis (Feeg et al. 2014). A survey conducted by the University of South Carolina asked 87 faculty members about their familiarity with mental disorders (Brockelman and Scheyett 2015). The researchers found that the least familiar mental disorders were personality disorders (43.5%), schizophrenia (42.3%), and paranoia (41.7%). Faculty often struggle with how to respond to students in distress. Brockelman and Scheyett (2015) found that the most common approach was to extend the deadline for assignments and discuss mental health concerns with the student. Nearly 80% consulted with the college's office of disability support or counseling center to gather more information about the resources available on campus. Although that number is encouraging, it is not known how many of those consultations resulted in referral to CSC or other specific early psychosis services for further management.

Another barrier to initiating psychiatric treatment is lack of empathy. For front-line student health professionals who are not experienced in caring for people with psychosis, it is often difficult to empathize with the student's experience, especially during active symptoms. Too often, individuals with serious mental illness feel blamed for their disorder or worry that their psychotic symptoms will be viewed as a sign of weakness or that they will be viewed as being "crazy." To address this issue, Bunn and Terpstra (2009) had medical students simulate the experience of auditory hallucinations by listening to headphones. The medical students had to continue with their daily activities while listening to the voices. The study found that this experience led to higher levels of empathy toward individuals with severe mental illness. A similar approach could be adapted to training for on-campus health professionals and faculty.

Given its distinct environment, college presents a unique opportunity to identify and treat serious psychopathology. Early intervention leads to better academic, social, health, and occupational outcomes. Reducing stigma and other treatment barriers is essential to improving the trajectory for students with serious mental illness.

Treatment Accommodations to Help Students With Psychosis Stay in School

College administrators and health officials often run into a significant dilemma when considering how best to help students once an episode of psychosis has been identified. There are often concerns about student privacy. Privacy laws can be difficult to understand and can present limitations because college students are generally over the age of majority and can make decisions for themselves yet often are still dependent on parents financially and emotionally. The two privacy laws at the center of the discrepancy are the Family Educational Rights and Privacy Act (FERPA), which protects student privacy, and the Health Insurance Portability and Accountability Act (HIPAA), which concerns privacy of medical information. In 2008, the U.S. Department of Health and Human Services and the U.S. Department of Education issued joint guidelines on the intersection of FERPA and HIPAA (U.S. Department of Education 2011; U.S. Department of Health and Human Services and U.S. Department of Education 2008). Student health records are specifically covered under FERPA; however, a mechanism exists for alerting parents to potential mental health crises. The exceptions for privacy are outlined in the *Code of Federal Regulations*, 34 *CFR* § 99.31(a); one exception is that information may be shared with parents in an emergency situation.

Once onset of psychosis has been identified in a student, administrators face a difficult decision regarding the suitability for continuing enrollment in school. At the heart of the dilemma is the need to balance risks for the student and the university if the student continues to be involved in a potentially high-pressure academic environment while also trying to find the best long-term solution for the student. Many schools have de facto policies mandating (or strongly recommending) medical leave after an initial episode. These policies are based in dated beliefs regarding the need for convalescence, often to the detriment of the student. Sending a student home is not without risk to the student because there may not be adequate mental health resources (such as a CSC clinic) in his or her hometown. Further, many college students who return home find themselves socially isolated while their peers remain at their respective universities. Students sent home then fall off their educational trajectory and are not given an opportunity to maintain their academic level. Lack of intellectual stimulation and structure can also undermine coping strategies for managing psychosis.

The Bazelon Center for Mental Health Law (2007) has proposed a set of guidelines for campus mental health treatment. The nearly 50 guidelines suggest that schools create a policy to support students to maintain their academic progress, providing counseling and voluntary leaves of absence when needed. In addition, schools should provide education to students and student health leaders on campus about mental health issues. College counseling centers should be available to students 24/7, including during school holidays. There should be access to emergency services when needed, and student health centers should make provisions for ongoing care to prevent crises from developing. When students need to take time away from school, they should be allowed to maintain contact with peers and professors, including continuing coursework remotely if possible. When involuntary leave is necessary, the head of the counseling center should be included in any committee making these case-by-case decisions. Ultimately, schools should provide the resources needed to help maintain students as close to the university as possible.

When students are able to stay enrolled, the college or university further has obligations under federal disability rights law—the same as for students with physical disabilities. These accommodations may take the form of increased time for exams or taking tests in a private area. Students should be allowed to retroactively withdraw from classes if their performance was significantly impacted by their psychiatric symptoms and they were unable to complete the necessary coursework to pass the class. Students should be allowed to select a reduced course load if full-time status is overwhelming. Housing accommodations should also be taken into consideration, including whether or not students should have roommates, depending on their specific psychiatric needs. These accommodations should be arranged in consultation with the treatment provider for the student because the university may require documentation of the illness and need for accommodation from a mental health professional (U.S. Department of Education 2011).

Recommendations

Because the college years are a time of transition when young people may experience a first episode of psychosis, it is critical for colleges and universities to provide training to staff in early identification of psychosis and make efforts to encourage students to use on-campus mental health services when they are in distress. Shared decision making, an individualized approach, and provision of reasonable accommodations are important aspects of treatment planning. A summary of recommendations is provided in Table 23–1.

Consider the following case in contrast to Sam's experience presented earlier. Perhaps we might have seen a different trajectory for Sam if there had been supports in place to identify psychosis earlier as in the case of Ronaldo.

Case Example 2

Ronaldo, an 18-year-old young man, enrolled in a university after a successful high school career. After several months of school, Ronaldo noticed decreased motivation and difficulty concentrating, which affected his athletic performance. He received his first C ever. Given the difficulty, he began to put in extra hours in the library and found himself working through the night on several occasions. Todd, the resident advisor in Ronaldo's dorm, received training during orientation on recognizing signs of early psychosis and was given information on how best to respond. He noticed a change in Ronaldo's behavior and talked to him about it. Although Ronaldo reassured Todd that everything was fine, they agreed to check in again in a couple of weeks. Todd informed the resident dean of the concerns and they agreed to monitor the situation.

When Todd and Ronaldo reconnect 2 weeks later, Ronaldo confides that he has been hearing things and worries that his roommate may be able to read his mind. Todd provides Ronaldo with information about auditory hallucinations, including information on how common these phenomena are and different reasons why they might occur (stress, sleep deprivation, psychosis, drugs). They agree to set up an appointment with a psychiatrist at the Wellness Center, and Todd accompanies Ronaldo to this appointment. The Wellness Center counselor conducts an assessment, in which Ronaldo reports that he has been hearing voices and thinks he is hearing the voice of his angel talking to him. The coun-

---

TABLE 23–1.   Summary of general guidelines

Basic principles

- Universities should make extra efforts to ensure that faculty and college counseling staff are trained in early identification of the signs of psychosis and use of early psychosis screening measures such as the Prodromal Questionnaire (PQ), PRIME Screen-Revised (PS-R), and Structured Interview for Psychosis-Risk Syndromes (SIPS).

- College faculty and staff members should encourage students to use on-campus mental health services if they exhibit academic, behavioral, and/or emotional difficulties that could be related to an underlying mental health condition.

- College counseling centers should make direct efforts to engage and encourage students to access mental health services.

- College counseling centers and emergency psychiatric services should be available 24/7.

Treatment planning

- Appropriate treatment and management should follow the coordinated specialty care model, which emphasizes having a shared decision-making and individualized treatment plan.

- Treatment care should involve a comprehensive approach that includes evidence-based psychotherapy, medication management for first-episode psychosis, family psychoeducation and support, case management, and housing and academic accommodations.

- If the student has been hospitalized, college counseling centers should obtain consent from the student to work closely with the hospital treatment team to ensure aftercare planning.

Accommodations and leaves of absence

- College and universities should provide reasonable housing and academic accommodations to allow students to maintain their academic progress and social relationships.

- If a medical leave of absence is necessary, students should be allowed to remain in contact with peers and professors to maintain a strong social support network.

- Absences for treatment and hospitalization should count as excused absences. Students should not be sanctioned or punished for missing classes because of a mental health condition.

Source.   Adapted from Bazelon Center for Mental Health Law 2007.

selor recommends that Ronaldo receive further evaluation at the local CSC program. He also suggests that Ronaldo reach out to his family for additional support. Ronaldo does this, and his family come to his next appointment at the CSC clinic. Ronaldo is accepted into the service and immediately meets with an educational support specialist. Together, Ronaldo and his family work with the college to establish a plan to support Ronaldo in his studies, including an amended schedule for the remainder of the semester, thus allowing him to continue to stay matriculated.

Students presenting with a recent onset of psychosis are heterogeneous and present with many different needs. Although many will have cognitive and social deficits at the onset of illness, this is not the case for all students. The overall panoply of symptoms that one can have, from hallucinations and delusions to primarily negative symptoms including cognitive difficulties and social isolation, means that careful attention must be paid to the specific needs of each individual student. Successful treatment of students in this age group requires an appreciation of the common symptoms and a unique and personalized approach to treatment. There is no "one size fits all" approach to treatment of psychotic illnesses.

KEY CONCEPTS

- College presents a unique opportunity for identifying students with early psychosis and shortening their duration of psychosis.

- With early intervention and appropriate educational supports, young people experiencing onset of psychosis while enrolled in college can access treatment and continue progress toward their educational goals.

- Providing strong institutional support that is easily accessible and free of stigma gives students with severe mental illness the best chance of continued academic success.

- Forced medical leaves should be used minimally after all other options have been exhausted. When students need to take time away from school, they should be allowed to maintain contact with peers and professors and continue coursework remotely.

Discussion Questions

1. What supports can best help students seek evaluation in a college setting? How can the process be simplified for students seeking psychiatric care? How do students ordinarily find their way to psychiatric treatment? What can be done to help lower the barriers for students seeking treatment for a potential psychotic disorder?

2. How can a university or college help support and treat students with new-onset psychosis? What is the process for the family to be involved, and when and how are they contacted? How are the treatment options discussed with students and families? How does your university typically handle a new-onset psychotic disorder? What are the treatment options for students?

3. How does your coordinated specialty program interface with colleges and universities in your area to support early identification and referral for students with emerging psychosis?

Suggested Readings

Books and Reports

Bazelon Center for Mental Health Law: Supporting Students: A Model Policy for Colleges and Universities. Washington, DC, Judge David L. Bazelon Center for Mental Health Law, May 15, 2007. Available at: www.bazelon.org/wp-content/uploads/2017/04/Supporting StudentsCampusMHPolicy.pdf. Accessed October 15, 2018.

National Collaborating Centre for Mental Health: Psychosis and schizophrenia in children and young people, in Psychosis and Schizophrenia in Children and Young People: Recognition and Management (NICE Clinical Guidelines No 155). Bethesda, MD, National Center for Biotechnology Information, 2013. Available at: www.bazelon.org/wp-content/uploads/2017/04/SupportingStudentsCampusMH Policy.pdf. Accessed January 26, 2019.

Roberts LW: Student Mental Health: A Guide for Psychiatrists, Psychologists, and Leaders Serving in Higher Education. Washington, DC, American Psychiatric Association Publishing, 2018

Websites and Social Media Resources

Students With Schizophrenia Facebook page: www.facebook.com/
   studentswithschizophrenia
Students With Schizophrenia website, www.sws.ngo

References

Amminger GP, Harris MG, Conus P, et al: Treated incidence of first-episode
   psychosis in the catchment area of EPPIC between 1997 and 2000. Acta Psychiatr Scand 114(5):337–345, 2006 17022793
Bazelon Center for Mental Health Law: Supporting Students: A Model Policy for
   Colleges and Universities. Washington, DC, Judge David L. Bazelon Center
   for Mental Health Law. May 15, 2007. Available at: www.bazelon.org/wp-
   content/uploads/2017/04/SupportingStudentsCampusMHPolicy.pdf. January 26, 2019.
Brockelman KF, Scheyett AM: Faculty perceptions of accommodations, strategies, and psychiatric advance directives for university students with mental illnesses. Psychiatr Rehabil J 38(4):342–348, 2015 26053532
Bunn W, Terpstra J: Cultivating empathy for the mentally ill using simulated
   auditory hallucinations. Acad Psychiatry 33(6):457–460, 2009 19933888
Cannon TD, Yu C, Addington J, et al: An individualized risk calculator for research
   in prodromal psychosis. Am J Psychiatry 173(10):980–988, 2016 27363508
Cohen AN, Hamilton AB, Saks ER, et al: How occupationally high-achieving individuals with a diagnosis of schizophrenia manage their symptoms. Psychiatr Serv 68(4):324–329, 2017 27842472
Feeg VD, Prager LS, Moylan LB, et al: Predictors of mental illness stigma and
   attitudes among college students: using vignettes from a campus common
   reading program. Issues Ment Health Nurs 35(9):694–703, 2014 25162192
Hardy KV, Gonzalez-Flores B, Ballon JS: Intervening early in first-episode psychosis in a college setting, in University Student Mental Health: A Guide
   for Psychiatrists, Psychologists, and Leaders Serving Higher Education.
   Edited by Roberts LW. Washington, DC, American Psychiatric Publishing,
   2018a pp 285–298
Hardy KV, Noordsy DL, Ballon JS, et al: Impact of age of onset of psychosis and
   engagement in higher education on duration of untreated psychosis. J Ment
   Health 27(3):257–262, 2018b 29707996
Kosyluk KA, Al-Khouja M, Bink A, et al: Challenging the stigma of mental illness
   among college students. J Adolesc Health 59(3):325–331, 2016 27324577
Loewy RL, Bearden CE, Johnson JK, et al: The prodromal questionnaire (PQ):
   preliminary validation of a self-report screening measure for prodromal
   and psychotic syndromes. Schizophr Res 79(1):117–125, 2005 16276559
Loewy RL, Pearson R, Vinogradov S, et al: Psychosis risk screening with the
   Prodromal Questionnaire—Brief version (PQ-B). Schizophr Res 129(1):42–
   46, 2011 21511440

U.S. Bureau of Labor Statistics: College enrollment and work activity of recent high school and college graduates summary. April 26, 2018. Available at: www.bls.gov/news.release/hsgec.nr0.htm. Accessed January 26, 2019.

U.S. Department of Education: Students with Disabilities Preparing for Postsecondary Education. Washington, DC, U.S. Department of Education, 2011. Available at: https://ed.gov/about/offices/list/ocr/transition.html. Accessed January 26, 2019.

U.S. Department of Health and Human Services; U.S Department of Education: Joint guidance on the application of the Family Educational Rights and Privacy Act (FERPA) and the Health Insurance Portability and Accountability Act of 1996 (HIPAA) to Student Health Records. Washington, DC, U.S. Department of Health and Human Services, November 2008. Available at: www2.ed.gov/policy/gen/guid/fpco/doc/ferpa-hipaa-guidance.pdf. Accessed October 15, 2018.

Index

Page numbers printed in **boldface** type refer to tables and figures.